AN ATLAS OF MORTALITY IN SCOTLAND

Including the Geography of Selected Socio-Economic Characteristics

International statistics on mortality and morbidity show Scotland to come out poorly, a fact which has been known by epidemiologists for some time. Scotland therefore provides a particularly interesting case study of a Western industrialised nation.

This book is based on data collected over three time spans: 1959–63, 1969–73 and 1979–83. Thus data are available for three five-year periods covering three decades, which permit a unique analysis of how mortality patterns associated with particular diseases can change over time. The book consists of approximately 100 maps with accompanying text, with maps printed in two colours. They show mortality in Scotland by small burgh, large burgh, city and landward areas, totalling 234 small communities. Certain socio-economic variables are also shown. The book contains an unrivalled amount of research data and should interest epidemiologists and medical geographers throughout the world, not just those with a particular interest in the Scottish situation.

AN ATLAS OF MORTALITY IN ◇ SCOTLAND ◇

Including the Geography of Selected Socio-Economic Characteristics

Edited by

O. Ll. Lloyd F. L. R. Williams

W. G. Berry C. du V. Florey

CROOM HELM
London • New York • Sydney

Croom Helm Ltd, Provident House, Burrell Row,
Beckenham, Kent, BR3 1AT
Croom Helm Australia, 44-50 Waterloo Road,
North Ryde, 2113, New South Wales

Published in the USA by
Croom Helm
in association with Methuen, Inc.
29 West 35th Street
New York, NY 10001

British Library Cataloguing in Publication Data

An Atlas of mortality in Scotland: including
the geography of selected socio-economic
characteristics.
1. Mortality — Scotland — Maps 2. Scotland
— Statistics, Vital — Maps
I. Lloyd, Owen Ll.
912'.130464'09411 G1826.E24

ISBN 0-7099-4122-6

Library of Congress Cataloging in Publication Data

ISBN 0-7099-4122-6

This atlas was typeset in 10 on 12-point Times Roman on a Monotype Lasercomp phototypesetter at Oxford University Computing Service.

TABLE OF CONTENTS

CONTRIBUTORS

W G Berry
Department of Geography
University of Dundee
Dundee DD1 4HN
(editor, cartography)

Professor C du V Florey
Department of Community Medicine
University of Dundee
Dundee DD1 9SY
(editor, bronchitis/emphysema/asthma)

Professor W M Garraway
Department of Community Medicine
University of Edinburgh
Edinburgh EH8 9AG
(cerebrovascular and other circulatory disease)

Dr C R Gillis
West of Scotland Cancer Surveillance Unit
Greater Glasgow Health Board
Ruchill Hospital
Glasgow G20 9NB
(lung cancer, lymphatic/haematopoietic cancers)

Professor Emeritus G Melvyn Howe
Department of Geography
University of Strathclyde
Glasgow G1 1XH
(history of disease mapping)

Dr D W Lamont
West of Scotland Cancer Surveillance Unit
Greater Glasgow Health Board
Ruchill Hospital
Glasgow G20 9NB
(lung cancer, lymphatic/haematopoietic cancers)

Dr M M Lloyd
Environmental Epidemiology and Cancer Centre
Department of Community Medicine
University of Dundee
Dundee DD1 9SY
(sex ratios of births)

Dr O Ll Lloyd
Environmental Epidemiology and Cancer Centre
Department of Community Medicine
University of Dundee
Dundee DD1 9SY
(editor, total cancers, breast cancer, gastric cancer, colorectal cancer, remainder cancers)

W R Lyster
33 Colville Gardens
London W11 2BL
(sex ratios of births)

Professor Emeritus A Mair
Department of Community Medicine
University of Dundee
Dundee DD1 9SY
(total cancers, remainder cancers)

Dr S M McIver
MRC Medical Sociology Unit
6 Lilybank Gardens
Glasgow G12 8QQ
(spatial variations in mortality)

Dr D Reid
Communicable Diseases (Scotland) Unit
Ruchill Hospital
Glasgow G20 9NB
(acute respiratory infection: influenza and pneumonia)

M S J Reilly
Department of Community Medicine
University of Dundee
Dundee DD1 9SY
(the geological environment and disease, fishing vessel losses and emergency survival at sea)

Dr D P Strachan
Department of Community Medicine
University of Edinburgh
Edinburgh EH8 9AG
(cerebrovascular and other circulatory disease)

Dr C H M Walker
Department of Child Health
University of Dundee
Dundee DD1 9SY
(mortality at early ages)

Dr P B West
MRC Medical Sociology Unit
6 Lilybank Gardens
Glasgow G12 8QQ
(spatial variations in mortality)

F L R Williams
Environmental Epidemiology and Cancer Centre
Department of Community Medicine
University of Dundee
Dundee DD1 9SY
(editor, methods, total mortality, coronary and other heart disease)

ACKNOWLEDGEMENTS

This atlas could not have been completed without the valuable help of several people, to whom we extend our thanks:

Dr M B Cottam (Department of Geography, Dundee University) for his time and expertise in assisting with the initial Lasercomp settings for the text;

to Mr I Bradbury (Inveresk International plc) and Mr S Ogston (Department of Community Medicine, Dundee University) for advice on statistics and computing;

to Miss J MacDonald (Paisley College of Technology) for her considerable contribution to the start of the project;

to Miss K Herschel, Mrs C Bain and Mr J Ford (Department of Geography, Dundee University) for their help with the cartography;

to Miss K Ireland and Miss E A Will (Department of Community Medicine, Dundee University) for their accurate and rapid processing of much of the data;

and finally to the staff of the Computing Centre of the University of Dundee who made diverse computing facilities available to us.

The Economic and Social Research Council has provided financial support for further work on the data used in the compilation of the atlas.

FOREWORD

For many decades, information on mortality in Scottish communities has been provided by the Registrar General for Scotland in his Annual Reports. Until 1973, the communities covered by the B list of the International Classification of Disease (ICD) were the traditional communities: the Cities, the Large Burghs (generally with populations over 25000), the Small Burghs (with populations mostly above 5000, but some even lower) and the Landward Areas (the remainders of the counties, containing mostly villages and some small towns). Spread widely throughout Scotland and demographically relatively stable, these communities provided a conveniently-available and detailed matrix for observing variations of mortality throughout Scotland. The width of the diagnostic classifications used in the B list allowed the contents of many categories to remain comparatively stable over several revisions of the ICD classifications, and also increased confidence that most of the deaths included in each category belonged there.

A question arose, some years ago, about the ranking for lung cancer mortality held by some small communities in Scotland. It was clear that the information in the Annual Reports could answer not only that question, but also any others which might arise about the mortality ranking of individual communities for a range of diseases. Equally clearly, the same information for all communities could be adapted to illustrate the geographical patterns of mortality from various diseases within Scotland during successive periods of time.

By taking two years on either side of the natural epidemiological 'anchorages' provided by the census years of 1961 and 1971, five year periods were created which gave reasonably large numbers of deaths for most causes in all but the smallest communities; hence the two periods chosen initially for the mapping survey were 1959-63 and 1969-73. After 1973, however, the reorganization of Local Government removed the Burghs as administrative units, so that the smallest areas for which mortality data were provided in the Annual Reports were the 56 Districts. To bring the patterns of mortality closer to present times, the period of 1979-83, which encompassed the 1981 census year, was taken as the third period for mapping, with the Districts forming the geographical units.

By illustrating mortality data as maps enclosing a timespan of almost 25 years, this atlas is primarily a record of the valuable work of the Registrar General for Scotland. But the subject matter has been widened by adding some environmental and socio-economic factors of potential aetiological relevance to the diseases illustrated. We also extended the Scottish geography to offshore areas by including a map of the recently investigated problem of mortality from fishing vessel losses amongst that highly neglected occupational group, fishermen. Lastly, epidemiologists were invited to contribute introductory texts for many of the diseases and for the environmental and social maps. Some of these topics are more complex and less familiar to the public than others, and so a uniform format by the contributors for the different texts was discarded in favour of a variety of approaches.

No atlas of reasonable dimensions can provide all the information which readers might wish. In this atlas, for example, the use of the small communities in two of the time-periods made it necessary for the mortality data for the communities to be presented for the sexes combined. The material in this atlas supplements in time, space and subject-matter the information presented in other studies (albeit prepared along different lines and for larger demographic units) such as the National Atlases of Disease Mortality in the United Kingdom by Melvyn Howe [1] and the Atlas of Cancer Incidence in Scotland produced in association with the World Health Organization [2].

Scotland's mortality rates and patterns, internationally notorious as they are, provide a potentially rich harvest of geographical clues about disease causation. It is our hope that medical practitioners, environmental health officers and others with epidemiological interests or responsibilities in Public Health will be encouraged by such maps and texts to think geographically and environmentally about disease causation, and then to explore the possibilities for disease prevention.

O.LL.LLOYD, F.L.R.WILLIAMS, W.G.BERRY, C.DU.V.FLOREY

HISTORY OF DISEASE MAPPING

'.... to obtain a view of the Geographical extent of the ravages of this disease, and to discover the local conditions that might influence its progress and its degree of fatality .... Geographical delineation is of the utmost value, and even indispensable; for while the symbols of the masses of statistical data in figures, however clearly they might be arranged in Systematic Tables, present but a uniform appearance, the same data, embodied in a Map, will convey at once the relative bearing and proportion of the single data (sic), together with their position, extent and distance, and thus, a Map will make visible to the eye the development and nature of any phenomenon in regard to its Geographical distribution'.
Augustus Petermann, 1852

Maps demonstrate with a unique efficiency the distributions of phenomena in space. Maps of disease, like other types of map, convey factual information. But, by illustrating disease distributions which either change over short time-periods or vary non-randomly in space, disease maps also inevitably stimulate the formation of causal hypotheses.

The earliest examples were stimulated by the search for clues about the origins of the dreaded infections. One early example of such mapping appeared in America in 1820, when Felix Pascalis-Ouvière drew a careful spot map to show the distribution of cases of yellow fever in New York, in an effort to establish causative factors. A map produced in 1826 of a locality in Mississippi linked environmental factors closely to an epidemic of disease: 'A damp climate, an eighty-degree temperature ..... combined with the special effluvia of rotting pork and oysters to envelop the community in a sort of pathogenic mist. The inevitable consequence was widespread yellow fever'. Born largely of experience with yellow fever in the United States and with cholera in Britain, disease mapping became relatively commonplace during the subsequent decades. For example, Dr. Robert Baker's Report of the Leeds Board of Health of 1833 was accompanied by a cholera plan of Leeds which indicated the districts in which cholera prevailed; it illustrated Baker's observation of '.... how exceedingly the disease has prevailed in those parts of the town where there is a deficiency, often an extreme want, of sewage, drainage and paving'. In 1849 a map within a book showed the distribution of deaths from cholera in Exeter between 1832 and 1834. By using differently shaped red symbols for each year, it showed where deaths took place, the localities where clothes were destroyed, the cholera burying grounds, the druggists, the soup kitchens, and it demonstrated that a high proportion of the deaths were in the low-lying, south-eastern quarter of the old walled city. One of the most famous maps to generate ideas about causation of disease appeared six years later - the 'spot map' produced by John Snow, showing the distribution of cases of cholera around the historic Broad Street (London) pump during September 1854. The weighty and positive evidence in the distribution map was strengthened by careful investigation of anomalous cases, such as the widow of a percussion-cap maker who lived in the Hampstead district, who was of 'the custom to take out a large bottle of the water from the pump in the Broad Street, as she preferred it'; and so she caught cholera without having lived in Broad Street. In 1866 a cholera map appeared in the Report of the Medical Officer of the Privy Council; in this map, the deaths from cholera in London in mid-1866 were superimposed on a map of the geological formations.

Because of the less dramatic nature of their manifestations, non-infectious diseases were mapped with less frequency. In 1875, Haviland published the first edition of a book which contained coloured plates of the distribution of heart disease, dropsy, cancer (females only) and phthisis (females only) in the eleven registration divisions and 44 registration counties of England and Wales. The areas with low crude death rates appeared in various shades of red and the areas with high rates in shades of blue, the red representing health by analogy with healthy arterial blood, and the blueness of cyanotic blood representing disease. During the 1880s maps were compiled to illustrate the findings of a study, sponsored by the British Medical Association, into the incidence of diseases such as rickets, rheumatism, chorea and cancer.

Conceptual developments in mapping included the 'poverty maps' of 1889 by Booth, which accompanied a systematic survey of social conditions in London. In the maps produced by Stocks in the 1920s and 1930s, the mortality rates of the counties of England and Wales were standardized by age and sex. The resulting patterns justified his contention that the mortalities 'vary over such wide limits and the counties group themselves into such definite regions of high and low prevalence, that there can be no question that geographical influences are in some way concerned'. The Atlas of Diseases produced on behalf of the American Geographical Society illustrated the distribution of a wide range of diseases such as poliomyelitis, cholera, malaria vectors, helminthiasis, and spirochaetal, rickettsial and nutritional diseases. In 1964, Brown used the proportional circles technique to illustrate the distribution of various tropical fevers in Nigeria. At about the same time in Britain, there appeared two editions of the National Atlas of Disease Mortality, the edition of 1963 covering the years 1954-58, and that of 1970 covering 1959-63 as well as the earlier period. For the second edition, a demographic base map was used to show mortality localized to dense populations of towns and cities, with urban populations shown as squares and rural populations as diamonds. The use of this technique avoided that potentially misleading prominence of mortality data which a geographical base map gives to extensive, but sparsely populated, areas of the United Kingdom. The second edition also provided possible explanations for the mortality distributions.

Technological innovations arrived. During the late 1960s and early 1970s, the increasing availability of modern data processing equipment heralded the introduction of computer-assisted techniques for producing disease maps. These techniques allowed repetitive processes such as the standardization of death rates to be undertaken speedily and plotted directly on to a map. The quality of the map itself was improved with the commercial introduction of the pen plotter, which met the needs of workers who wanted maps speedily and in camera-ready format. There has followed a flood of disease atlases, mainly concentrating on the modern problems of cancer and degenerative disease, from countries as scattered as the United States, Japan, West Germany, Canada, Taiwan, Mainland China, the Netherlands, Belgium, Uganda, Australia, the Soviet Union and Brazil.

This burgeoning of the popularity of mapping for epidemiological purposes constitutes an acknowledgement of the potential value of the product. Maps provide instant visual impressions of the relation of diseases to their appropriate geographical position. With reservations such as the likelihood of an element of chance, variations in medical diagnosis, and differences in the application of the rules of disease coding, disease maps can reveal spatial variations and distributional patterns not previously discernible nor suspect from the examination of tables of statistics. They provide essential descriptive information relating to geographical variations in disease incidence or mortality. They answer the question 'Where?'. They can be used to facilitate the allocation and re-allocation of health care services, or they can be used for planning, evaluating and monitoring services provided by the community.

The map is also a research tool in associative studies in medical geography or analytical epidemiology. High risk communities are highlighted, within which in-depth local studies may be conducted. By helping to relate diseases to environmental factors which might contribute to their causation, valuable pointers are offered. But there is never proof of causation; for the map is a factual document, and geographical associations can prove nothing other than the necessity for analytical work such as case-control studies and environmental investigations.

The association of disease with topographical factors of aetiology has been recognized since the earliest days of medical practice. Yet there is still much work to be done. Each disease must be studied in time and space; and for this, maps are essential.

As the late Sir Dudley Stamp said tersely, 'Put it on a map'.

(Adapted in part from 'The Mapping of Disease in History' [3])

METHODS

General Methods. Until 1973, the Annual Reports of the Registrar General for Scotland (ARRG) provided mortality data for the Cities, the Large and Small Burghs (a burgh was the equivalent of an English town), and the Landward Areas encompassing those communities, normally small, which did not have burgh or city status. For the years 1959-63, the ARRG provided information on mortality for 231 communities: 4 Cities, 20 Large Burghs, 174 Small Burghs and 33 Landward Areas. For the years 1969-73, one Large Burgh (East Kilbride) and two Small Burghs (Bishopbriggs and Cumbernauld) were added, giving a total of 234 communities. Following local government boundary changes in 1974, the ARRG provided data only for the 56 local government Districts.

The Standardized Mortality Ratio (SMR) for each cause of mortality in the communities was calculated using the Scottish figures as the standard population. There are many options on the choice of the standard population: a world standard population [4] which has been used in atlases both of mortality [5] and morbidity [2]; a European standard population [6]; and traditionally, a standard population based on the national figures of the country being studied [7,8]. Advantages and disadvantages are associated with all standard populations. For example, the world population, when used with European data, overestimates the numbers in the younger age groups, and similar disadvantages are present with the use of the European population. Clearly, the use of the supranational populations allows the mortality and morbidity values in different countries to be compared directly. However, since one of the main aims of this atlas was to initiate hypotheses concerning the variability of the distribution of disease within Scotland, a standard population based on the actual Scottish experience was considered to be the most appropriate.

The groups of years mapped (1959-63, 1969-73 and 1979-83) were chosen for three reasons. Firstly, population figures (by age and sex) for each community were available only for the census years of 1961, 1971 and 1981. Groups of years centred on a census year minimized the effects in the inter-census years of changes in population structure due to births, deaths and migration; the larger the number of years within the grouping, the greater the probability that the population structure selected for that period may not be representative of large parts of it. Secondly, calculating an SMR over several years increased the stability of the observed mortality, which was particularly important when determining the mortality experience of Small Burghs. Thirdly, the presentation of Scotland's mortality experience in three separate periods allowed cautious speculation on the secular trends for some diseases.

The numbers of combined male and female deaths for each cause in each of the communities were obtained from the ARRG. The expected numbers of deaths were derived from the product of the appropriate mean Scottish cause-specific death rates (by 5-year age-group and sex) and the relevant populations at the appropriate census year; hence, communities with SMRs of less than 100 have age-standardized death rates lower than the national rate, and vice-versa. The statistical test for significance was the Exact test described by Liddell [9], which is based upon the link between the Poisson and Chi-square distributions. A community's SMR was considered to be significantly different from Scotland at the five percent level of statistical significance. Mean SMRs were calculated for the three periods 1959-63, 1969-73 and 1979-83. Because inaccurate diagnoses (as recorded on death certificates) are more likely in older age groups [10], the use of truncated age-rates is sometimes considered appropriate. However, truncation does not appear to markedly alter the geographical distribution [11,12], but information is lost about the mortality in the older ages. For example, in Scotland during 1979-83, 75 percent of deaths from coronary heart disease occurred in persons over 65 years. Hence all age-groups were used in this atlas.

In the ARRG, mortality data for the individual communities were available only under the ICD B listing. This list included relatively wide disease categories, which minimized the problem associated with analyzing and interpreting the mortality of small populations. For the years 1959-63 and 1969-73, the data were provided for males and females combined; during the years 1979-83, the data were provided separately, but to maintain consistency the combined mortality for these years was mapped.

The categories of mortality included within the ICD rubrics were not identical over the three periods; between the seventh (1959-63) and eighth (1969-73) revisions the changes were substantial; but only small changes were present between the eighth and the ninth (1979-83) revisions.

Lung Cancer. The category of malignant neoplasm of the trachea, bronchus and lung was largely unchanged between the revisions. But in 1959-63 the rubric also included: malignant neoplasms of the nose, nasal cavities, middle ear and accessory sinuses, and larynx; lung cancer unspecified as primary or secondary;

mediastinal cancer; and secondary cancer of the thoracic organs. These accounted for about five percent of the lung cancer rubric.

Lymphatic/Haematopoietic Cancers. In addition to small changes between the seventh and eighth revisions, the eighth revision included the two new categories of polycythaemia vera and myelofibrosis. Only in the ninth revision was it possible to extract data for leukaemia which had formed about 37 percent of the lymphatic/haematopoietic cancers of the previous revisions.

Remainder Cancers. For the periods 1959-63, 1969-73 and 1979-83, this category was formed by the subtraction of malignant neoplasms of the respiratory system and of lymphatic/haematopoietic tissues (during the two earlier periods, and leukaemia for the last period) from the total cancer figures. The major components of total cancer within this category were gastric, colorectal, breast and genito-urinary.

Breast Cancer. Breast cancer was not available in the ICD B list during the seventh revision. The differences between the eighth and ninth revisions were very small, with male breast cancer being included only in the eighth revision.

Gastric Cancer. Gastric cancer was not available in the ICD B list during the seventh revision. Only small differences were present between the eighth and ninth revisions, with the ninth revision allowing more detailed classification.

Colorectal Cancer. Cancers of the colon and rectum appeared in the ICD B list only in the ninth revision.

Coronary Heart Disease. During 1959-63, coronary heart disease (CHD) was included within the category of arteriosclerotic and degenerative heart disease, of which it formed 63 percent. During 1969-73 and 1979-83, however, it formed an exclusive category. During the earliest period only, the rubric also included chronic endocarditis not specified as rheumatic, other myocardial degeneration, fatty degeneration of the heart, myocardial degeneration with arteriosclerosis and other myocardial degeneration. Asymptomatic ischaemic heart disease appeared only in 1969-73 and 1979-83. The differences between the eighth and ninth revisions were minor, with chronic ischaemic heart disease in the eighth revision (ICD 412) included in the ninth revision under other forms of heart disease (ICD 429).

Other Heart Disease. Major differences exist between the seventh and eighth revisions. Chronic disease of the endocardium, cardiomyopathy, some pulmonary heart disease and other myocardial insufficiency were excluded in the seventh revision. The changes were smaller between the eighth and ninth revisions: more detailed classification, with cardiomegaly, functional disturbances following cardiac surgery, and other and unspecified acute pericarditis, for example, included in the ninth but not the eighth revisions.

Cerebrovascular Disease. Only very slight differences arose in the classification of cerebrovascular diseases between the three revisions. Occlusion of pre-cerebral arteries was included in the eighth and ninth revisions but not in the seventh revision; and late effects of cerebrovascular disease and other more specific diagnoses were included in the ninth but not earlier.

Other Circulatory Disease. The eighth revision was expanded slightly from the seventh revision to encompass conditions allied to polyarteritis nodosa and diseases of the capillaries. However, some of the inclusions within polyarteritis nodosa were subsequently dropped in the ninth revision, along with chilblains and gangrene.

Bronchitis, Emphysema and Asthma. During 1959-63, bronchitis (ICD 500-502) was coded separately, with emphysema included under Remainder Respiratory Disease (ICD 470-527) and asthma under ICD 241. However, during 1969-73, bronchitis was coded together with emphysema and asthma (ICD 490-493) and accounted for 91-93 percent of the mortality. Only slight variations occurred between the eighth and ninth revisions.

Pneumonia. Only slight differences in coding arose. During 1959-63 it was coded separately as pneumonia (ICD 490-493) and as pneumonia of the newborn (ICD 763-768). Of the total figures for newborn, infections other than pneumonia accounted for 16-30 percent. During 1969-73 and 1979-83 pneumonia and pneumonia of the newborn were recorded together.

Other Respiratory Disease. The largest single component of Other Respiratory Disease was influenza, which during 1969-73 accounted for 34 percent of the mortality. Other diseases included were: occupational diseases such as silicosis, asbestosis and pneumoconiosis, and acute bronchitis. Emphysema was included in 1959-63 but not in 1969-73 and 1979-83. Hay fever was excluded in 1959-63 but included in the later periods.

Definitions of infant mortality, stillbirths, neonatal and perinatal mortality.

Infant mortality	the ratio of the annual number of deaths of children less than 1 year old, to the number of live births in the same year;
Stillbirths	the ratio of the annual number of fetal deaths (over 28th week of gestation), to the number of live and stillbirths in same year;
Neonatal mortality	the ratio of the annual number of deaths of liveborn infants within 28 days of birth, to the number of live births in the same year;
Perinatal mortality	the ratio of the annual number of deaths (over 28 weeks of

Definitions (continued)

gestation) + early neonatal deaths (first week), to the number of live and stillbirths in the same year.

Reliability of death certification. In the construction of mortality tables, the Registrar General uses the diagnosis given for the underlying cause of death (cause 1c on the death certificate). All Scottish death certificates are processed in Edinburgh, and the death certificate may be recoded in specified circumstances. However, the coder may be merely recoding chaos if the sequence of the cause of death on the certificate is biologically implausible. In recent years the accuracy of death certification has been discussed frequently [10,13-16]. The disagreement between the pathologist's certificate (after necropsy) and the clinical diagnosis has been as high as 39 percent [13]. The divergence of opinion increases with age at death 'especially when neoplasms of cardiovascular or respiratory diseases were thought in life to have been responsible for the last illness' [10]. Although the Registrar General recodes all certificates in response to information derived from necropsy, necropsies are performed on only about 30 percent of deaths in Scotland, and hence the accuracy of the diagnoses on the remaining certificates is not checked. Nevertheless, the value of death certification in epidemiology is recognized [17], for although some diagnoses are completely altered as a result of necropsy, in most cases the revised certificate is only altered by a digit (Registrar General for Scotland, personal communication). In this atlas, therefore, the effects of misclassification were mitigated by the use of ICD rubrics which often encompassed several integers.

Socio-economic and environmental variables. These variables were compiled from the ARRG and from census publications, with the exceptions of geological substrata and surface temperature of the sea. The map of geological substrata was compiled in the Geography Department of the University of Dundee; and surface temperature of the sea was prepared in the University's Department of Community Medicine from data published by the Meteorological Office.

Symbols used in mapping. Red symbols indicated communities experiencing high mortality, and black symbols those experiencing low or 'normal' mortality. The Cities have been denoted by triangles, the Large Burghs by squares, the Small Burghs by circles and the Landward Areas by diamonds. During the last period, when only one category of community was mapped (the Districts), only one symbol was required; a square was chosen because of its cartographic clarity in the potentially congested area around Glasgow, and also to prevent a solid block of colour in a large District from having a greater impact than a similar block of colour in a smaller District.

Mortality maps. To allow readers with diverse interests to interpret the significance - whether statistical or otherwise - of the communities with high or low SMRs, the mortality maps have been produced using seven, mutually exclusive, categories:

1) large red symbols (triangle, square, circle or diamond): the SMRs were significantly high ($p<0.05$) and within the top tenth of the communities;
2) medium-sized, cross-hatched red symbols: the SMRs were significantly high ($p<0.05$) but not within the top tenth;
3) medium-sized red symbols: the SMRs were within the top tenth but not significantly high;
4) small black symbols: the SMRs were neither significantly high nor low, and did not lie within the top or bottom tenth;
5) medium-sized black symbols: the SMRs were within the bottom tenth but not significantly low;
6) medium-sized, cross-hatched black symbols: the SMRs were significantly low but not within the bottom tenth;
7) large black symbols: the SMRs were significantly low and within the bottom tenth.

The same mapping categories were used throughout the three periods; however, during the period 1979-83, the influence of small numbers of deaths in the calculation of the SMR was diminished, and consequently many of the disease distributions did not include SMRs within categories 3 and 5.

Socio-economic and environmental maps. The data for socio-economic maps were plotted according to seven categories, the ranges of which varied according to the characteristic mapped. These maps were plotted with the categories selected to show the natural groupings of the Districts. This method was chosen because the aim of including socio-economic data was to allow those Districts with extreme values to be clearly distinguished, rather than to enable absolute comparisons to be made between the Districts over time. Also, it was planned to facilitate the generation of hypotheses on possible associations between socio-economic status and mortality within a District. As a result, some of the socio-economic maps showed distributions which appeared implausible at first. For example, in the map illustrating the percentage of the population involved in construction, the percentage was high in the western Highlands but low in the Glasgow conurbation; it must be remembered that the percentage is a relative measurement which does not take into account the differences in the population size of the two Districts.

DISEASES MAPPED BY ICD CODE

Disease	*7th Revision*	*8th Revision*	*9th Revision*
Total cancers	140-205	140-209	140-208
Lung cancer	160-165	162	162
Lymphatic and haematopoietic cancer	200-205	200-209	-
Leukaemia	-	-	204-208
Remainder cancer	140-159, 170-199	140-161, 163-200	140-161, 163-203
Breast cancer	-	174	174
Gastric cancer	-	151	151
Colorectal cancer	-	-	153,154
Coronary heart disease	420-422	410-414	410-414
Other heart disease	430-434	420-429	415-429
Cerebrovascular disease	330-334	430-438	430-438
Other circulatory disease	450-468	440-458	440-459
Bronchitis, emphysema, asthma	500-502	490-493	490-493
Pneumonia	490-493, 763	480-486	480-486
Other respiratory disease	470-475, 480-483, 510-527	460-479, 487-489, 494-519	460-479, 487-489, 494-519

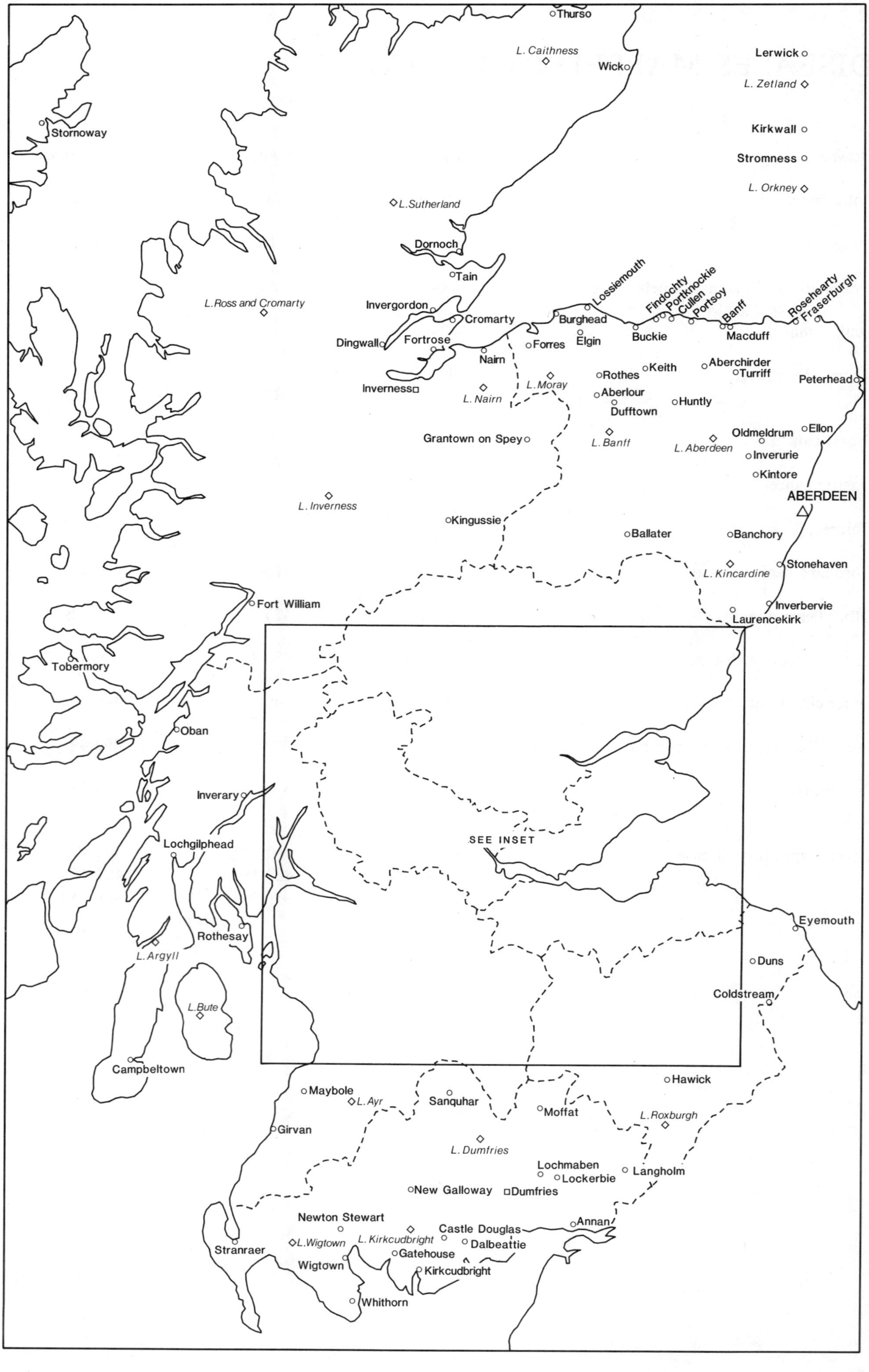
Thurso
L. Caithness
Wick
Lerwick
L. Zetland
Kirkwall
Stromness
L. Orkney
Stornoway
L. Sutherland
Dornoch
Tain
L. Ross and Cromarty
Invergordon
Cromarty
Dingwall
Fortrose
Nairn
Inverness
L. Nairn
Lossiemouth
Burghead
Forres
Elgin
L. Moray
Findochty
Portknockie
Cullen
Portsoy
Banff
Buckie
Macduff
Rosehearty
Fraserburgh
Rothes
Keith
Aberchirder
Turriff
Peterhead
Aberlour
Dufftown
Huntly
Grantown on Spey
L. Banff
L. Aberdeen
Oldmeldrum
Ellon
Inverurie
Kintore
ABERDEEN
L. Inverness
Kingussie
Ballater
Banchory
L. Kincardine
Stonehaven
Fort William
Inverbervie
Laurencekirk
Tobermory
Oban
Inverary
SEE INSET
Lochgilphead
Rothesay
L. Argyll
L. Bute
Eyemouth
Duns
Coldstream
Campbeltown
Maybole
L. Ayr
Sanquhar
Moffat
Hawick
Girvan
L. Roxburgh
L. Dumfries
Lochmaben
Lockerbie
Langholm
New Galloway
Dumfries
Newton Stewart
Castle Douglas
Annan
L. Wigtown
L. Kirkcudbright
Dalbeattie
Stranraer
Gatehouse
Wigtown
Kirkcudbright
Whithorn

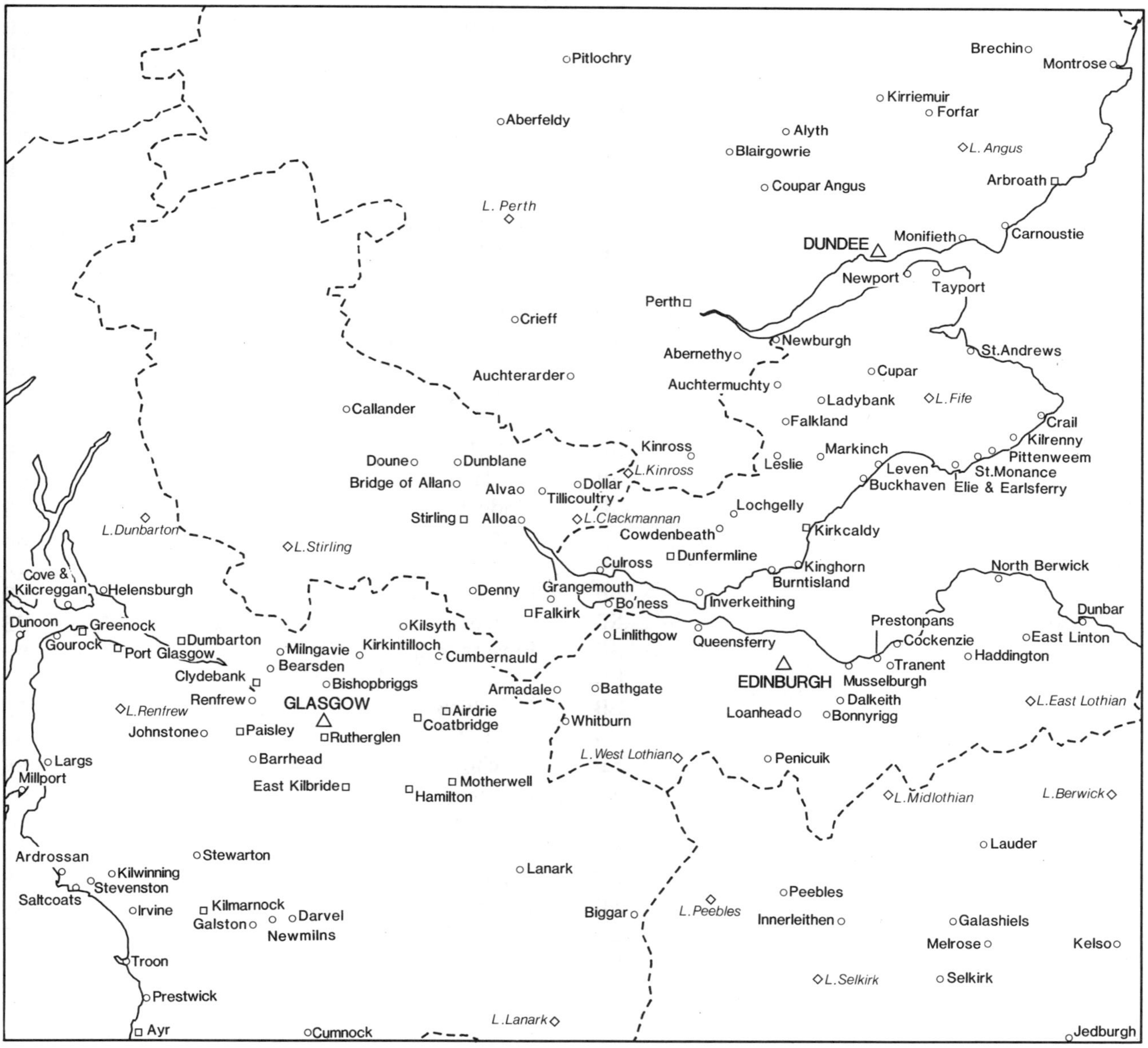

Pitlochry
Brechin
Montrose
Kirriemuir
Forfar
Aberfeldy
Alyth
Blairgowrie
L. Angus
Coupar Angus
Arbroath
L. Perth
Monifieth
Carnoustie
DUNDEE
Newport
Tayport
Perth
Crieff
Newburgh
Abernethy
St.Andrews
Cupar
Auchterarder
Auchtermuchty
Ladybank
L. Fife
Callander
Falkland
Crail
Kinross
Kilrenny
Markinch
Pittenweem
Doune
Dunblane
L.Kinross
Leslie
Leven
St.Monance
Bridge of Allan
Alva
Dollar
Tillicoultry
Buckhaven
Elie & Earlsferry
Lochgelly
Stirling
Alloa
L.Clackmannan
L.Dunbarton
Cowdenbeath
Kirkcaldy
L.Stirling
Dunfermline
Culross
Kinghorn
North Berwick
Cove &
Kilcreggan
Helensburgh
Denny
Grangemouth
Burntisland
Dunbar
Bo'ness
Inverkeithing
Falkirk
Dunoon
Greenock
Kilsyth
Prestonpans
Dumbarton
Linlithgow
Queensferry
Cockenzie
East Linton
Gourock
Port Glasgow
Milngavie
Kirkintilloch
Cumbernauld
Tranent
Haddington
Bearsden
Clydebank
Bishopbriggs
Armadale
Bathgate
EDINBURGH
Musselburgh
Renfrew
GLASGOW
Airdrie
Dalkeith
L.Renfrew
Coatbridge
Whitburn
Loanhead
Bonnyrigg
L.East Lothian
Johnstone
Paisley
Rutherglen
Largs
Barrhead
L.West Lothian
Penicuik
Millport
East Kilbride
Motherwell
Hamilton
L.Midlothian
L.Berwick
Lauder
Ardrossan
Stewarton
Kilwinning
Stevenston
Lanark
Saltcoats
Kilmarnock
Peebles
Irvine
Galston
Darvel
Newmilns
Biggar
L.Peebles
Innerleithen
Galashiels
Melrose
Kelso
Troon
L.Selkirk
Selkirk
Prestwick
Ayr
Cumnock
L.Lanark
Jedburgh

PLACE NAMES

SB Small Burgh, **LB** Large Burgh, **C** City

Aberchirder	SB
Aberdeen	C
Aberfeldy	SB
Aberlour	SB
Abernethy	SB
Airdrie	LB
Alloa	SB
Alva	SB
Alyth	SB
Annan	SB
Arbroath	LB
Ardrossan	SB
Armadale	SB
Auchterarder	SB
Auchtermuchty	SB
Ayr	LB
Ballater	SB
Banchory	SB
Banff	SB
Barrhead	SB
Bathgate	SB
Bearsden	SB
Biggar	SB
Bishopbriggs	SB
Blairgowrie and Rattray	SB
Bo'ness	SB
Bonnyrigg and Lasswade	SB
Brechin	SB
Bridge of Allan	SB
Buckhaven and Methil	SB
Buckie	SB
Burghead	SB
Burntisland	SB
Callander	SB
Campbeltown	SB
Carnoustie	SB
Castle Douglas	SB
Clydebank	LB
Coatbridge	LB
Cockenzie and Port Seaton	SB
Coldstream	SB
Coupar Angus	SB
Cove and Kilcreggan	SB
Cowdenbeath	SB
Crail	SB
Crieff	SB
Cromarty	SB
Cullen	SB
Culross	SB
Cumbernauld	SB
Cumnock and Holmhead	SB
Cupar	SB
Dalbeattie	SB
Dalkeith	SB
Darvel	SB
Denny and Dunipace	SB
Dingwall	SB
Dollar	SB
Dornoch	SB
Doune	SB
Dufftown	SB
Dumbarton	LB
Dumfries	LB
Dunbar	SB
Dunblane	SB
Dundee	C
Dunfermline	SB
Dunoon	SB
Duns	SB
East Kilbride	LB
East Linton	SB
Edinburgh	C
Elgin	SB
Elie and Earlsferry	SB
Ellon	SB
Eyemouth	SB
Falkirk	LB
Falkland	SB
Findochty	SB
Forfar	SB
Forres	SB
Fort William	SB
Fortrose	SB
Fraserburgh	SB
Galashiels	SB
Galston	SB
Gatehouse	SB
Girvan	SB
Glasgow	C
Gourock	SB
Grangemouth	SB
Grantown-on-Spey	SB
Greenock	LB

SB Small Burgh, **LB** Large Burgh, **C** City

Haddington	SB
Hamilton	LB
Hawick	SB
Helensburgh	SB
Huntly	SB
Innerleithen	SB
Inverary	SB
Inverbervie	SB
Invergordon	SB
Inverkeithing	SB
Inverness	LB
Inverurie	SB
Irvine	SB
Jedburgh	SB
Johnstone	SB
Keith	SB
Kelso	SB
Kilmarnock	LB
Kilrenny etc	SB
Kilsyth	SB
Kilwinning	SB
Kinghorn	SB
Kingussie	SB
Kinross	SB
Kintore	SB
Kirkcaldy	SB
Kirkcudbright	SB
Kirkintilloch	SB
Kirkwall	SB
Kirriemuir	SB
Ladybank	SB
Lanark	SB
Langholm	SB
Largs	SB
Lauder	SB
Laurencekirk	SB
Lerwick	SB
Leslie	SB
Linlithgow	SB
Loanhead	SB
Lochgelly	SB
Lochgilphead	SB
Lochmaben	SB
Lockerbie	SB
Lossiemouth and Branderburgh	SB
Macduff	SB
Markinch	SB
Maybole	SB
Melrose	SB
Millport	SB
Milngavie	SB
Moffat	SB
Monifieth	SB
Montrose	SB
Motherwell and Wishaw	LB
Musselburgh	SB
Nairn	SB
New Galloway	SB
Newburgh	SB
Newmilns and Greenholm	SB
Newport-on-Tay	SB
Newton Stewart	SB
North Berwick	SB
Oban	SB
Old Meldrum	SB
Paisley	LB
Peebles	SB
Penicuik	SB
Perth	LB
Peterhead	SB
Pitlochry	SB
Pittenweem	SB
Port Glasgow	LB
Portknockie	SB
Portsoy	SB
Prestonpans	SB
Prestwick	SB
Queensferry	SB
Renfrew	SB
Rosehearty	SB
Rothes	SB
Rothesay	SB
Rutherglen	LB
Saltcoats	SB
Sanquhar	SB
Selkirk	SB
St Andrews	SB
St Monance	SB
Stevenson	SB
Stewarton	SB
Stirling	LB
Stonehaven	SB
Stornoway	SB
Stranraer	SB
Stromness	SB
Tain	SB
Tayport	SB
Thurso	SB

SB Small Burgh, **LB** Large Burgh, **C** City

Tillicoultry	SB	Whitburn	SB
Tobermory	SB	Whithorn	SB
Tranent	SB	Wick	SB
Troon	SB	Wigtown	SB
Turriff	SB		

Landward	Aberdeen
Landward	Angus
Landward	Argyll
Landward	Ayr
Landward	Banff
Landward	Berwick
Landward	Bute
Landward	Caithness
Landward	Clackmannan
Landward	Dumfries
Landward	Dunbarton
Landward	East Lothian
Landward	Fife
Landward	Inverness
Landward	Kincardine
Landward	Kirkcudbright
Landward	Kinross
Landward	Midlothian
Landward	Moray
Landward	Nairn
Landward	Orkney
Landward	Peebles
Landward	Perth
Landward	Renfrew
Landward	Ross and Cromarty
Landward	Roxburgh
Landward	Selkirk
Landward	Stirling
Landward	Sutherland
Landward	West Lothian
Landward	Wigtown
Landward	Zetland

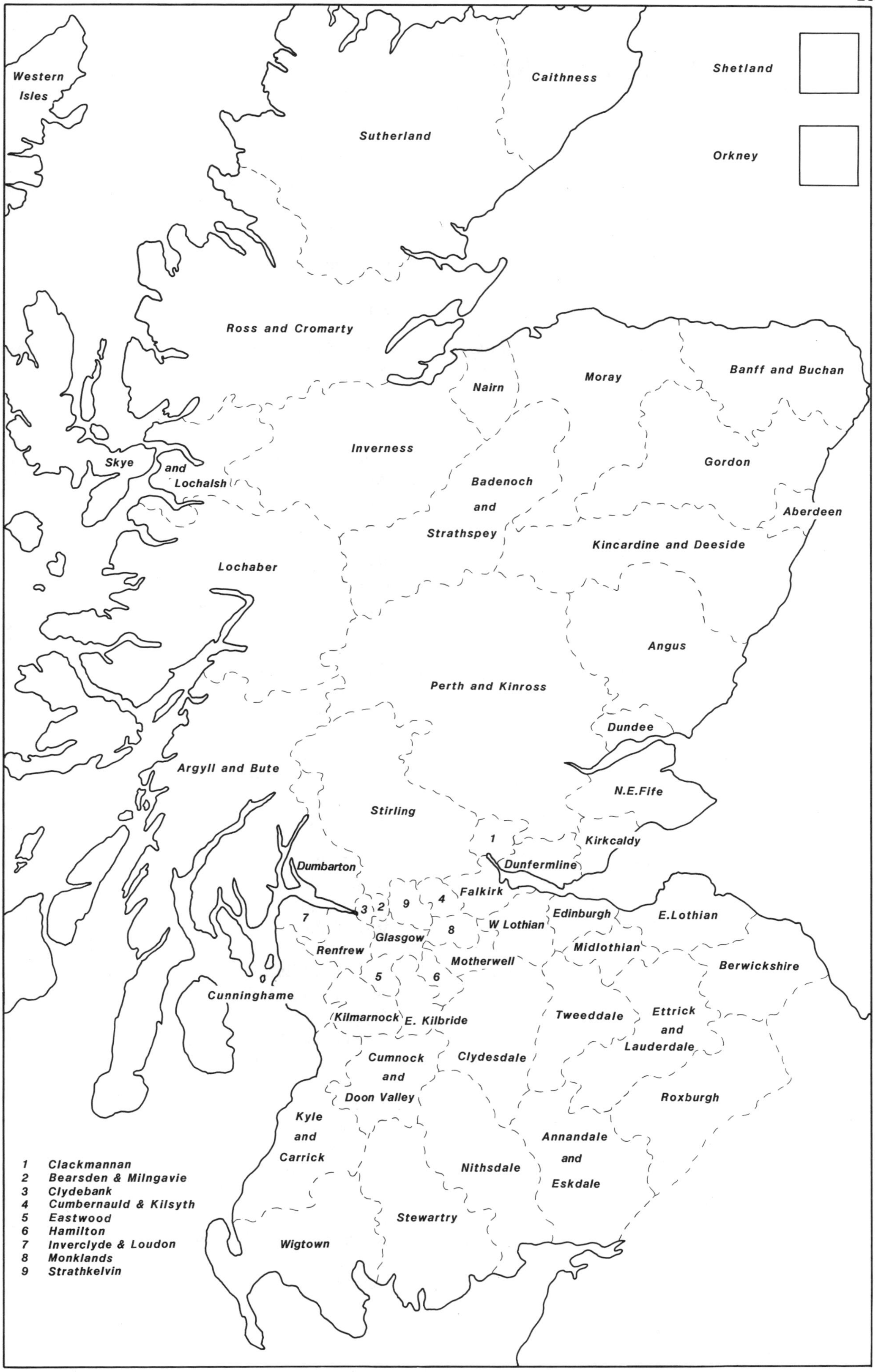
Western Isles
Caithness
Shetland
Sutherland
Orkney
Ross and Cromarty
Nairn
Moray
Banff and Buchan
Inverness
Skye and Lochalsh
Badenoch and Strathspey
Gordon
Aberdeen
Kincardine and Deeside
Lochaber
Angus
Perth and Kinross
Dundee
Argyll and Bute
N.E.Fife
Stirling
1
Kirkcaldy
Dunfermline
Dumbarton
Falkirk
3
2
9
4
7
Edinburgh
E.Lothian
W Lothian
8
Glasgow
Renfrew
Midlothian
Motherwell
Berwickshire
5
6
Cunninghame
Tweeddale
Ettrick and Lauderdale
Kilmarnock
E. Kilbride
Cumnock and Doon Valley
Clydesdale
Roxburgh
Kyle and Carrick
Annandale and Eskdale
Nithsdale
Stewartry
Wigtown
1 Clackmannan
2 Bearsden & Milngavie
3 Clydebank
4 Cumbernauld & Kilsyth
5 Eastwood
6 Hamilton
7 Inverclyde & Loudon
8 Monklands
9 Strathkelvin

REGIONS AND DISTRICTS

BORDERS	Berwickshire Ettrick and Lauderdale Roxburgh Tweeddale
CENTRAL	Clackmannan Falkirk Stirling
DUMFRIES AND GALLOWAY	Annandale and Eskdale Nithdale Stewartry Wigtown
FIFE	Dunfermline Kirkcaldy North East Fife
GRAMPIAN	Aberdeen Banff and Buchan Gordon Kincardine and Deeside Moray
HIGHLAND	Badenoch and Strathspey Caithness Inverness Lochaber Nairn Ross and Cromarty Skye and Lochalsh Sutherland
LOTHIAN	East Lothian Edinburgh Midlothian West Lothian
STRATHCLYDE	Argyll and Bute Bearsden and Milngavie Clydebank Cumbernauld and Kilsyth Cumnock and Doon Valley Cunninghame Dumbarton East Kilbride Eastwood Glasgow City Hamilton Inverclyde Kilmarnock and Loudoun Kyle and Carrick Lanark (now Clydesdale)

STRATHCLYDE (cont.)	Monklands Motherwell Renfrew Strathkelvin
TAYSIDE	Angus Dundee City Perth and Kinross
ISLAND AREAS	Orkney Shetland Western Isles

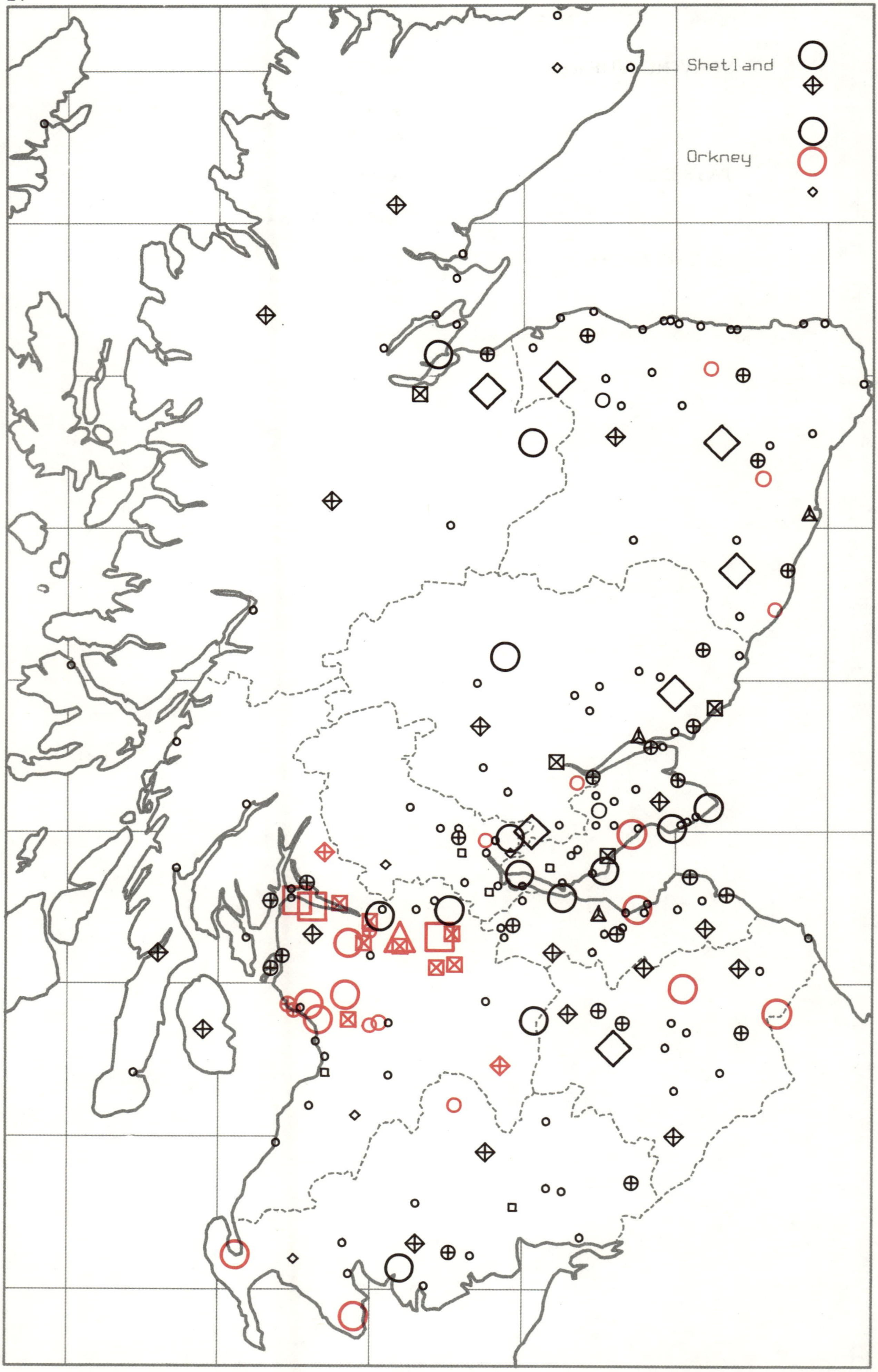
Shetland
Orkney

TOTAL MORTALITY 1959-63

SMR significantly high ($p < 0.05$) and within the top tenth

SMR significantly high ($p < 0.05$) not within the top tenth

SMR not significantly high but within the top tenth

SMR not significantly high or low and not within the top or bottom tenth

SMR not significantly low but within the bottom tenth

SMR significantly low ($P < 0.05$) not within the bottom tenth

SMR significantly low ($P < 0.05$) and within the bottom tenth

City | Large Burgh | Small Burgh | Landward Area

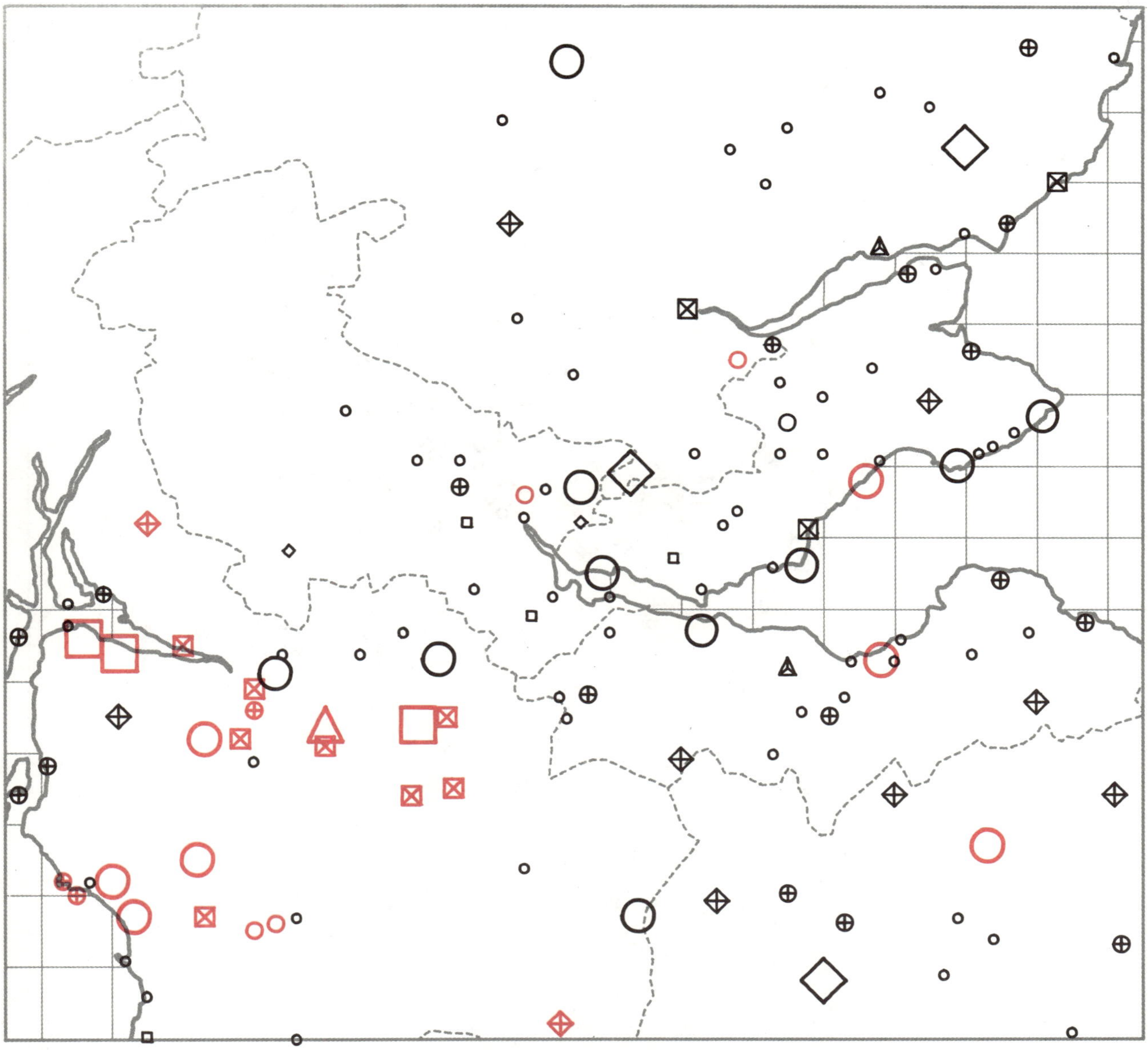

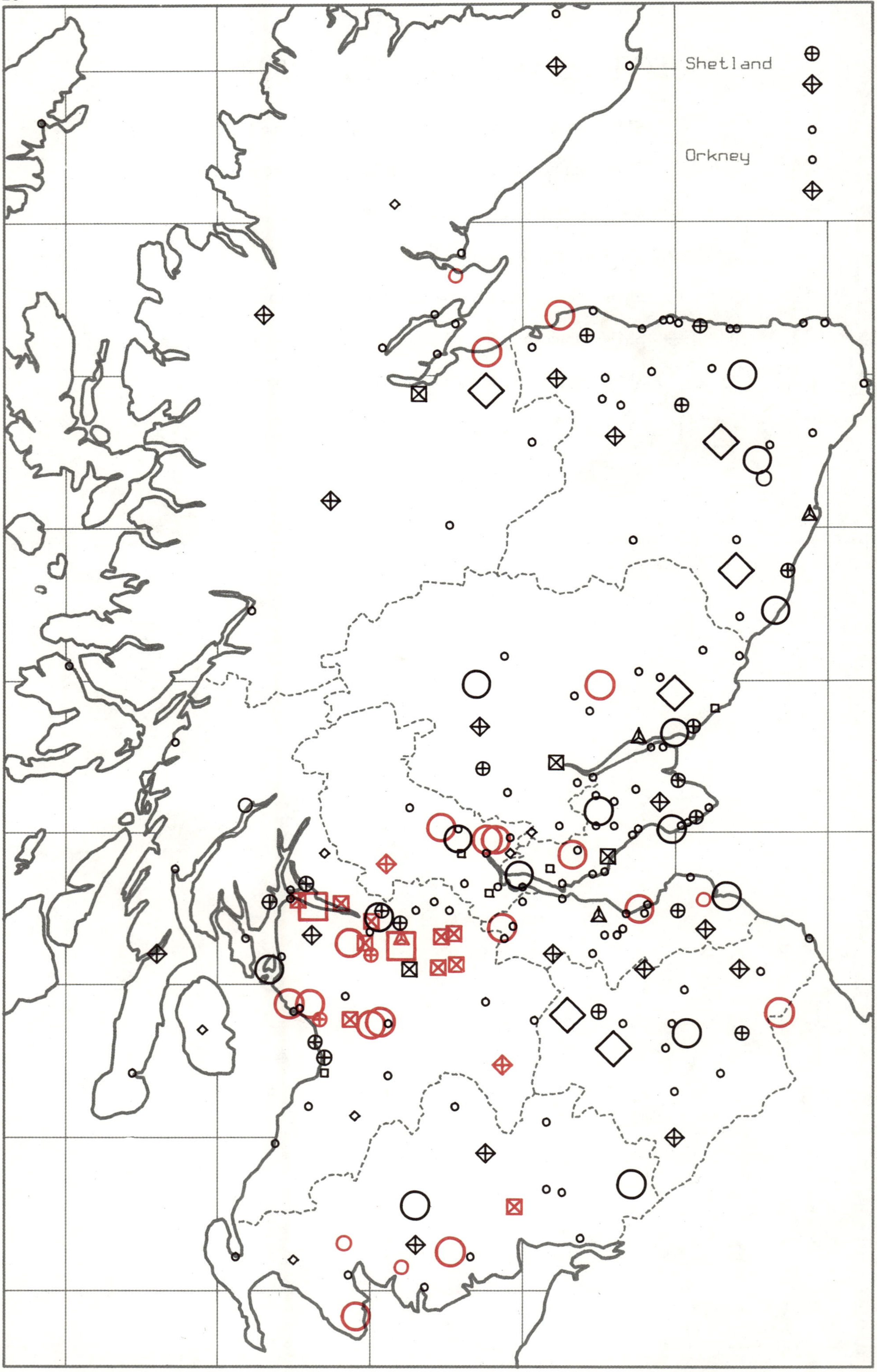
Shetland
Orkney

TOTAL MORTALITY 1969-73

SMR significantly high ($p < 0.05$) and within the top tenth

SMR significantly high ($p < 0.05$) not within the top tenth

SMR not significantly high but within the top tenth

SMR not significantly high or low and not within the top or bottom tenth

SMR not significantly low but within the bottom tenth

SMR significantly low ($P < 0.05$) not within the bottom tenth

SMR significantly low ($P < 0.05$) and within the bottom tenth

City △ Large Burgh □ Small Burgh ○ Landward Area ◇

A SQUARE SYMBOL IS USED FOR THE DISTRICTS ON THE MAP OVERLEAF FOR 1979-83.

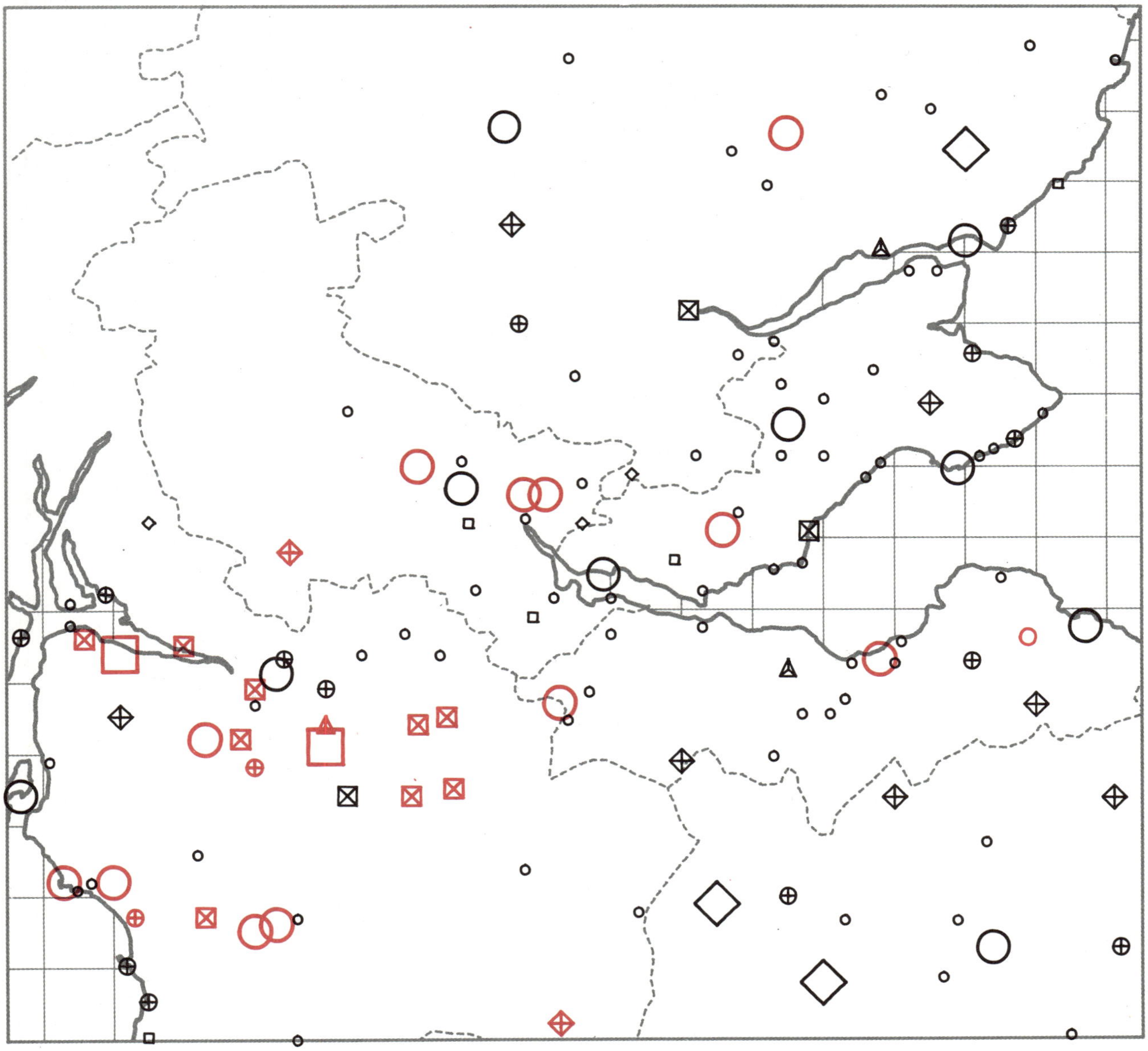

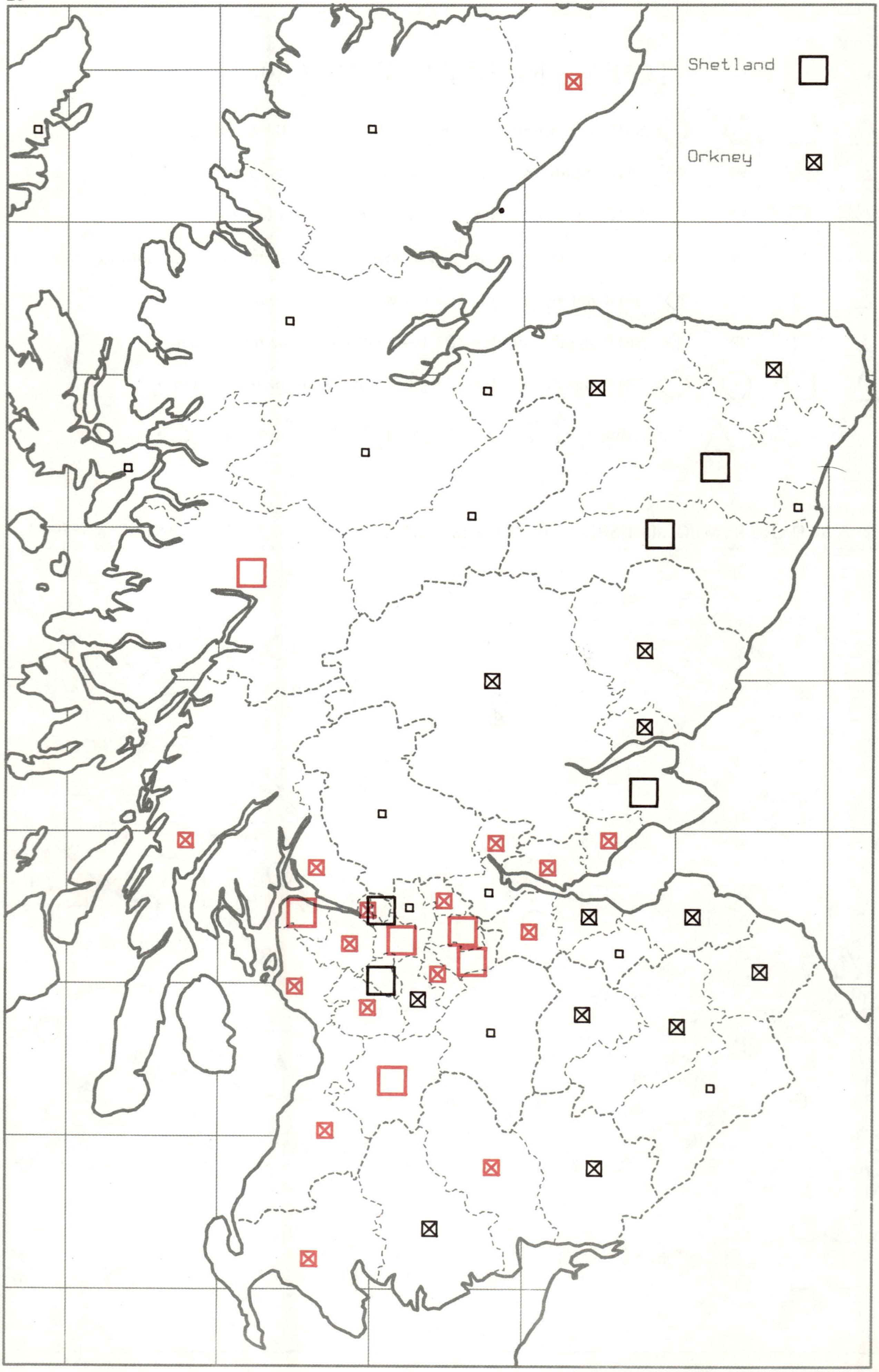
Shetland
Orkney

TOTAL MORTALITY

Rates for Total Mortality have been falling steadily in Britain since the 1850s, a phenomenon mostly attributable to the decline in deaths in the younger age-groups. Following the impact of the successful control of many of the infectious diseases - through a combination of advances in sanitation, preventive medicine and effective chemotherapy - the present-day major causes of death are coronary and cerebrovascular diseases, lung cancer and bronchitis, many of which have environmental causes.

In international comparisons [18], Scotland has an unenviable record of Total Mortality. Expressed as rates per 100,000 population of males aged 40-69 years, only Hungary (1842), Czechoslovakia (1702) and Poland (1701) had rates exceeding those of Scottish men (1542) in 1980. Scottish women in the same age-group were ranked more highly, their rates (866) only exceeded by those of Hungarian women (917).

Analysis of the secular trends between 1972 and 1982 suggests that the Scottish rates are declining in line with most Western European countries. Males show a decline of four percent between 1972 and 1977, and of nine percent between 1978 and 1982, while women show an increase of two percent and a decline of ten percent respectively over the same periods.

Within Britain, the male mortality rates vary from north to south: 1267 per 100,000 for England and Wales, 1492 for Northern Ireland and 1542 for Scotland. For women the pattern is the same, with England and Wales showing the lowest rates (687) followed by Northern Ireland (802) and Scotland (866).

Within Scotland, there is a consistent pattern throughout the three periods, with high mortality in the west and south and low mortality in the east and north. Clearly, the distribution of the communities' SMRs for Total Mortality should reflect the patterns of those diseases which contribute the highest numbers of deaths, i.e. cardiovascular diseases and cancers. And indeed, the distributions of Coronary and Other Heart Diseases are very similar (qv). The patterns for all cancers, however, are not particularly similar, with the 'usual' predilection for high SMRs in the region around Glasgow not being in evidence.

In the search for environmental factors which may affect (unfavourably) communities' SMRs, the maps of Total Mortality can provide a useful starting point - especially for the Small Burghs, where the numbers of deaths in the sub-categories may be low. Even a cursory look at these maps reveals anomalies. For example, why do the Small Burghs of Prestonpans, Coldstream and Whithorn experience significantly raised SMRs during both 1959-63 and 1969-73? They are, after all, small rural communities which theoretically would be expected to show favourable mortality ratios. Similarly, it is intriguing that the District of Caithness during 1979-83 should show high mortality: it is largely a rural area with a complete absence of Large Burghs and Cities, and the mortality ratios of Thurso, Wick and Landward Caithness (which together make up the District) were unexceptional during the two earlier periods. Only very general hypotheses may be generated using solely the distributions shown in the maps, but an obvious follow-up would be to formulate a disease profile for the community in question. Caithness District, for example, shows significantly high SMRs for coronary heart and cerebrovascular diseases, a significantly low SMR for lung cancer and average SMRs for all the other diseases mapped: the mortality ratios for the categories of death encompassed within the first year of life again show average values with the exception of high stillbirth mortality in 1979-83. Together, these profiles suggest that environmental characteristics - whether behavioural or general - associated with coronary and cerebrovascular diseases (qv) are unusually clustered in the District of Caithness. The raised stillbirth ratio may indicate the presence of toxic factors in the environment [19] or distance from hospital facilities, or may merely highlight the problems encountered with the interpretation of data which are based upon the analysis of a small number of cases.

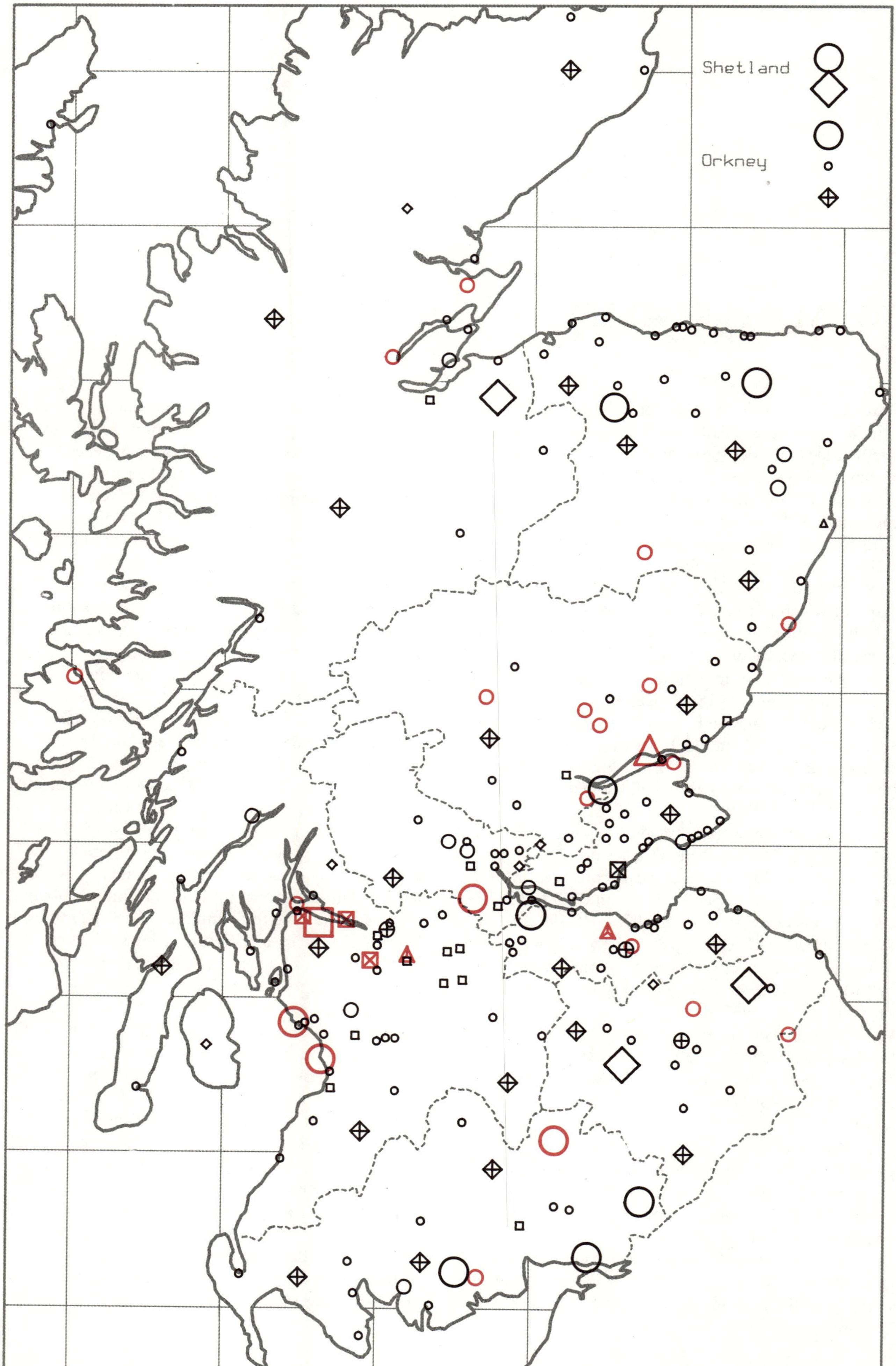
Shetland
Orkney

TOTAL CANCERS 1959-63

- SMR significantly high ($p < 0.05$) and within the top tenth
- SMR significantly high ($p < 0.05$) not within the top tenth
- SMR not significantly high but within the top tenth
- SMR not significantly high or low and not within the top or bottom tenth
- SMR not significantly low but within the bottom tenth
- SMR significantly low ($P < 0.05$) not within the bottom tenth
- SMR significantly low ($P < 0.05$) and within the bottom tenth

City △ Large Burgh □ Small Burgh ○ Landward Area ◇

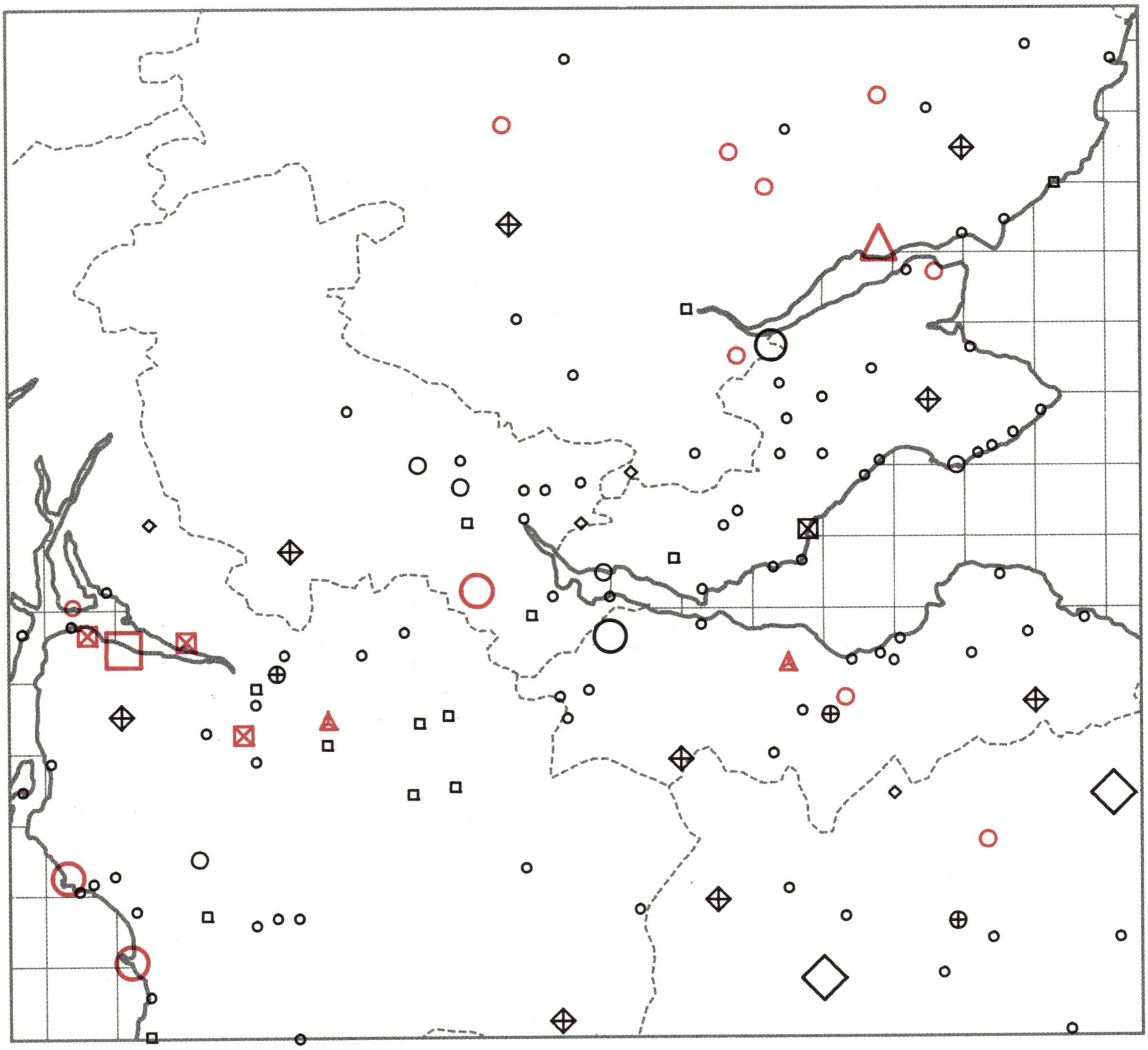

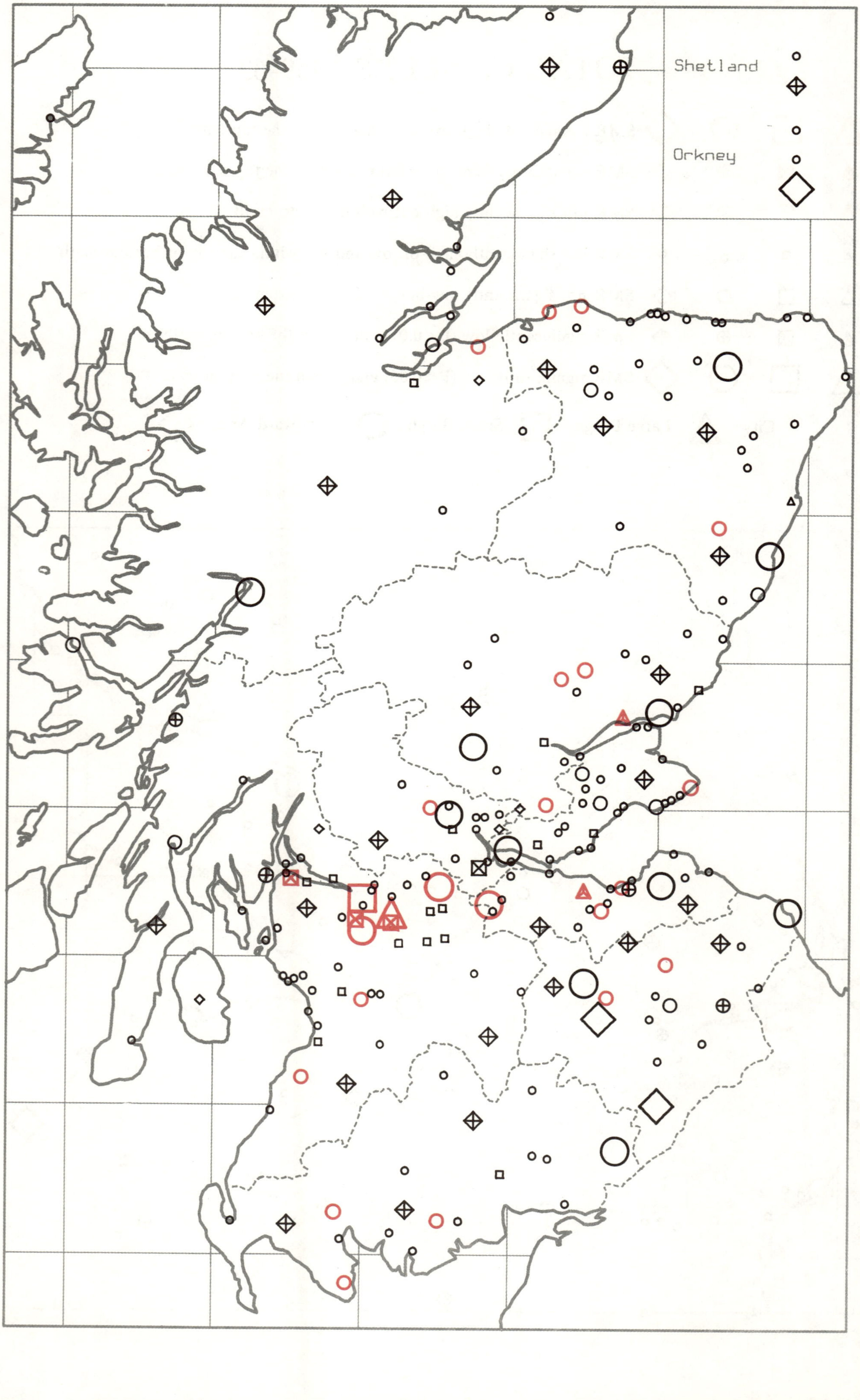
Shetland
Orkney

TOTAL CANCERS 1969-73

- SMR significantly high ($p < 0.05$) and within the top tenth
- SMR significantly high ($p < 0.05$) not within the top tenth
- SMR not significantly high but within the top tenth
- SMR not significantly high or low and not within the top or bottom tenth
- SMR not significantly low but within the bottom tenth
- SMR significantly low ($P < 0.05$) not within the bottom tenth
- SMR significantly low ($P < 0.05$) and within the bottom tenth

City △ Large Burgh □ Small Burgh ○ Landward Area ◇

A SQUARE SYMBOL IS USED FOR THE DISTRICTS ON THE MAP OVERLEAF FOR 1979-83.

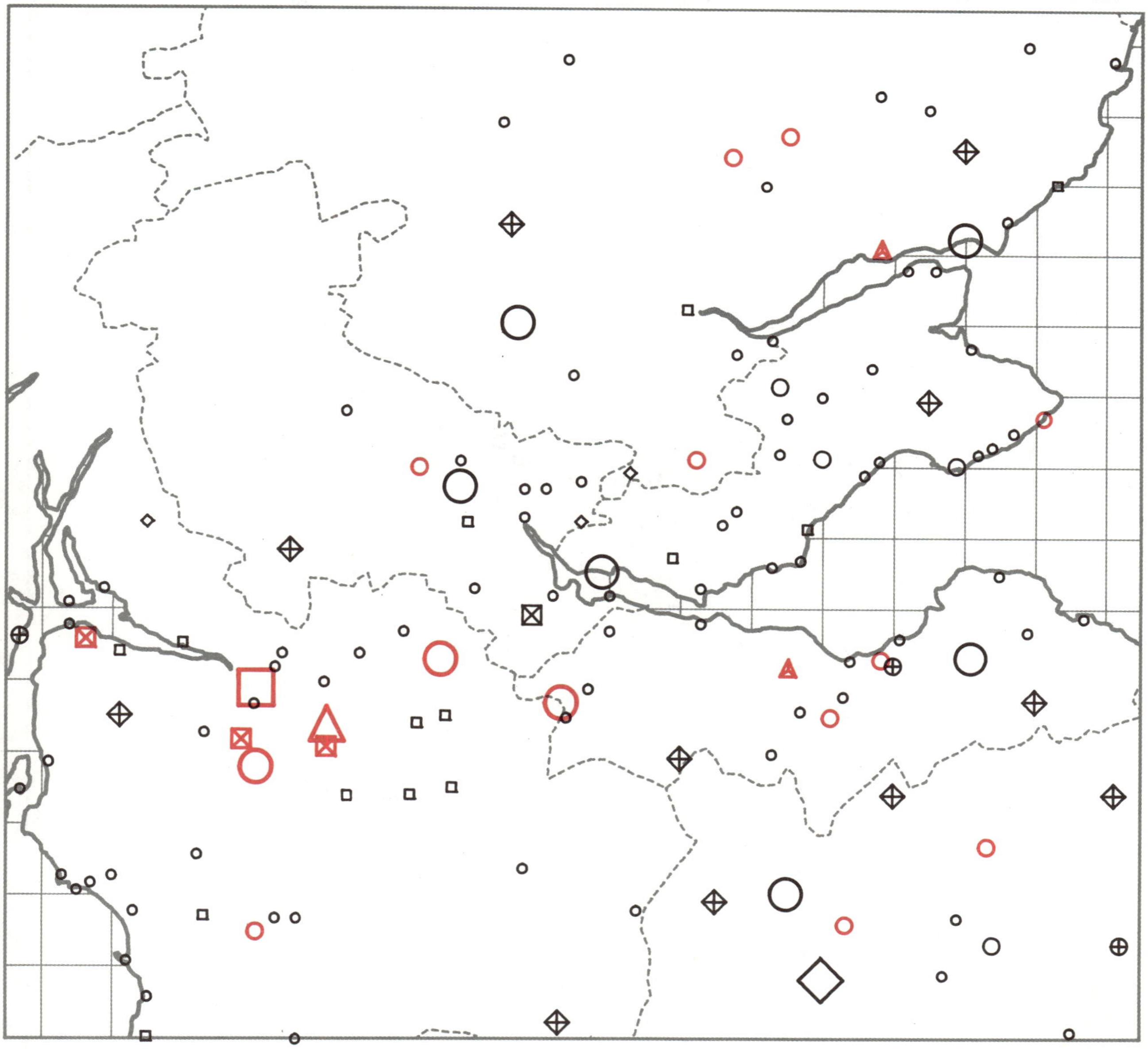

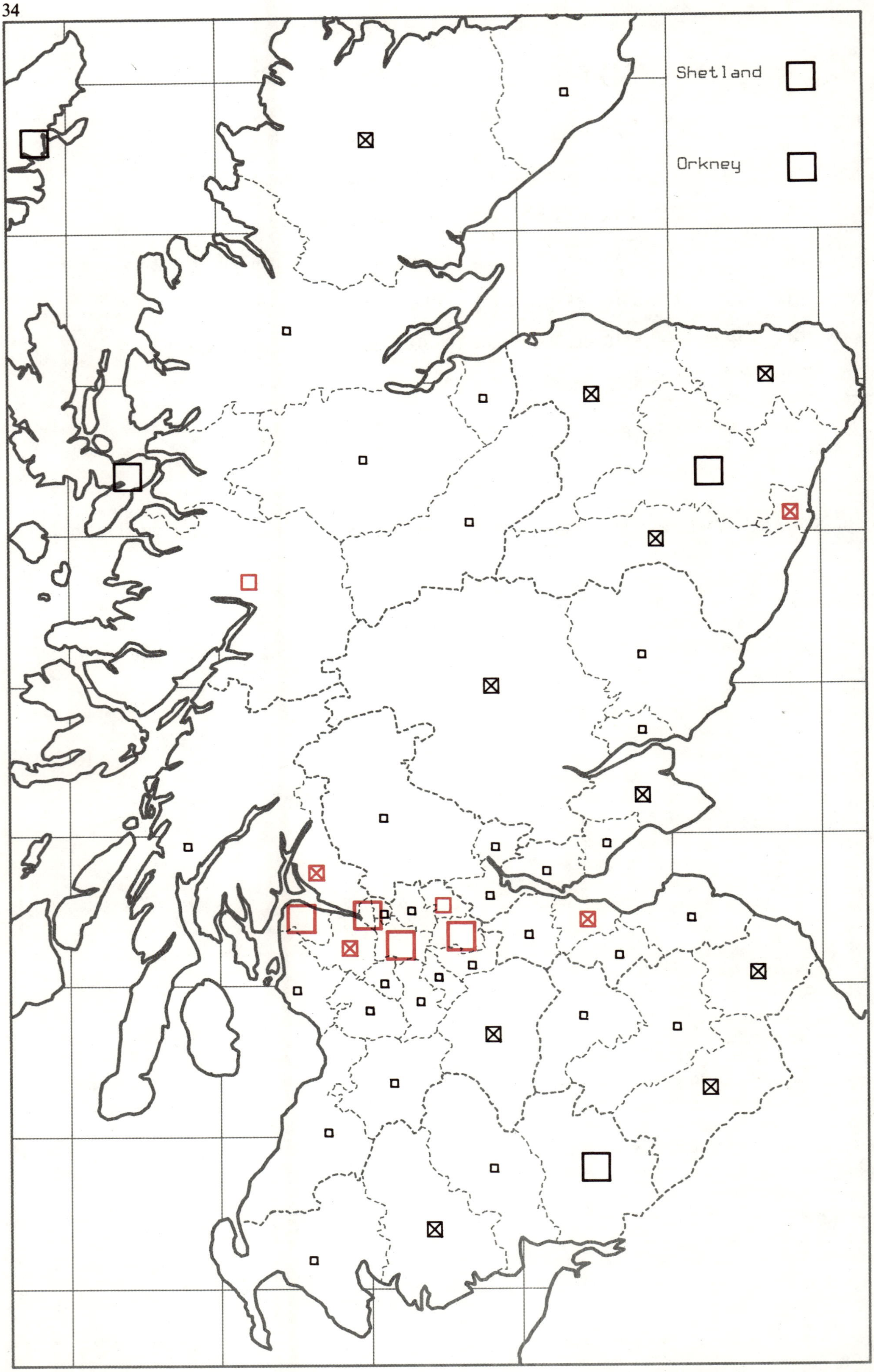
Shetland
Orkney

TOTAL CANCERS

On a global basis, the most common cancers in males are lung, stomach, colon and rectum, mouth and pharynx, prostate, and oesophagus, with the annual numbers of new cases of these cancers estimated at 464,000, 422,000, 251,000, 233,000, 198,000 and 194,000 respectively [20]. For women, the correspondingly common cancers and annual numbers of new cases are breast (541,000), uterine cervix (459,000), stomach (262,000), colon and rectum (256,000), lung (127,000), and mouth and pharynx (107,000). 'These figures represent a desert of human misery and of premature death'[20].

Over many years, Segi and his colleagues [4] have demonstrated the international differences in the age-adjusted mortality rates for various cancers, with Scotland often at the top of the list. In 1978-79, for example, the male rates (per 100,000 population) for total cancer ranged from 206 in Scotland to 130 in Israel; amongst the female rates, Scotland was again highest at 135, but the lowest was 85 in Portugal. Even greater ranges of the rates are found amongst cancers at individual sites: for lung cancer in males they varied from 85 in Scotland to under 20 in Portugal and Chile, and for male cancer of the liver from almost 15 in Japan to below two in Norway. For female breast cancer, the rates varied from about 28 in England and Wales, and Scotland to five in Japan. Even more striking differences in the rates of some cancers can be found if one examines the records of regions within the countries; cancer of the oesophagus in parts of Iran, China and France are an example [21,22]. Because the incidence of some cancers in migrants and in their offspring can differ dramatically from the incidence in their countries of origin, genetic factors are thought to play only a minor role in the aetiology of most cancers; hence environmental carcinogenic risk factors must be of differing importance in different environments. In Scotland risk factors have had an exceptional impact.

The primacy of environmental agents in the causation of cancer gives Preventive Medicine the urgent task of identifying the risk-factors in the human environment, and then of eliminating them. The practice of preventive oncology, stimulated by Percival Pott's observation of the association between scrotal cancer and the occupation of chimney sweep, has accumulated evidence linking many cancers to specific components of the environment. An example is cancer of the urinary bladder, first linked with the aniline dye industry in Germany at the end of the 19th Century, and for which the aromatic amines are the well-recognized industrial hazards. For other cancers such as respiratory cancer, a far wider range of environmental factors has been incriminated, and in many cases the evidence has been more circumstantial. The pace of detecting and 'convicting' new carcinogens has been slow, largely because of difficulties in understanding the precise mechanisms which transform a normal cell into a malignant one. Such uncertainties are found in many processes: the roles of 'initiators' and 'promoters' in neoplasia are unclear; intrinsically harmless solvents and 'carrier' substances may introduce biologically dormant carcinogens into tissues. The host's own metabolism may convert previously-inactive molecules into active carcinogens, or substances may be prevailed upon by other substances to retard or accelerate the neoplastic process. A chemical may be carcinogenic only within certain limits of concentration, or alternatively may inhibit the carcinogenic properties of other substances. Humoral or tissue antibodies of the host to the cancer may retard its neoplastic progress; and these immune responses in turn may be under hormonal, sex-linked or other genetic cellular control.

Epidemiological analysts must penetrate the many layers of confounding variables in their search for the causal agents: genetic variability between and within ethnic groups; the complexity of the environment to which an individual is exposed during the four decades preceding the years when he is most prone to cancer; the wide variation (five-45 years) in the 'lag-phases' between carcinogenic insult and overt carcinogenesis ('lag-phases' may be shorter where a carcinogen contacts tissues which have been damaged already by toxins, irritants and weak carcinogens). Indeed, so complex is the physico-chemical environment of modern urban and industrial life that many epidemiologists hesitate to identify any single, self-sufficient carcinogenic substance amongst the multitude of suspected carcinogens [23]. The emphasis is now placed on the interacting (additive or synergistic) carcinogenic effects of several such substances. When associations between environmental risk-factors and a cancer are discovered, well-known Criteria for Causation [24] provide useful guidelines in assessing the evidence for causality.

A major problem repeatedly encountered in trying to discover factors is the ignorance of the extent of previous exposure to them. Examples can be cited from both the occupational and the general environmental fields. In the occupational field, ignorance of a worker's past history (both occupational and social) is almost routine in many industrial settings. And so, when alarms are raised over the incidence of cancer in an industry, the worker's records may not provide adequate information on previous types of work performed in the same factory and previously, or on the worker's tobacco habits. In the general environmental field, information about patterns of air pollution in the neighbourhood of polluting industries is usually absent. Yet both types of information could be obtained readily and cheaply. In the occupational field, practical experience has demonstrated that workers are willing to complete questionnaires on their occupational and social histories before any question of morbidity has arisen; these questionnaires can be stored, and updated as necessary, until they are required for investigations. In the general environmental field, methods of low technology sampling can reveal, at negligible cost, the detailed patterns of air pollution by metals in residential areas around industries [25-28].

Currently unsuspected carcinogens are more likely to be identified, or identified at smaller cost, in the following favourable circumstances: the exposed population is culturally and genetically homogeneous, and within a compact geographical area; the mobility of the workers and other inhabitants in the community is low; the inhabitants attend one hospital; the mortality data on cancer can be corroborated by information from a Cancer Register and from hospital statistics; important changes in industrial processes are documented; and the industrial and health data are accessible. Hence, when deciding whether or not to start an investigation to detect possible carcinogens, the cost-benefit equation is affected by the number of these circumstances present.

The search for risk-factors is the major task of preventive oncology. This sentiment is well expressed in these words from over 300 years ago. 'Hee is a better physician that keepes diseases off us, than hee that cures them being on us. Prevention is so much better than healing because it saves the labour of being sick [20].'

When studying the distribution of total cancer in a country, a discussion of risk-factors is limited by the knowledge of the heterogeneity of the links between various sites of cancer and risk factors. Different histological types of tumour are found at some sites (for example the skin, lung and stomach) and these histological differences can result from different risk-factors. Nevertheless, the epidemiological features of total cancer are of interest, and its distribution is described in some atlases of mortality [5,7]. For some risk-factors can be common to several cancers: tobacco, alcohol, natural radiation, and some pollutants in occupational and social environments [22,29,30]. In particular, tobacco has links with cancers at several sites, and is generally recognized as the most widespread carcinogen today. About 30 percent of all cancer deaths in the United States, and 15 percent in the world, are probably due to cigarette smoking; globally, over 60 percent of cancers of the lung are attributable to tobacco [20]. Hence the elimination of this hazard would be the most effective single measure for reducing the incidence of cancer in most parts of the world. Moreover, were tobacco removed from society, the cryptic carcinogenic actions of many other substances, at present concealed by (and attributed to) the well-publicized effects of tobacco, might become clear: an example is the link between asbestosis and lung cancer.

The data for total cancer can be of particular value when communities of the size of the smallest of the Scottish Small Burghs are being examined. In such circumstances, the data for total cancer may provide the only statistically useful numbers. Where burghs have only a single major industry, total cancer may be the most appropriate parameter to investigate, at least in the earliest stages of a search for potential carcinogenic consequences of that industry.

In Scotland, the high values for total cancer in the traditional communities during 1959-63 and 1969-73 did not follow any striking geographical pattern, although many of the Large Burghs directly to the west of Glasgow showed high values, as did all the Cities except Aberdeen. Of the Small Burghs, only Blairgowrie (in Perthshire) and Lauder (south-east of Edinburgh) were high in both periods. There were no Landward Areas with high SMRs in either period. Although it is always difficult to interpret the biological significance of elevated values of mortality in small communities, particularly when the values are not maintained over some time, one cannot dismiss as statistical artefact those Small Burghs where the mortality was high in one period only. For example, although Armadale (in West Lothian) had a high SMR only in 1969-73, the burgh was the scene of extraordinarily bad and wide-ranging problems during those years and later [28,31].

Most of the Districts with high values for total cancer in 1979-83 were to the east and west of Glasgow. Of the Cities, Glasgow and Edinburgh continued to have high values, but Aberdeen replaced Dundee as the third city. Of the more rural Districts only Lochaber had a high SMR.

Most of the communities with low SMRs during both 1959-63 and 1969-73 were Landward Areas. The Large Burghs were represented only by East Kilbride and Kirkcaldy in 1959-63 and by Falkirk in 1969-73. During 1979-83 most of the Districts with low values were those along the southern border and in the north-east and north-west of Scotland.

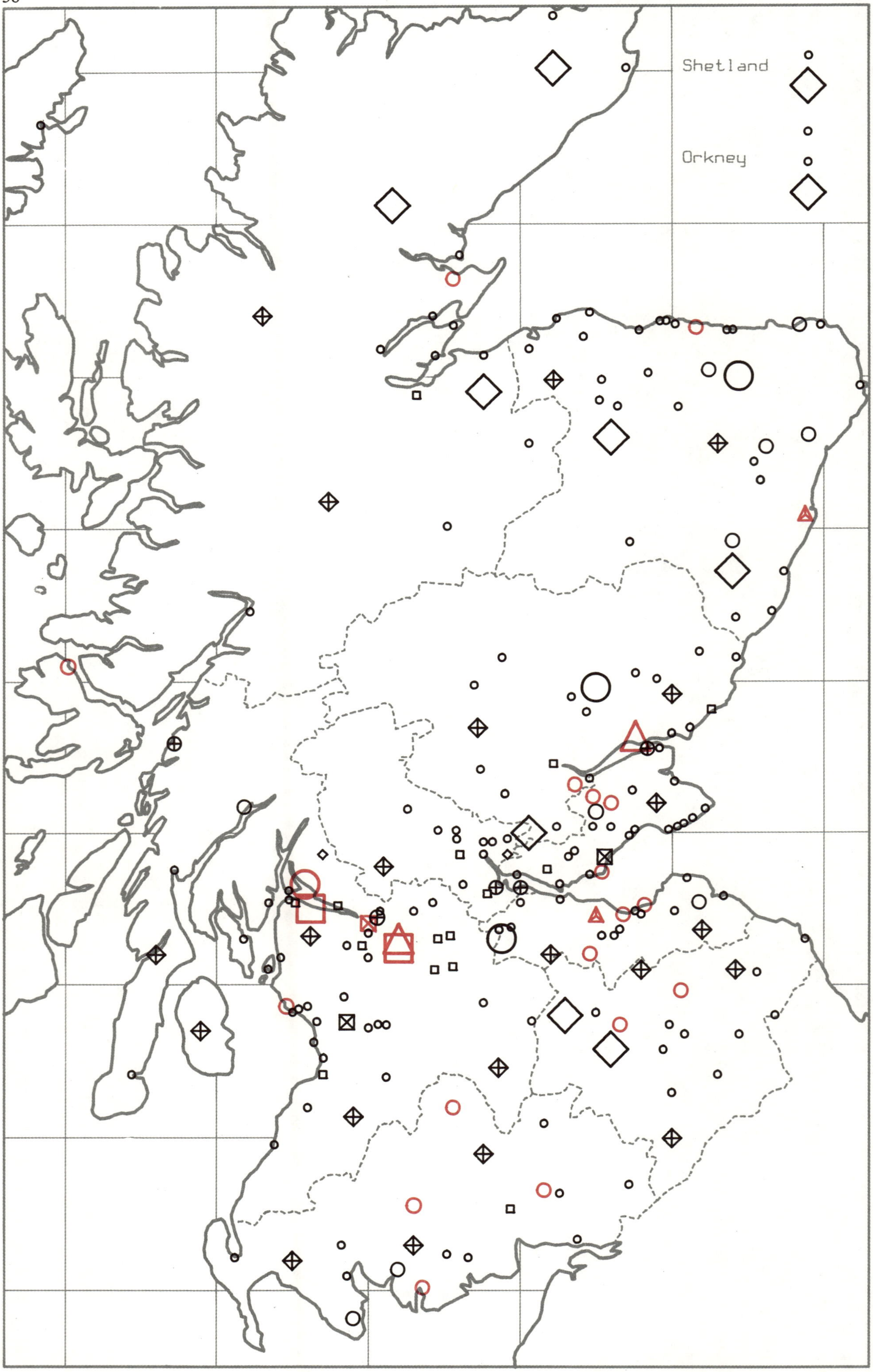
Shetland
Orkney

LUNG CANCER 1959-63

SMR significantly high (p < 0.05) and within the top tenth

SMR significantly high (p < 0.05) not within the top tenth

SMR not significantly high but within the top tenth

SMR not significantly high or low and not within the top or bottom tenth

SMR not significantly low but within the bottom tenth

SMR significantly low (P < 0.05) not within the bottom tenth

SMR significantly low (P < 0.05) and within the bottom tenth

City △ Large Burgh □ Small Burgh ○ Landward Area ◇

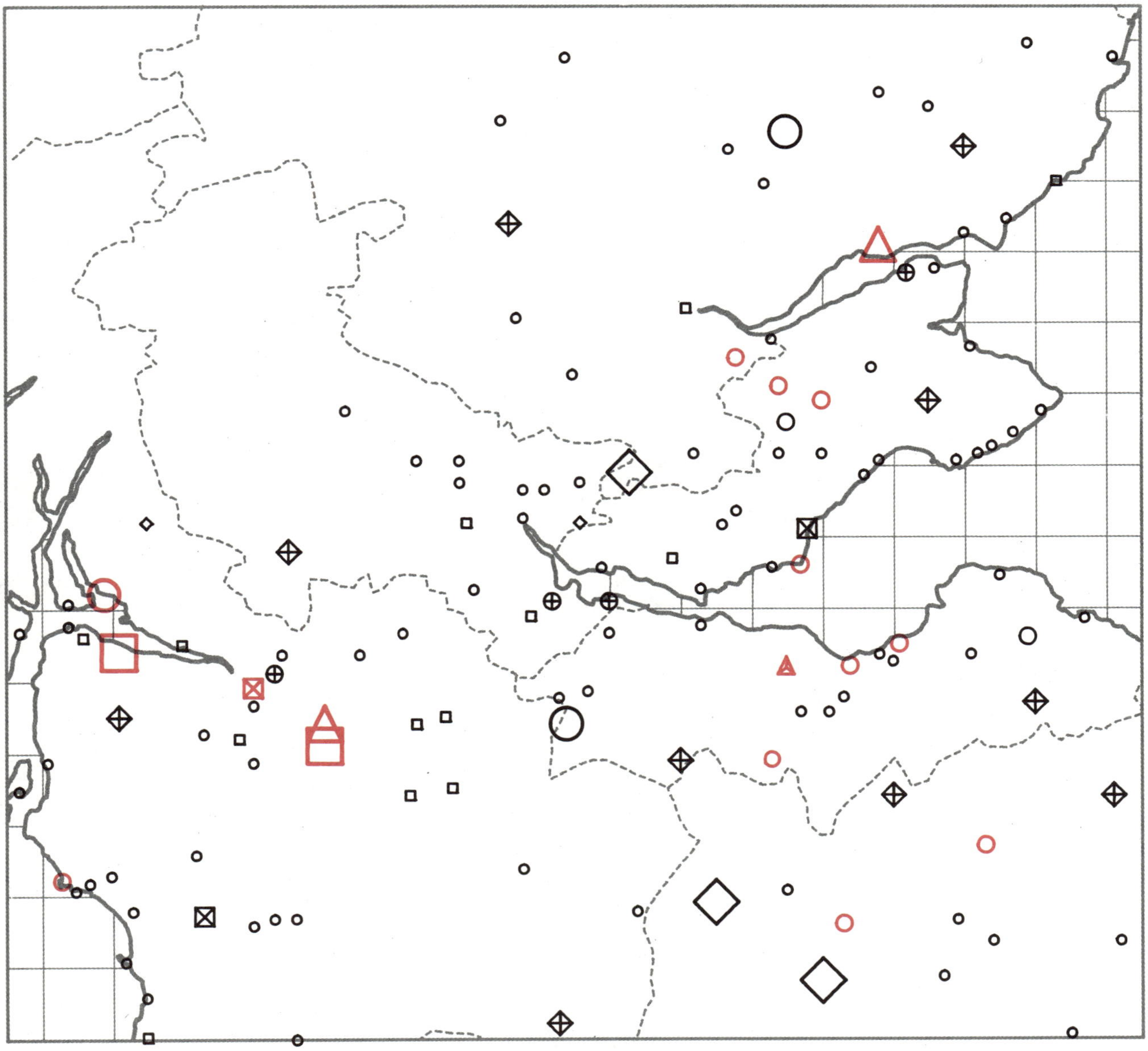

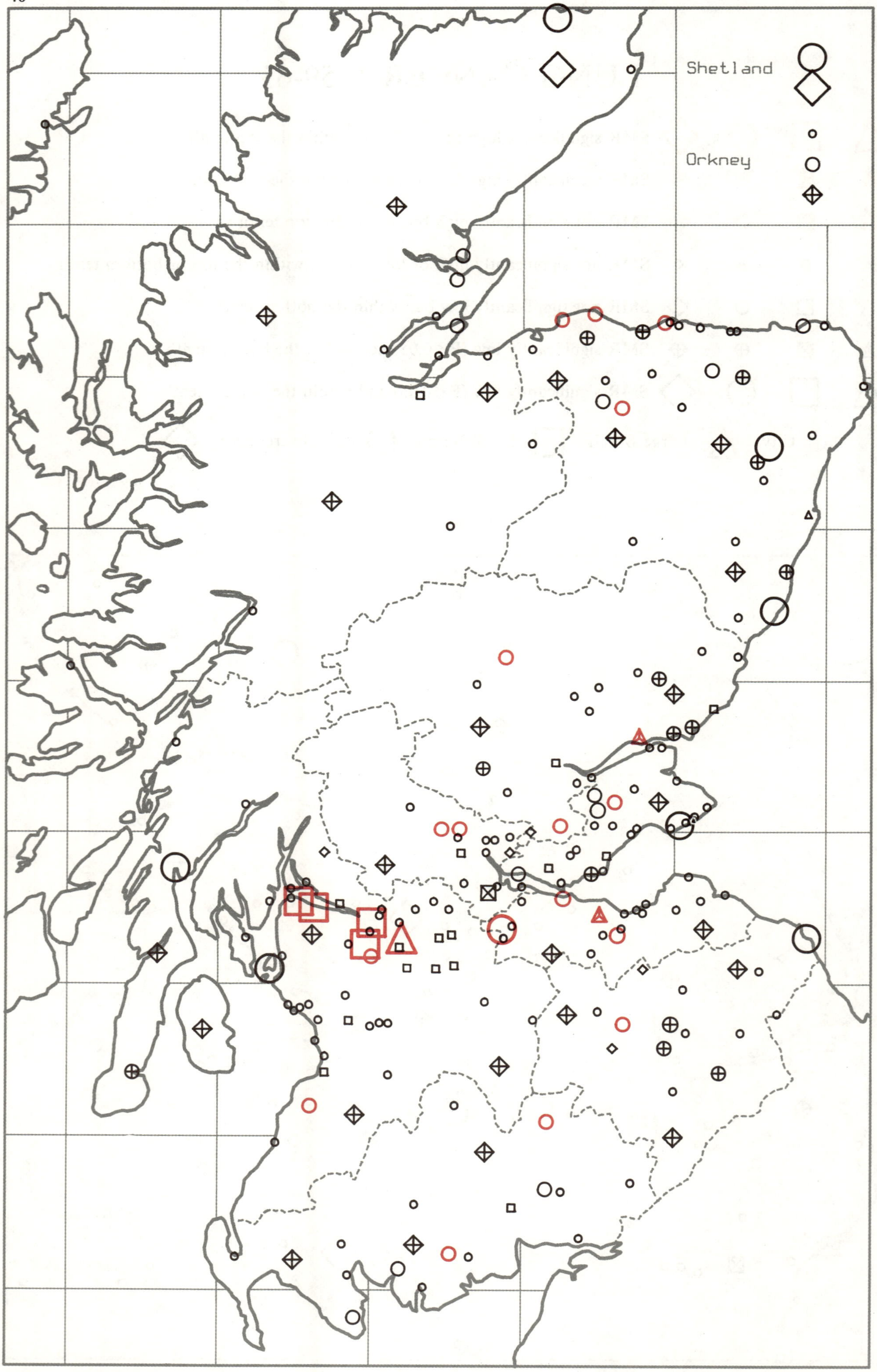
Shetland
Orkney

LUNG CANCER 1969-73

- SMR significantly high ($p<0.05$) and within the top tenth
- SMR significantly high ($p<0.05$) not within the top tenth
- SMR not significantly high but within the top tenth
- SMR not significantly high or low and not within the top or bottom tenth
- SMR not significantly low but within the bottom tenth
- SMR significantly low ($P<0.05$) not within the bottom tenth
- SMR significantly low ($P<0.05$) and within the bottom tenth

City △ Large Burgh □ Small Burgh ○ Landward Area ◇

A SQUARE SYMBOL IS USED FOR THE DISTRICTS ON THE MAP OVERLEAF FOR 1979-83.

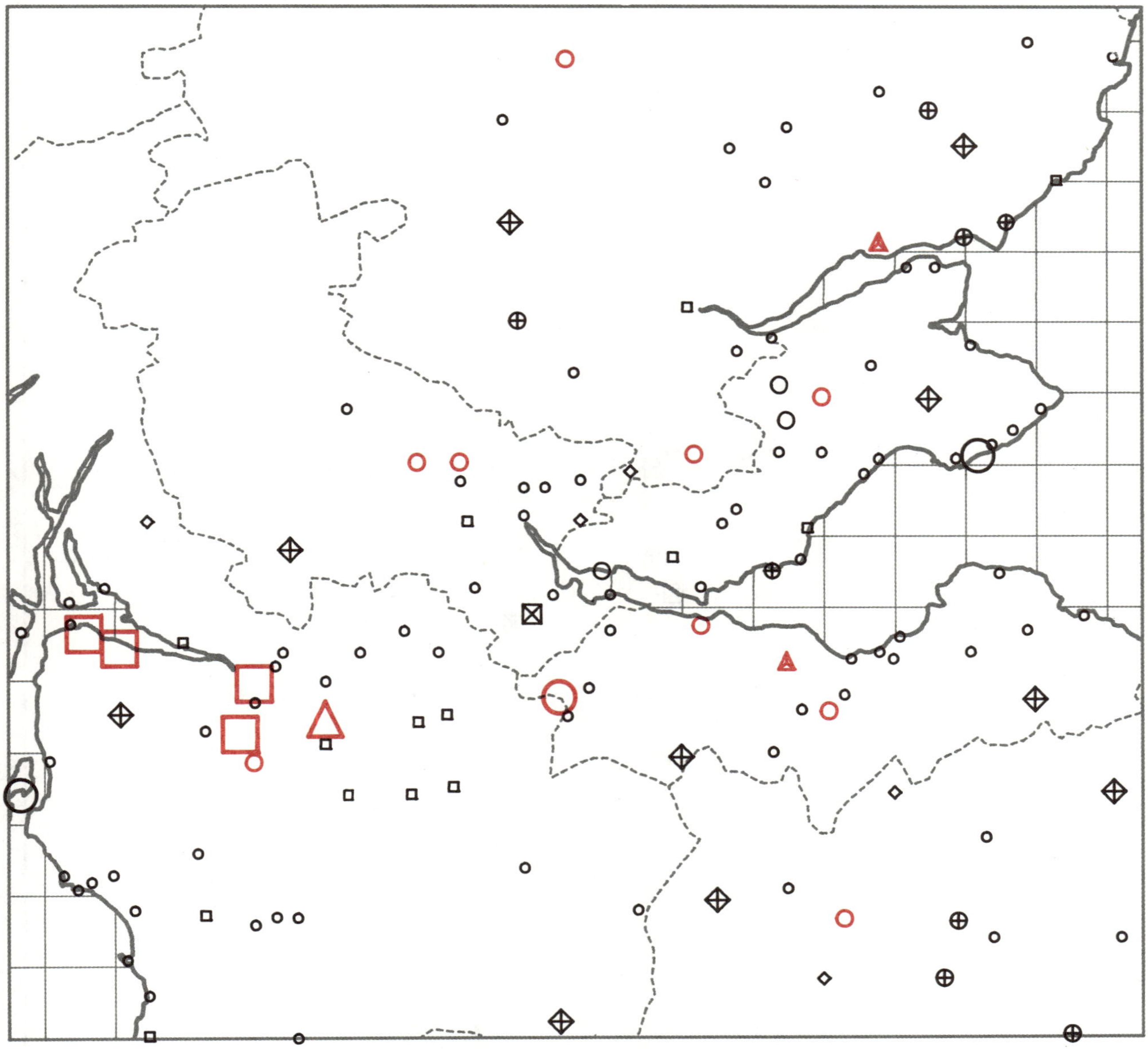

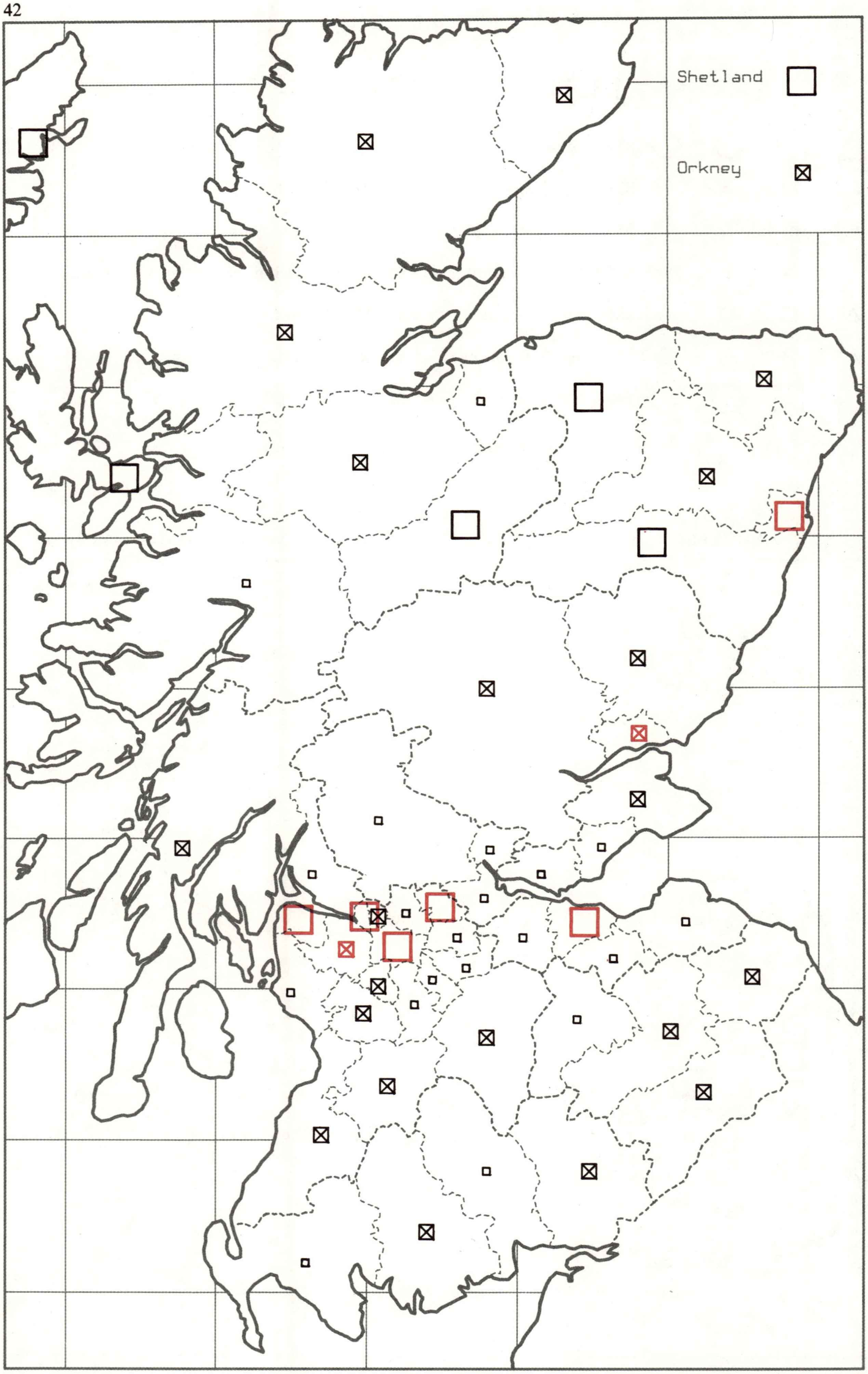
Shetland
Orkney

LUNG CANCER

For many years, cancer of the lung has been the commonest cancer in men. In Scotland in 1984, it overtook breast cancer to become the commonest cause of cancer mortality in women. In Segi's international comparisons [4], Scotland has shown exceptionally high mortality rates - and very frequently the highest rates - in both males and females since the early 1950s. It is the only major cancer where the cause in over ninety percent of cases is known and avoidable, namely cigarette smoking [32]. Despite a recent decline in morbidity from lung cancer amongst males aged under 50 in Scotland, female rates are rising to an alarming degree; recent surveys have shown that young Scottish women are increasing their consumption of cigarettes. A wide variety of occupations is also involved in adding to the lung cancer risk, but occupation usually only plays an important part in that risk if those occupationally exposed also smoke cigarettes.

The Scottish Cities, and especially Glasgow, generally have very high SMRs. In terms of morbidity Glasgow has the highest rate recorded [2], and has been described by the media as the 'world capital' of lung cancer. Passive smoking is possibly one factor in explaining the exceptionally high Glasgow mortality, especially when overcrowding in Central Glasgow in the earlier part of this century is taken into account.

The period 1959-63 saw significantly high SMRs recorded in the City of Glasgow and three other communities in west central Scotland (Rutherglen, Renfrew and Port Glasgow). High SMRs were also apparent in Tayside and in the Edinburgh area. Significantly low SMRs were apparent in the more rural parts of Scotland, particularly in the North-East, the northern Highlands and Islands and the Western Borders. Some parts of central Scotland outside the large towns also had low ratios, including East Kilbride, the Small Burgh of Whitburn in West Lothian, and Kinross.

By 1969-73 the highest SMRs were still found in the Glasgow/Rutherglen, Renfrew/Paisley and Greenock/Port Glasgow areas, and in the Cities of Edinburgh and Dundee. The significantly low SMRs found in East Kilbride and Whitburn ten years earlier had disappeared, to be replaced in the case of West Lothian by a significantly high ratio. Low ratios continued to be recorded by local authorities located in north-east Scotland, Caithness, Shetland and Borders.

The spatial distribution of SMRs for the period 1979-83 continued to show that significantly high ratios were characteristic of all four Scottish Cities and of communities to the west of Glasgow (the Districts of Inverclyde, Clydebank and Renfrew). A significantly high ratio was also recorded in Cumbernauld and Kilsyth District. Significantly low ratios were again found outside the central belt of Scotland, in the more rural Districts of Highland Region, Argyll and Bute, and in north-east and south-west Scotland and the Borders. Bearsden and Milngavie, a suburban District north of Glasgow, also recorded a significantly low SMR for this period.

The earliest time period illustrated came just after the promulgation of the Clean Air Act in 1956, and thus if atmospheric pollution were a major cause of lung cancer a decrease in mortality would be ultimately expected. The map for 1979-83 shows this is unlikely, as the ratio for the District including the new town of Cumbernauld, constructed on a former green field site, is now significantly high. The SMR for the District including the new town of East Kilbride, which similarly experienced substantial in-migration from the City of Glasgow over the period illustrated, appears also to have increased since 1959.

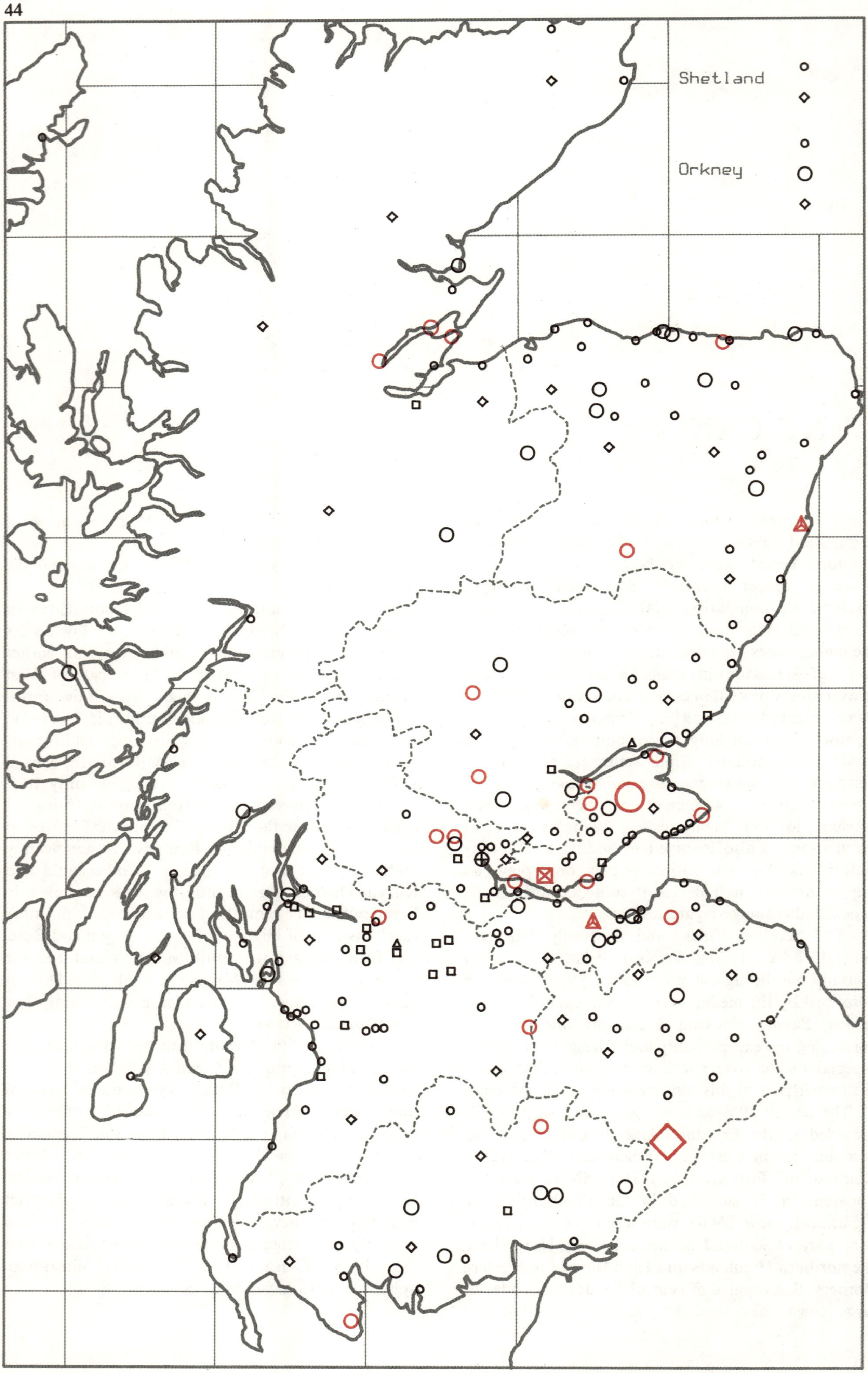
Shetland
Orkney

LYMPHATIC/HAEMATOPOIETIC CANCERS 1959-63

SMR significantly high ($p < 0.05$) and within the top tenth

SMR significantly high ($p < 0.05$) not within the top tenth

SMR not significantly high but within the top tenth

SMR not significantly high or low and not within the top or bottom tenth

SMR not significantly low but within the bottom tenth

SMR significantly low ($P < 0.05$) not within the bottom tenth

SMR significantly low ($P < 0.05$) and within the bottom tenth

City △ Large Burgh □ Small Burgh ○ Landward Area ◇

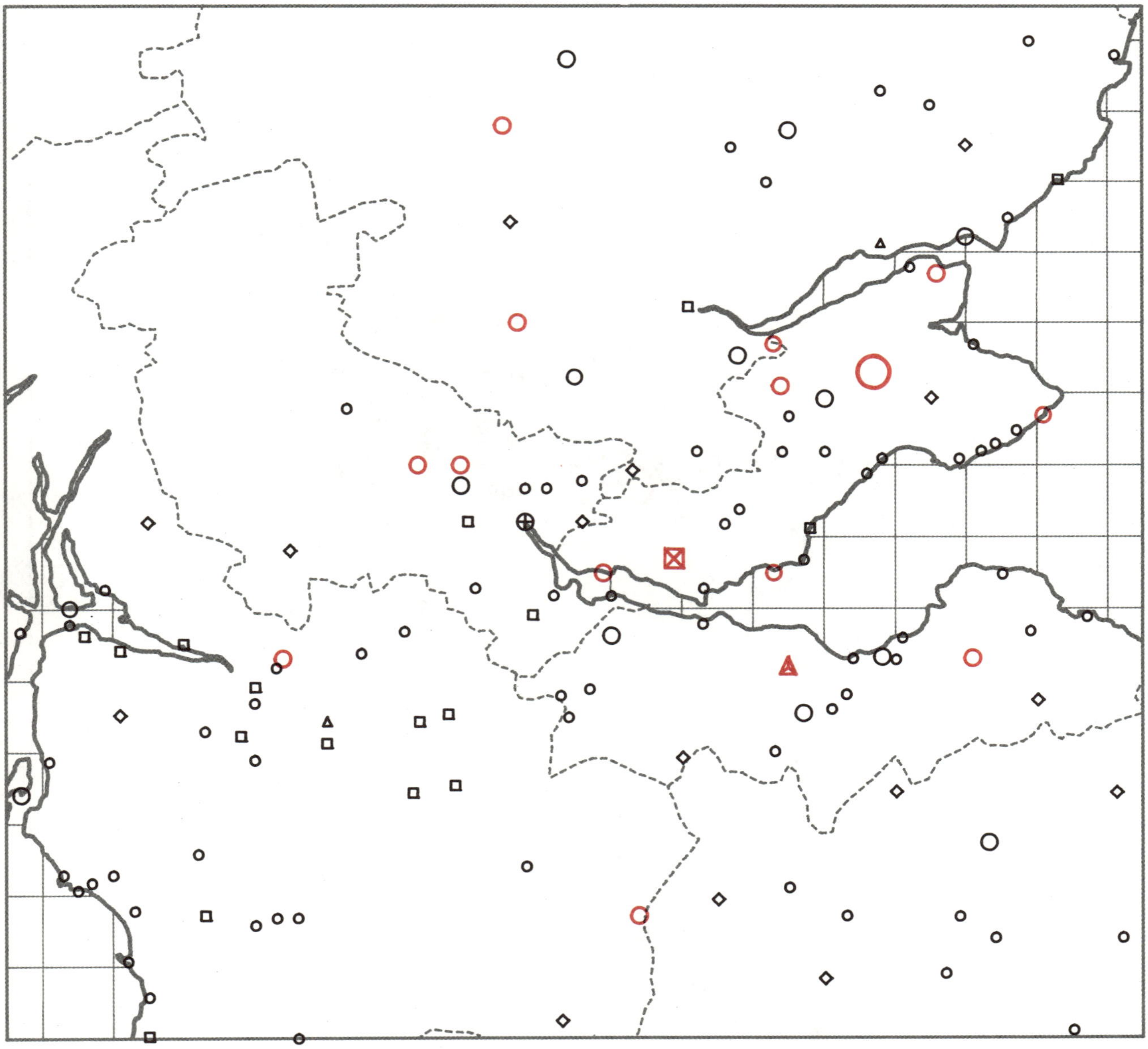

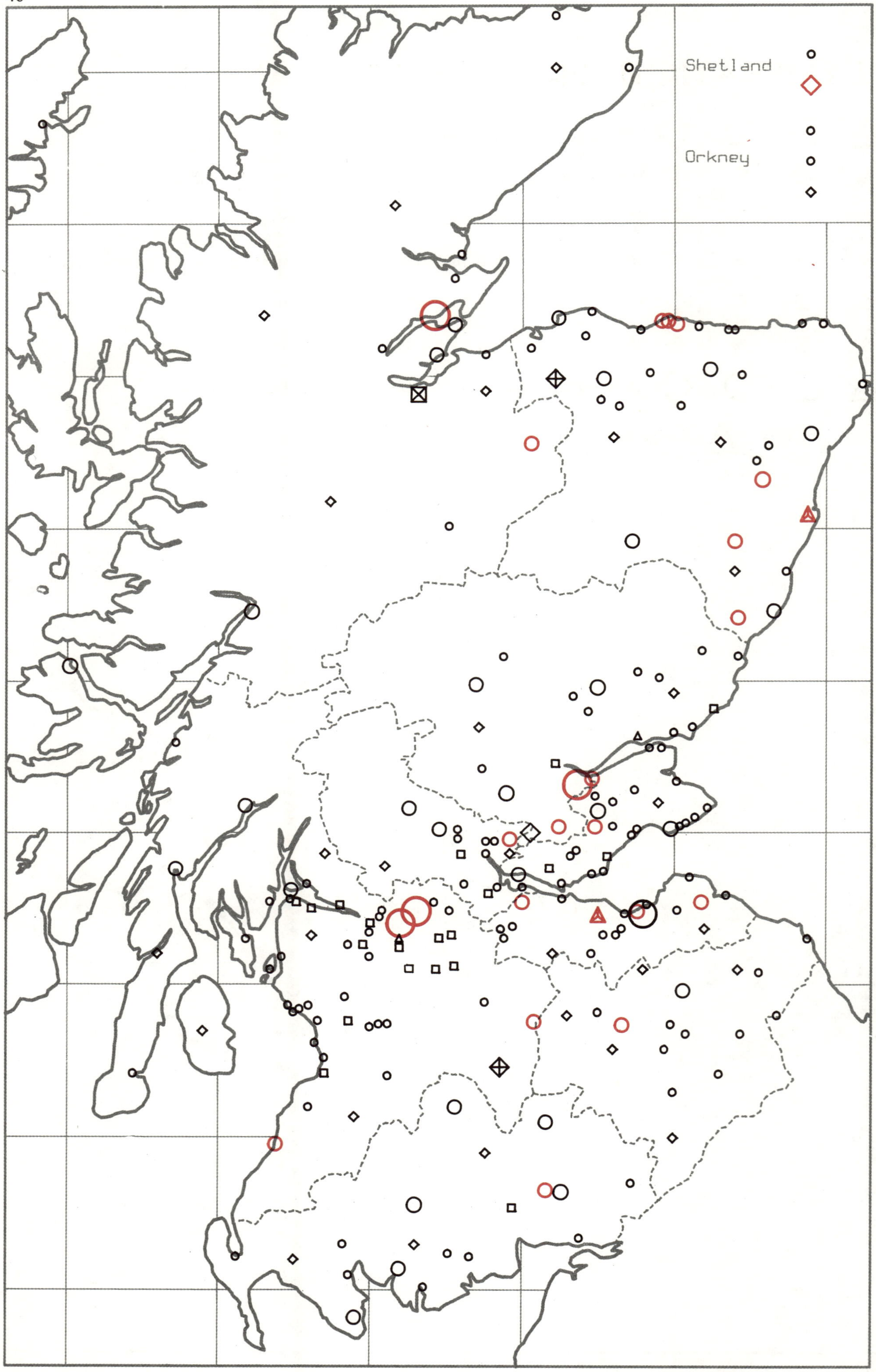
Shetland
Orkney

LYMPHATIC/HAEMATOPOIETIC CANCERS 1969-73

SMR significantly high ($p < 0.05$) and within the top tenth

SMR significantly high ($p < 0.05$) not within the top tenth

SMR not significantly high but within the top tenth

SMR not significantly high or low and not within the top or bottom tenth

SMR not significantly low but within the bottom tenth

SMR significantly low ($P < 0.05$) not within the bottom tenth

SMR significantly low ($P < 0.05$) and within the bottom tenth

City △ Large Burgh □ Small Burgh ○ Landward Area ◇

A SQUARE SYMBOL IS USED FOR THE DISTRICTS ON THE MAP OVERLEAF FOR 1979-83.

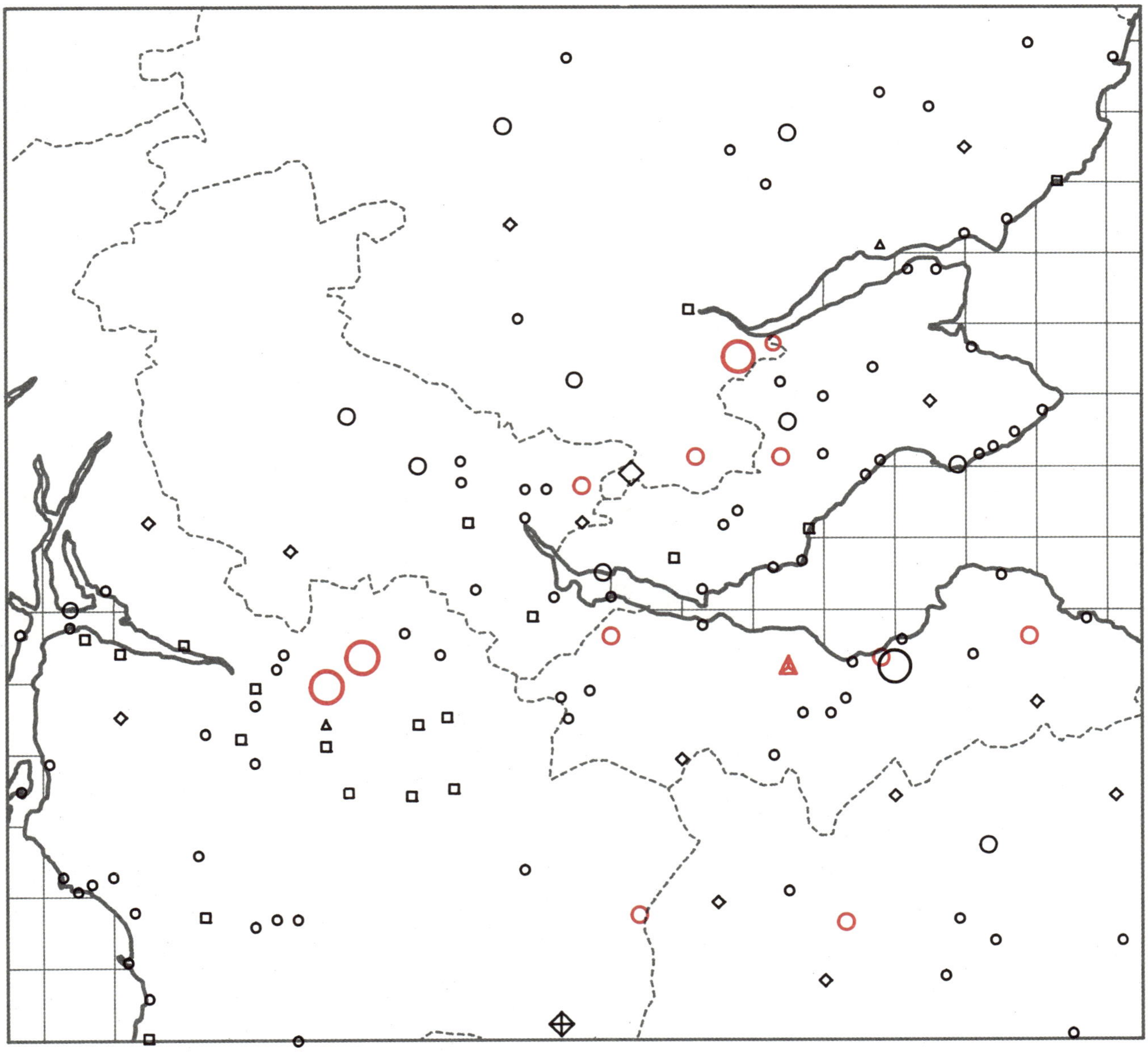

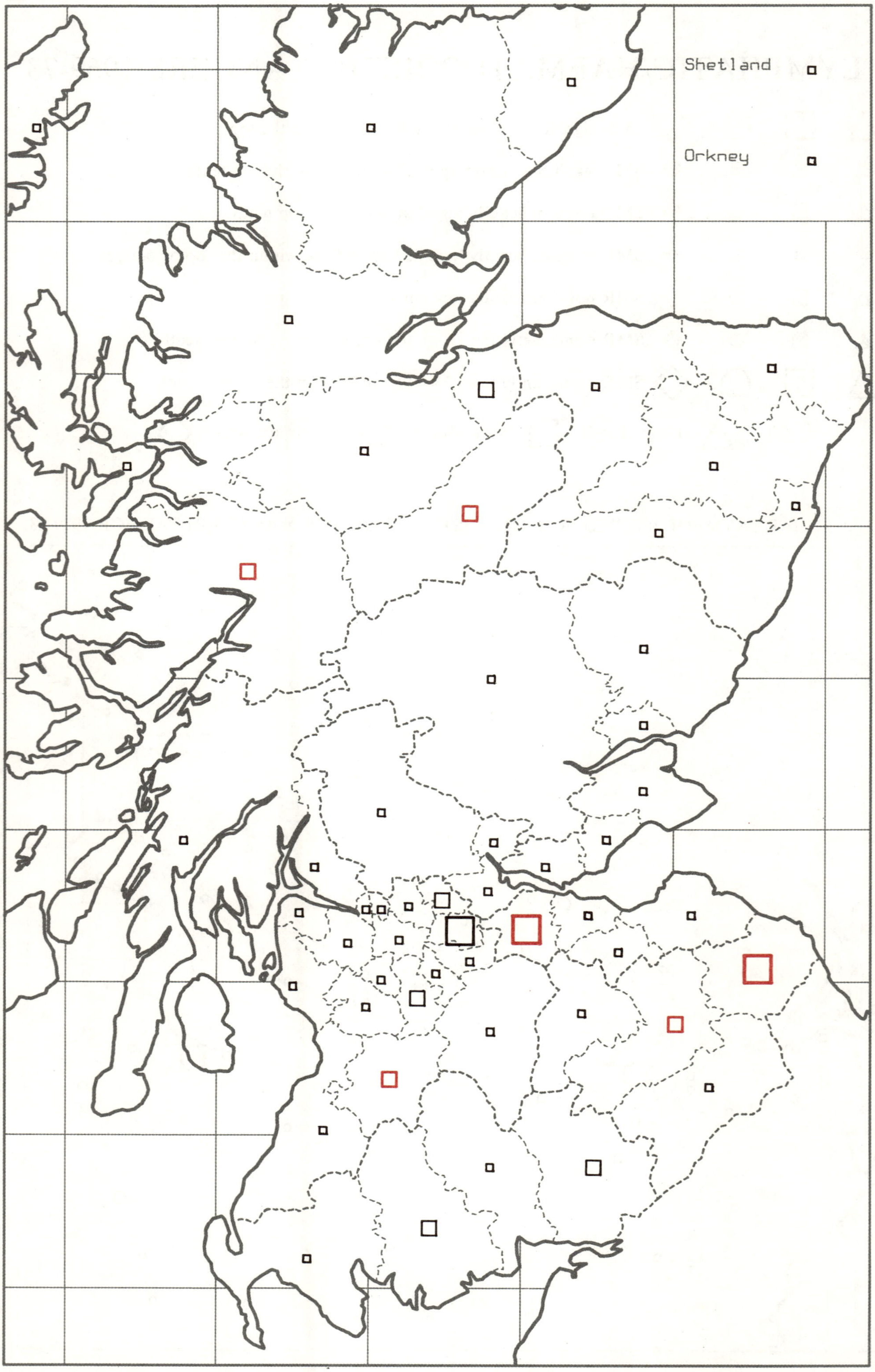
Shetland
Orkney

LYMPHATIC/HAEMATOPOIETIC CANCER (LEUKAEMIA ALONE 1979-83)

Malignant neoplasms of the lymphatic and haematopoietic tissue form a heterogeneous category of which leukaemia is the largest component. Since the mid 1970s problems of classification both clinically and pathologically have made any interpretation of data in this broad category extremely difficult. The leukaemias alone have been illustrated for 1979-83. Even here, however, problems of classification remain, particularly the problem of the categorization of non-Hodgkin's lymphoma outside the childhood age group.

Leukaemia in children and young adults has been a source of public concern in recent years, particularly in relation to possible emissions of radioactivity from the nuclear power station at Sellafield [33,34]. Before this, aetiological factors other than ionizing radiation were largely unknown, but suspicion now centres mainly on viruses and to a lesser extent on chemicals. Prolonged treatment with some drugs and also with radiotherapy may result in a secondary leukaemia. Because of the dramatic increase in survival, especially in children, due to recent improvements in treatment, mortality data are less satisfactory than morbidity data for epidemiological studies. In the elderly, where myelodysplastic syndromes are common, categorization according to the International Classification of Disease is uncertain. These same problems of classification make it difficult to compare data from previous years with those in this present time period. Knowledge of whether the SMR in a District is high or low is not necessarily helpful in trying to examine causal hypotheses in the Scottish population. The spatial distributions support the view, due to the small number of cases recorded in many of these Districts and to the heterogeneous nature of the disease itself (particularly in adults), that no firm conclusions can be drawn from this evidence as to the role of environmental factors.

Examination of the spatial pattern of mortality from leukaemia for the period 1979-83 indicates that the SMRs for all but 12 Districts are not significantly high or low, nor are they in the top or bottom deciles of District scores. This category includes all Districts in the north east of Scotland (Tayside and Grampian Regions) and the northern part of Highland Region, together with all of Fife and Central Regions and the western part of Strathclyde.

Two Districts in the east of Scotland, Berwickshire and West Lothian, possess significantly high SMRs which are also in the top decile. A further four Districts, two in Highland Region (Badenoch and Strathspey and Lochaber) and two in the south of Scotland (Roxburgh and Cumnock and Doon Valley), have SMRs either significantly high statistically or in the top decile.

Conversely, five Districts in the West of Scotland (Monklands, Strathkelvin, East Kilbride, Stewartry and Annandale), and Nairn in Highland Region, have SMRs which are either significantly low or in the bottom decile of District scores. The SMR for Monklands is both significantly low and in the bottom decile.

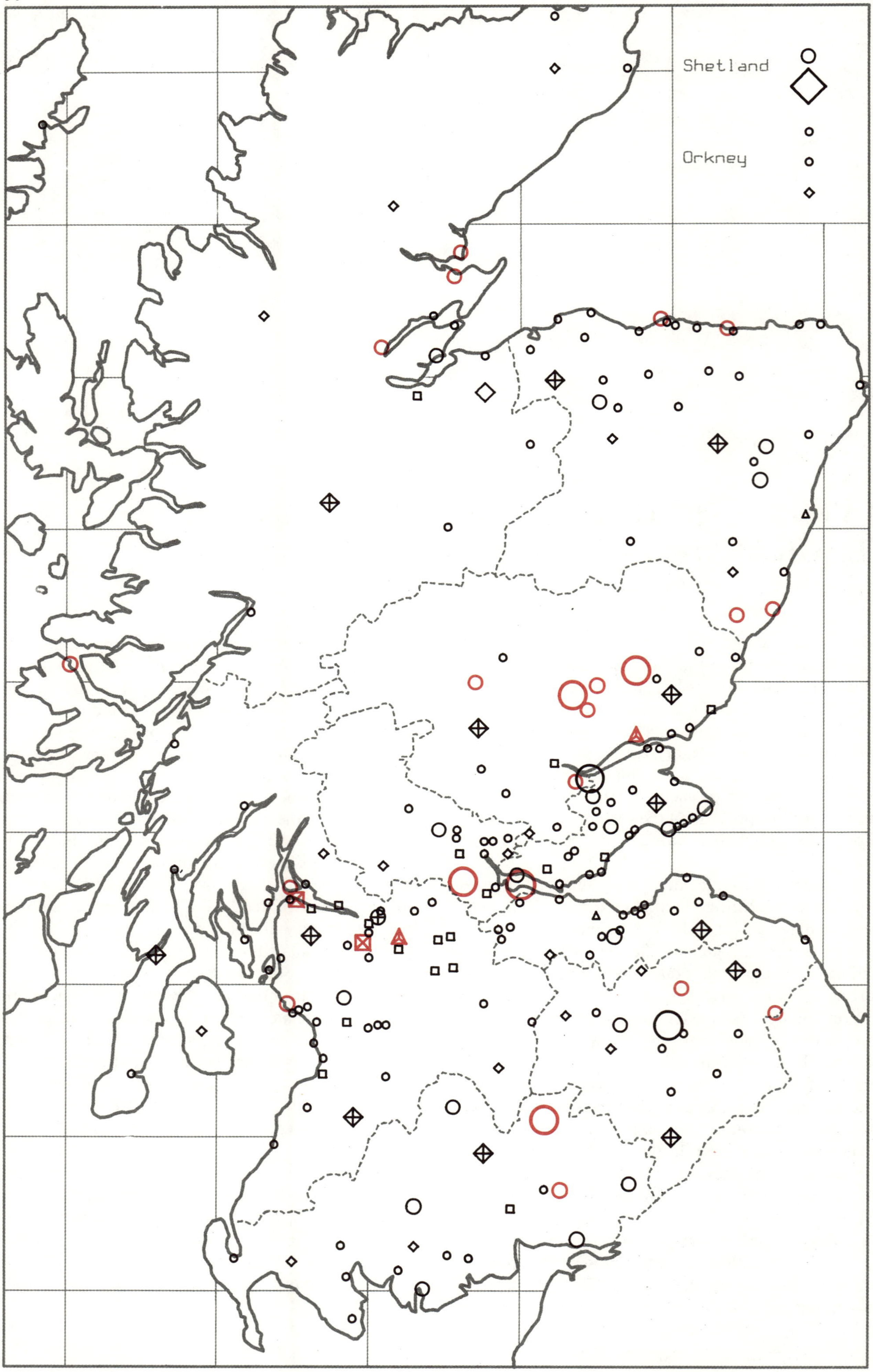
Shetland
Orkney

REMAINDER CANCERS 1959-63

SMR significantly high ($p < 0.05$) and within the top tenth

SMR significantly high ($p < 0.05$) not within the top tenth

SMR not significantly high but within the top tenth

SMR not significantly high or low and not within the top or bottom tenth

SMR not significantly low but within the bottom tenth

SMR significantly low ($P < 0.05$) not within the bottom tenth

SMR significantly low ($P < 0.05$) and within the bottom tenth

City | Large Burgh | Small Burgh | Landward Area

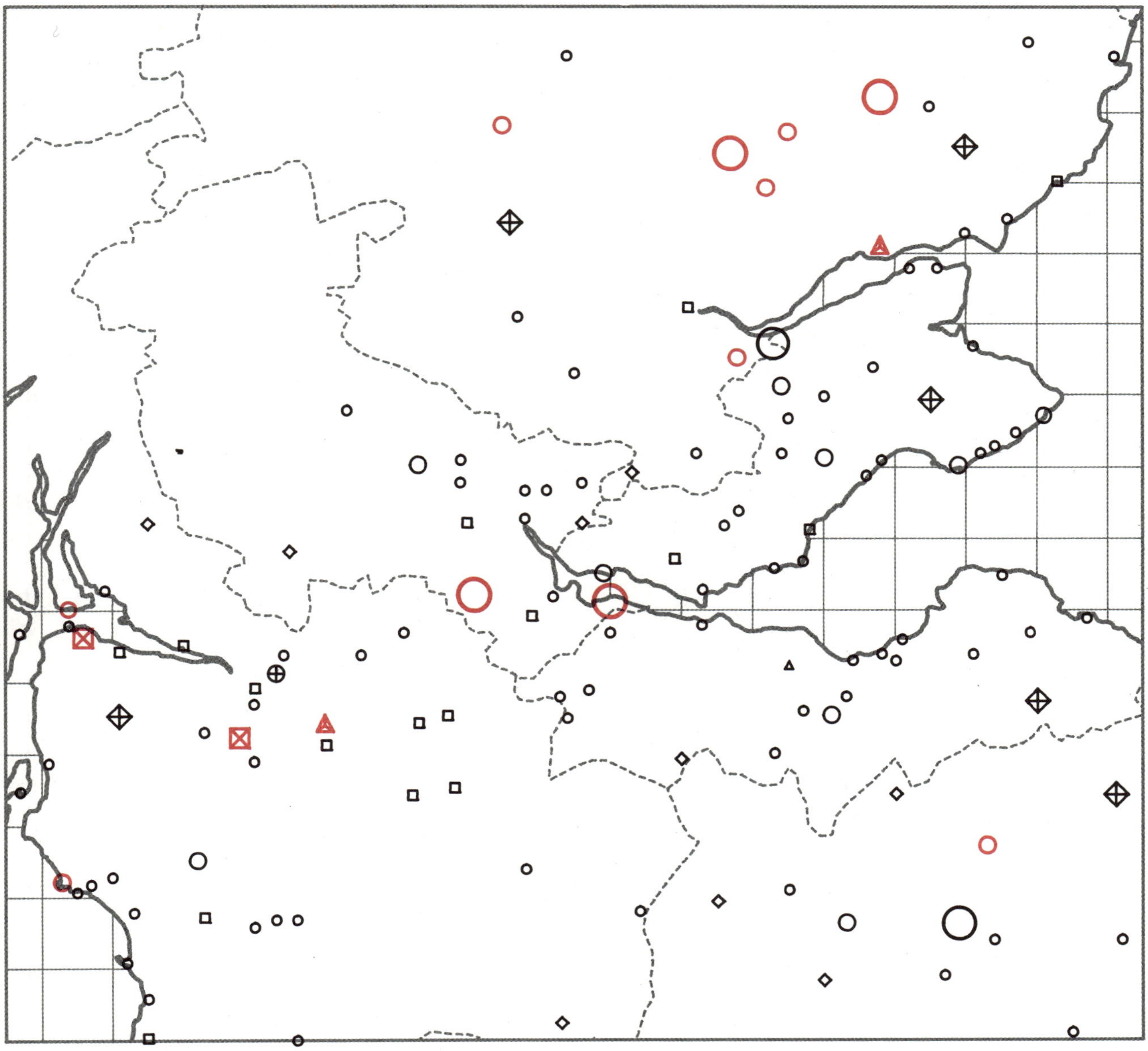

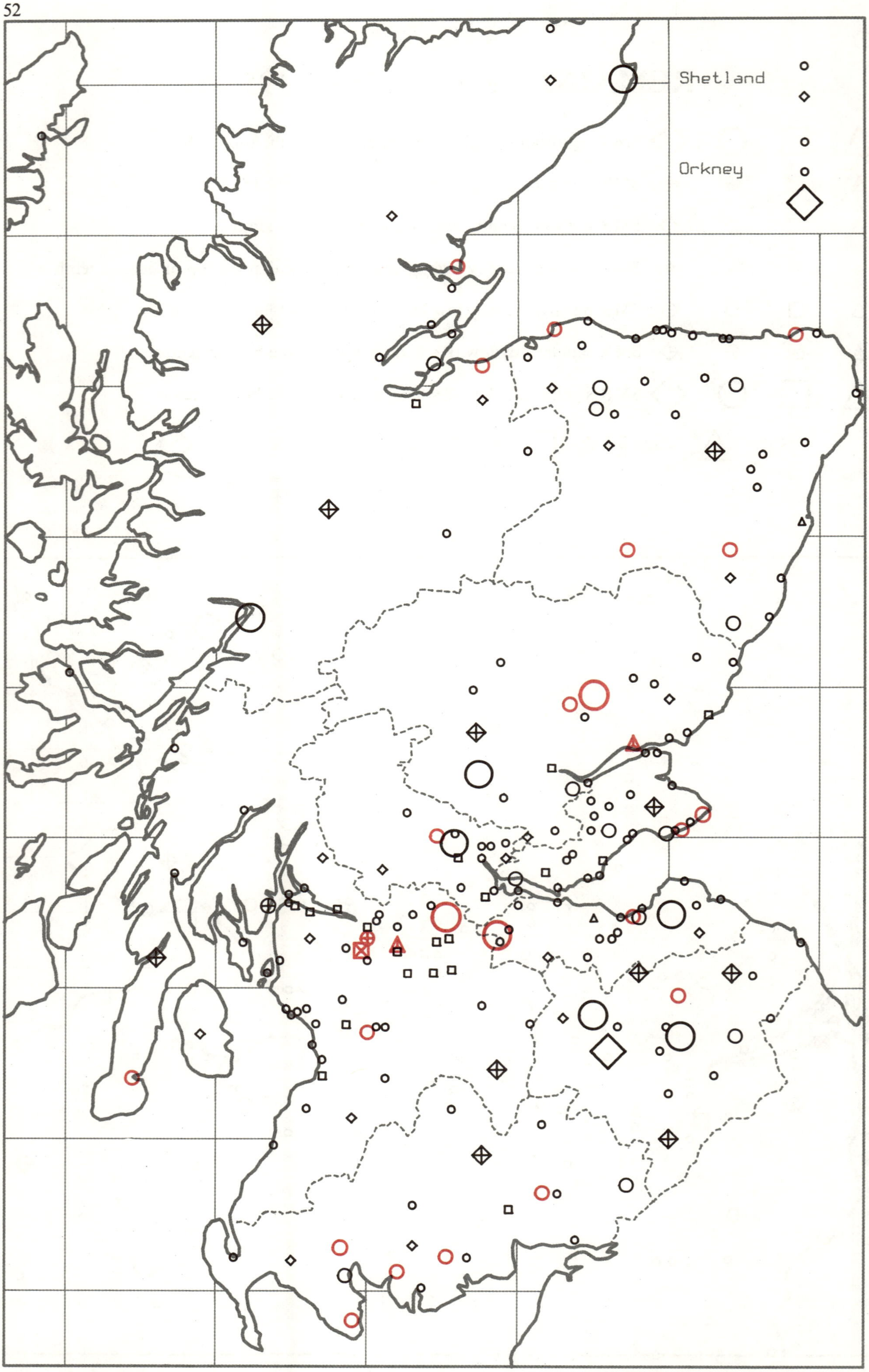
Shetland
Orkney

REMAINDER CANCERS 1969-73

SMR significantly high ($p < 0.05$) and within the top tenth

SMR significantly high ($p < 0.05$) not within the top tenth

SMR not significantly high but within the top tenth

SMR not significantly high or low and not within the top or bottom tenth

SMR not significantly low but within the bottom tenth

SMR significantly low ($P < 0.05$) not within the bottom tenth

SMR significantly low ($P < 0.05$) and within the bottom tenth

City △ Large Burgh □ Small Burgh ○ Landward Area ◇

A SQUARE SYMBOL IS USED FOR THE DISTRICTS ON THE MAP OVERLEAF FOR 1979-83.

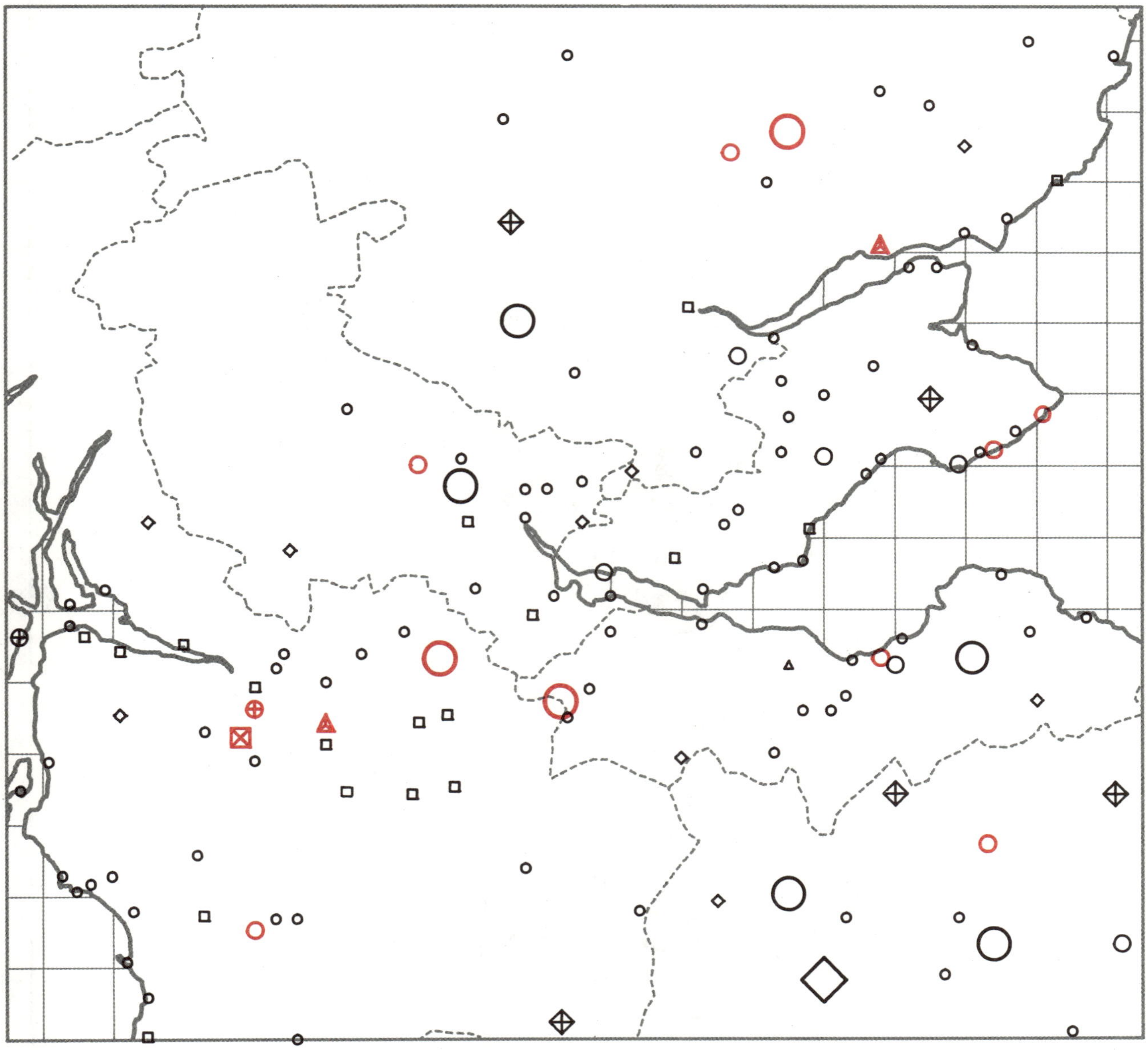

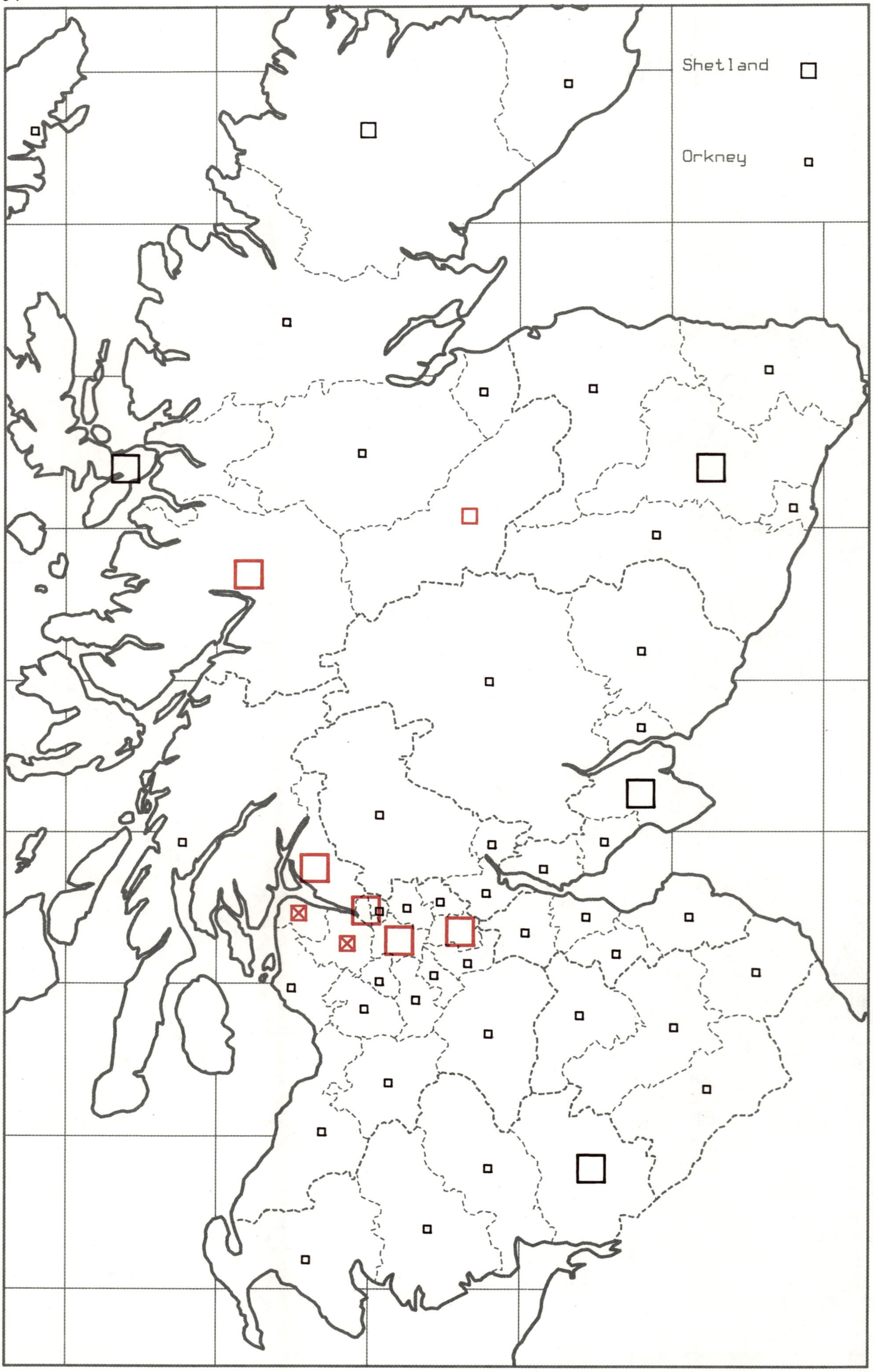
Shetland
Orkney

REMAINDER CANCERS

This category excludes the two categories of cancer for which separate data were available in the Annual Reports of the Registrar General for Scotland as far back as 1959: respiratory and lymphatic and haematopoietic cancers. Of these, the latter was a small part of total cancer mortality (six percent in 1969-73); respiratory cancer, however, formed a major component of total malignant disease in Scotland (27 percent in 1969-73), and its exclusion from Remainder Cancer removed the bias of the strong urban-rural gradient of respiratory cancer from the Remainder Cancer's maps. For 1979-83, Remainder Cancer differed from the earlier periods in excluding leukaemia rather than the older and wider category of lymphatic and haematopoietic cancer.

The principal components of Total Cancer falling within Remainder Cancer were gastric, colorectal and genito-urinary (each between ten percent and 15 percent) and breast (five percent).

During the first two periods, the relatively few communities with high SMRs were mostly found along the central belt of territory connecting the Forth and Clyde estuaries. Of the Cities, the values for Glasgow and Dundee were high in both periods. Of the Large Burghs, only Paisley was high in both periods. The Small Burghs with high values in both periods were Dornoch, Alyth and the adjacent town of Blairgowrie in Perthshire, and Lauder in the Border country. In 1969-73, the SMR for the Small Burgh of Armadale in West Lothian was high, (at the same time as its SMR for respiratory cancer was the highest in Scotland). During 1979-83, the pattern of the Districts with high SMRs broadly resembled that of the Total Cancers, with a horizontal band of Districts centred on Glasgow, and with the outlying District of Lochaber.

The largest proportion of low SMRs among the traditional communities was in the Landward Areas. The Small Burghs with low values in both periods included Fortrose and Aberlour in the north, Elie, Markinch and Culross in Fife, and Langholm in the Scottish Borders; but there were no Large Burghs or Cities. During 1979-83, all of the six Districts with low SMRs were peripherally situated.

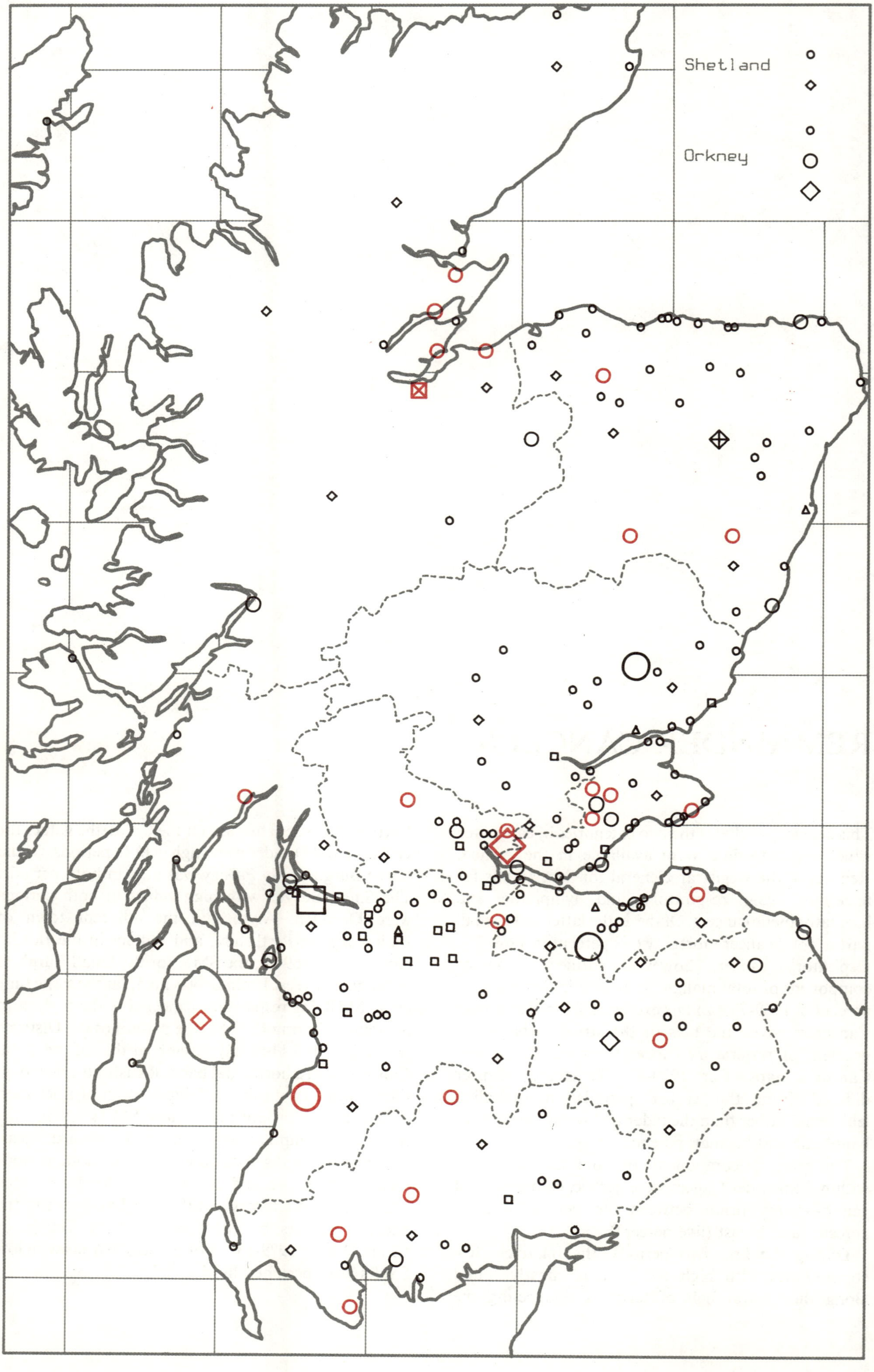
Shetland
Orkney

BREAST CANCER 1969-73

SMR significantly high ($p<0.05$) and within the top tenth

SMR significantly high ($p<0.05$) not within the top tenth

SMR not significantly high but within the top tenth

SMR not significantly high or low and not within the top or bottom tenth

SMR not significantly low but within the bottom tenth

SMR significantly low ($P<0.05$) not within the bottom tenth

SMR significantly low ($P<0.05$) and within the bottom tenth

City △ Large Burgh □ Small Burgh ○ Landward Area ◇

A SQUARE SYMBOL IS USED FOR THE DISTRICTS ON THE MAP OVERLEAF FOR 1979-83.

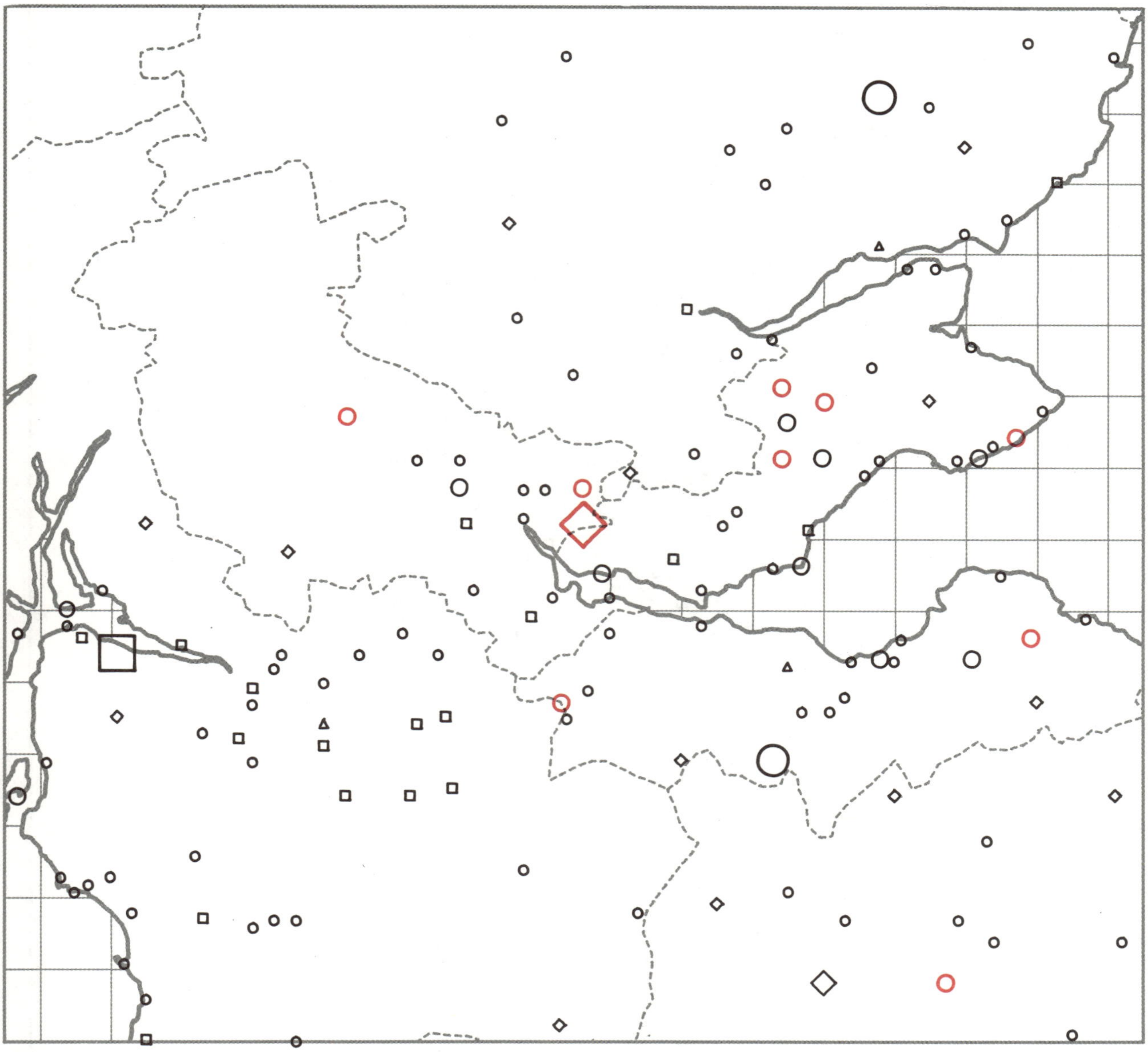

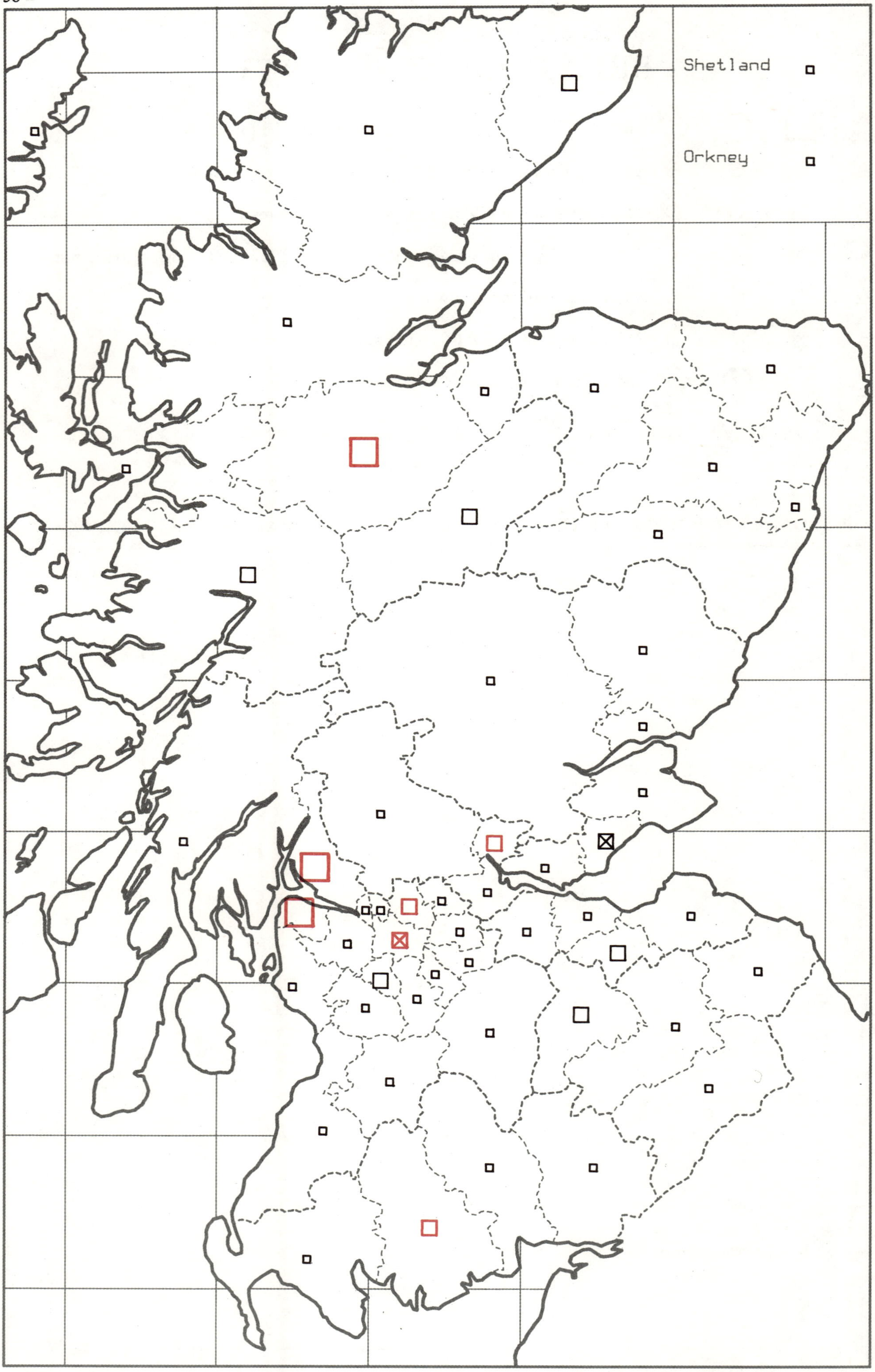
Shetland
Orkney

BREAST CANCER

In general, the lowest rates of this cancer are in developing countries in Asia, Africa and elsewhere. The highest rates are in the affluent and urbanized countries of Western Europe and the United States of America; it is the most frequent form of female cancer in the western hemisphere. In Scotland during 1969-73, it formed just under 20 percent of all female deaths from malignant disease. Migrant studies showed that, when populations move from areas of low to high incidence, they adopt the rates of the host area within a few generations. An example of the transition is the contrast between the low rates in Japan and the higher rates found in Japanese who have emigrated to areas with raised rates such as Hawaii [21,22]. Residence in areas of low risk, such as Japan, appears to carry a better prognosis for patients [35].

The age-adjusted annual mortality rates in Segi's international listing [4] have risen gradually between 1950-51 and 1978-79. In the earlier period, the highest rates per 100,000 were for Denmark (24.4), Netherlands (23.3) and England and Wales (23.2); the lowest rates were for Japan (4.0) and Chile (7.7); the Scottish rate was 22.0. In the later period, the two highest rates were for England and Wales (27.7) and Scotland (27.6); the rates for Denmark and Netherlands were 24.7 and 25.8 respectively; for Japan and Chile the rates were 5.2 and 11.4 respectively.

Incidence rates for breast cancer increase with age between menarche and menopause. Thereafter they usually increase slowly in high-risk countries, but decrease slowly in low-risk countries. The histological appearance of breast cancer is heterogeneous, and the various histological types have different epidemiological distributions and prognoses [35].

Suspected causal factors come under several headings. Of prime importance are the metabolic processes involved with endogenous sex hormones: oestrogen, prolactin and progesterone. Early menarche, short ovulatory cycles, late first full-term pregnancy, late menopause and raised post-menopausal weight are more frequently found in patients with breast cancer than in control groups [22,35]. Diets rich in fat and animal protein are also strongly implicated, particularly in older patients. Medical radiology of the chest is another influence, especially in younger or nulliparous patients; here the latency can lie between five and 40 years [35]. Genetic factors have been implicated because of family histories of the cancer which are more frequently found with younger patients and with bilateral disease; also, twin studies have shown that monozygotic twins have a higher degree of concordance for the disease than is found with dizygotic twins [22,35]. The processes of initiation and promotion probably take place in breast cancer as in other cancers. Apart from ionizing radiation, however, the initiating factors remain obscure and may be mostly of low-level potency. Ovarian hormones and dietary factors may be the major promoting factors.

The social class gradient is unusual for a cancer, in that the higher social classes have the higher mortality [36]. An urban-rural gradient has been described, with the higher rates for urbanization [22].

In Scotland during 1969-73, the figures for the mean death rates per 100,000 in the aggregates of the Cities, Large Burghs, Small Burghs and Landward Areas were 23, 21, 22 and 19 respectively, demonstrating a slight but irregular urban-rural gradient.

During 1969-73, high SMRs were present almost exclusively in Small Burghs; these were found in all parts of Scotland. Of the other communities with high SMRs, Inverness was the only Large Burgh, and Clackmannan and Bute were the only Landward Areas. Communities with low SMRs included the Large Burgh of Port Glasgow. During 1979-83, high SMRs were found in several Districts in the central-west of Scotland (Dumbarton, Inverclyde, Strathkelvin and the City of Glasgow), and also in Clackmannan and Inverness to the north and in Stewartry to the south. The Districts with low SMRs were more evenly dispersed.

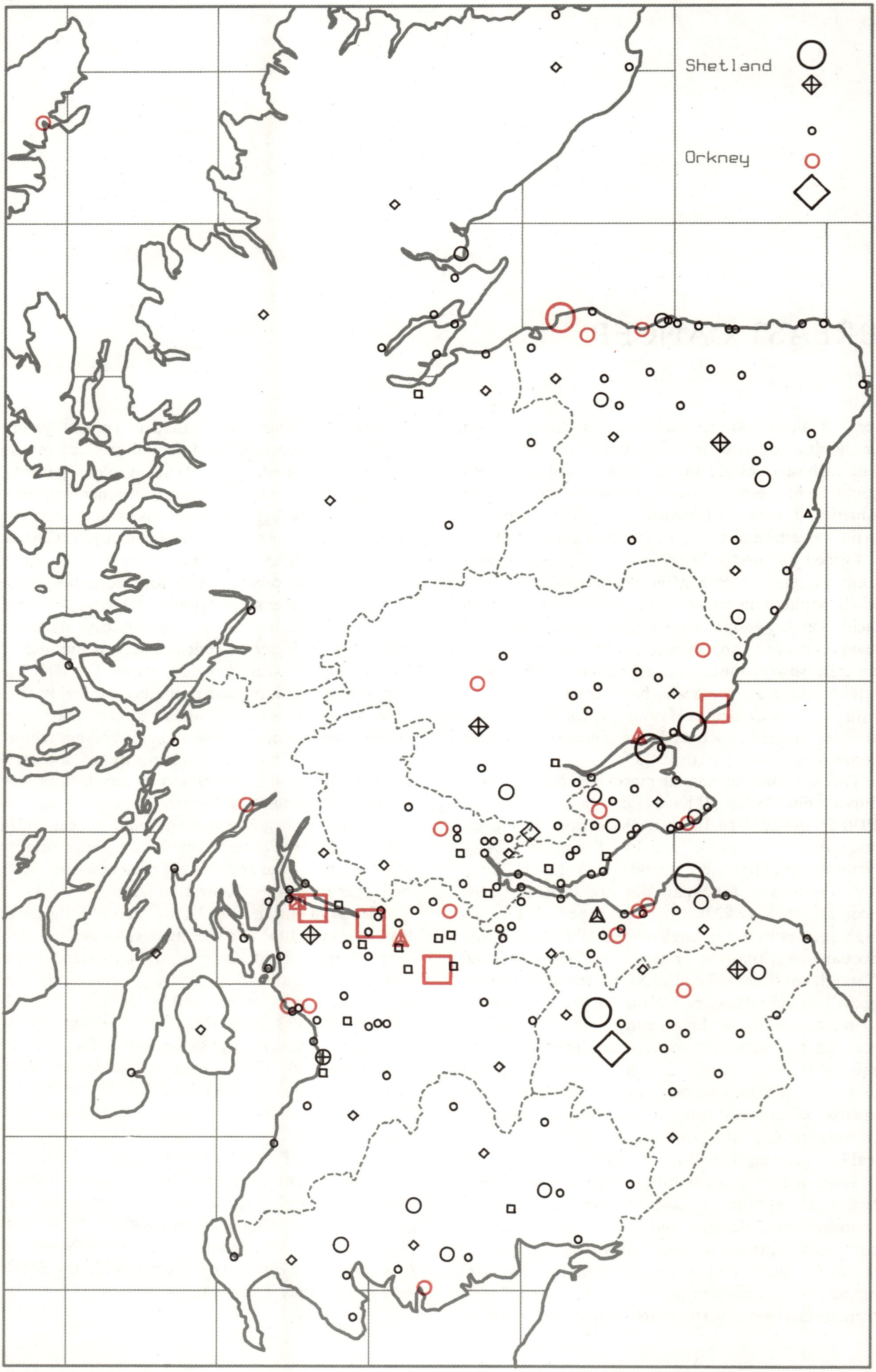
Shetland
Orkney

GASTRIC CANCER 1969-73

SMR significantly high ($p < 0.05$) and within the top tenth

SMR significantly high ($p < 0.05$) not within the top tenth

SMR not significantly high but within the top tenth

SMR not significantly high or low and not within the top or bottom tenth

SMR not significantly low but within the bottom tenth

SMR significantly low ($P < 0.05$) not within the bottom tenth

SMR significantly low ($P < 0.05$) and within the bottom tenth

City △ Large Burgh □ Small Burgh ○ Landward Area ◇

A SQUARE SYMBOL IS USED FOR THE DISTRICTS ON THE MAP OVERLEAF FOR 1979-83.

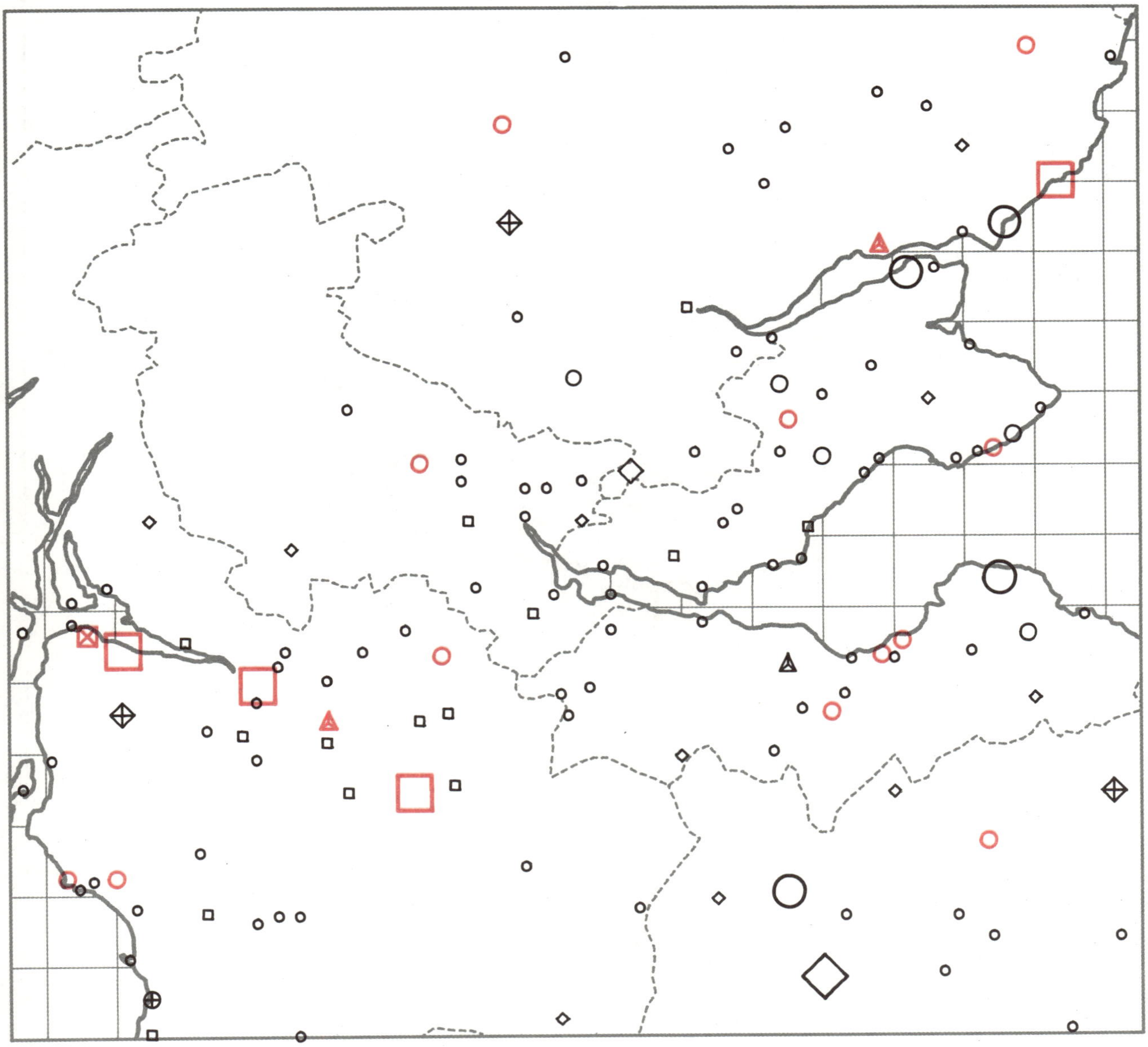

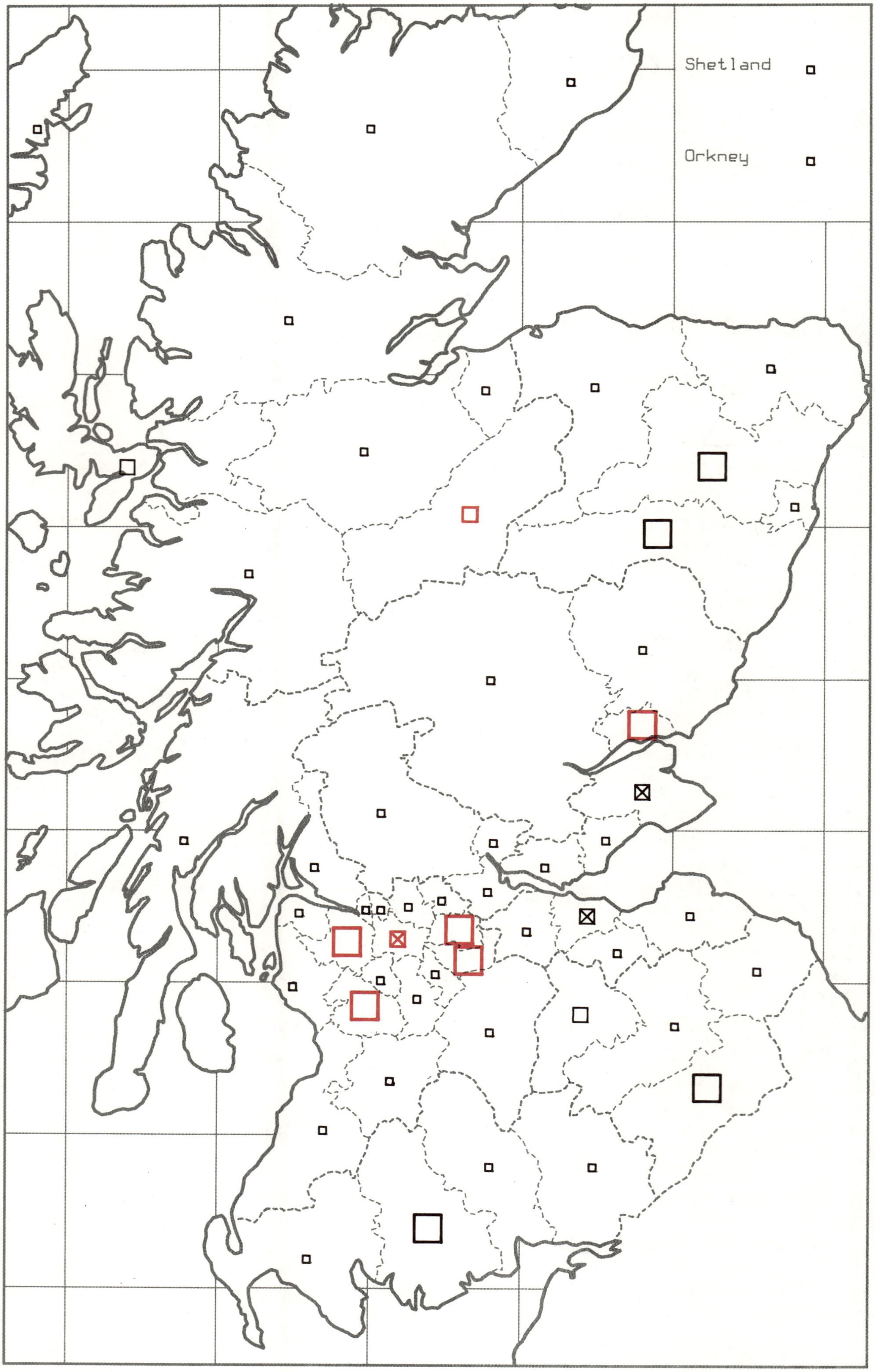
Shetland
Orkney

GASTRIC CANCER

In Segi's list of 24 countries [4], the rates for gastric cancer show two points of epidemiological importance: striking differences between countries, and convincing declines between the years 1950-51 and 1978-79. In 1950-51, the male rates per 100,000 ranged from 64.4 and 73.6 for Japan and Chile respectively to 25.5 for Canada. In the later period, the rates were 49.7 and 45.7 for Japan and Chile and 11.1 for Canada. Comparable patterns are found for female rates: the highest rates in 1950-51 were 52.1 in Chile and 35.2 in Japan, while Canada showed the low rate of 13.4; by the later period these rates had declined to 20.4, 25.2 and 4.8 respectively. Between 1950-51 and 1978-79, the Scottish rates for males declined from 31.1 to 18.2; for females, the decline was from 22.2 to 8.8. In both periods, these Scottish values were close to the rates for England and Wales and Northern Ireland.

In Britain a social class gradient of mortality is present, members of classes 4 and 5 being particularly vulnerable [36]. Occupational associations have been recorded, the dusty environments in some of the following occupations perhaps being a risk factor: ceramic, stone and textile workers, miners, fishermen, clerical workers, printers, painters and employees in the metal, construction and chemical industries. A genetic association with blood group A has been noted [22].

The role of tobacco carcinogenesis is not as sharply defined as for other organs. Dietary factors suspected of playing a part in the causation of gastric cancer include salted fish and pickled or smoked foods, dietary nitrosamines, and diets deficient in milk, fruit and vegetables. Environmental exposure during early life to such agents may be important [22]. The decline in gastric cancer during recent decades might have resulted in part from the change from chemical preservatives to refrigeration for maintaining the freshness of foodstuffs. Another factor may have been the increasingly effective distribution networks of the modern food industries which have extended the range of fresh fruit and vegetables available to the housewife throughout most of the year. The strong negative correlation between national rates for gastric and colon cancers may result from major dietary factors increasing the induction of the one cancer but inhibiting the development of the other [37].

The unusual geographical distributions found within many countries have provided ample scope for speculation about causal mechanisms. For example, districts with very high mortality among both males and females are found in the south east of West Germany [5]. In Newfoundland, an association has been found with fish factories and seagull colonies [38]. In Scotland, registrations of gastric cancer during 1975-80 were high in the industrial areas around Glasgow [2]. Peculiar geographical distributions in other countries, and their possible environmental causes, have been well reviewed [21].

In Scotland, gastric cancer during 1969-73 accounted for ten percent of total cancer mortality. The mortality rates show a slight urban-rural gradient: for the aggregated Cities, Large Burghs, Small Burghs and Landward Areas, the mean rates per 100,000 for 1969-73 were 29, 26, 23 and 23 respectively.

During 1969-73, many of the communities with high SMRs were industrial: the Cities of Dundee and Glasgow, and the Large Burghs of Clydebank, Port Glasgow, Greenock and Hamilton. The Large Burgh of Arbroath also had a high SMR but is noted for its fishing and fish-smoking activities. There were relatively few Small Burghs with high SMRs, and no Landward Areas. The communities with low SMRs followed no obvious pattern.

During 1979-83, high SMRs were found mainly in industrial areas: the Cities of Glasgow and Dundee, and the four Districts of Renfrew, Kilmarnock, Monklands and Motherwell around Glasgow. The only rural District was Badenoch and Strathspey in the central Highlands. The low SMRs were scattered: Edinburgh, Fife, two Districts adjacent to Aberdeen, Tweeddale and two of the most southern Districts, and Skye and Lochalsh on the north west coast.

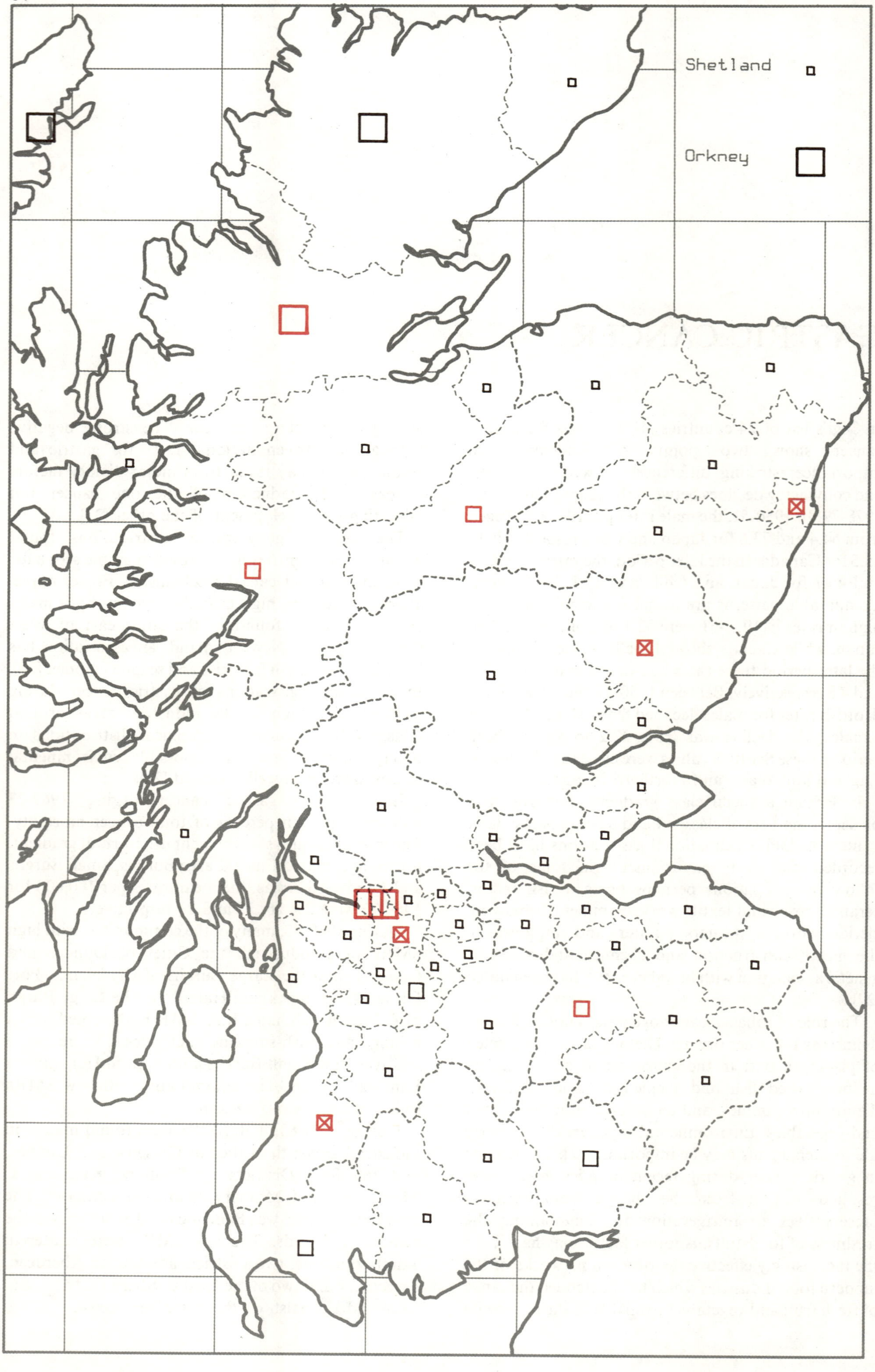
Shetland
Orkney

THE MAP OPPOSITE SHOWS THE DISTRIBUTION OF COLORECTAL CANCER FOR 1979-83.

COLORECTAL CANCER

The two categories of colon and rectum can be difficult to separate on anatomical grounds [22]. International mortality rates for colon and for rectal cancers have been shown to be positively and significantly correlated [37], and these two categories have been thought to share common aetiological factors [5]. For these reasons, they have sometimes been combined as colorectal cancer [2]. Elsewhere they have been considered separately, as in Segi's international comparison of age-adjusted mortality rates [4]. In international comparisons, the rank order of cancer of the colorectum in males is closely correlated with that of females [22].

In Segi's tables, Scotland had the highest rates in 1950-51 for colon cancer in both males and females: 20.3 and 19.8 per 100,000 respectively. By 1978-79, the male and female Scottish rates had declined to 14.1 and 13.5; the male rate had been surpassed (but only slightly) by males in Ireland, Australia, New Zealand, Canada, Belgium and U.S. whites; the Scottish female rate had been surpassed by New Zealand and Ireland.

For rectal cancer, in 1950-51 the rate for Scottish males was 11.7, second only to that of England and Wales (13.2). In 1978-79, it was 8.1, which is close below the rates for Denmark, Austria, West Germany, New Zealand, and England and Wales. In females, Scotland (6.1) in 1950-51 was again second to England and Wales (6.7); in the later period, Scotland (4.6) followed New Zealand and several other countries.

In the aetiology of colorectal cancer, dietary factors are probably of primary importance. In particular, an excess of dietary meat, animal fat and beer, and deficiencies of vegetables and fibre have been implicated. Positive associations with high social class and with occupations involved with leather, textiles and metals are described [22,36]; acrylonitrile, used in plastics and synthetic fibres, may be a carcinogen. Colorectal cancer is positively associated with cancers of the breast, uterus and ovary, and with ulcerative colitis and Crohn's disease [22].

In 1979-83, Scottish Districts with high SMRs for colorectal cancer included the Cities of Aberdeen and Glasgow, two Districts adjacent to Glasgow, and individual Districts in the southern, Highland and northern parts of the country. Low SMRs were present in East Kilbride, which is directly south of Glasgow, and in two Districts in the far north and two in the far south.

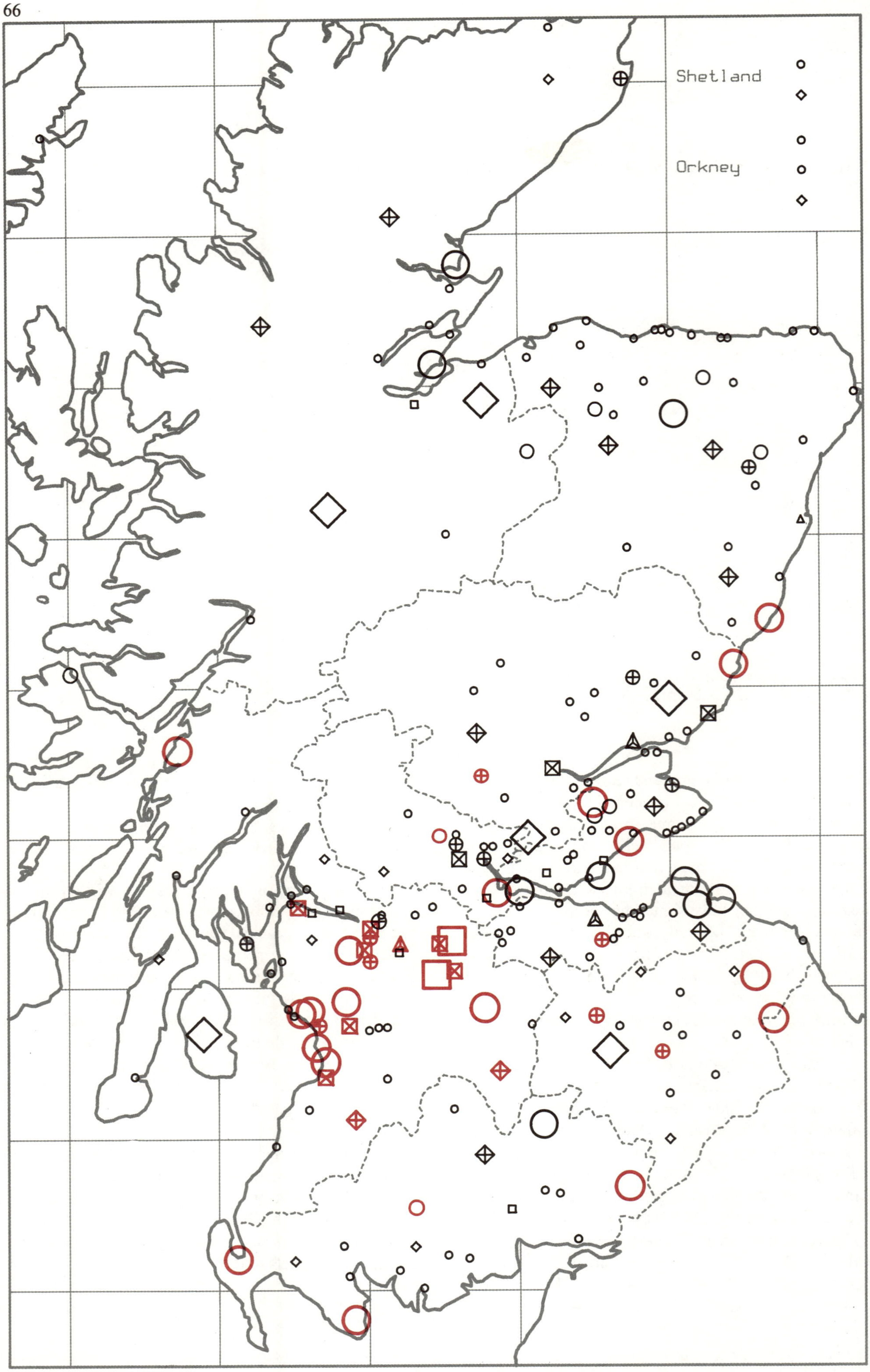
Shetland
Orkney

CORONARY HEART DISEASE 1959-63

SMR significantly high ($p < 0.05$) and within the top tenth

SMR significantly high ($p < 0.05$) not within the top tenth

SMR not significantly high but within the top tenth

SMR not significantly high or low and not within the top or bottom tenth

SMR not significantly low but within the bottom tenth

SMR significantly low ($P < 0.05$) not within the bottom tenth

SMR significantly low ($P < 0.05$) and within the bottom tenth

City Large Burgh Small Burgh Landward Area

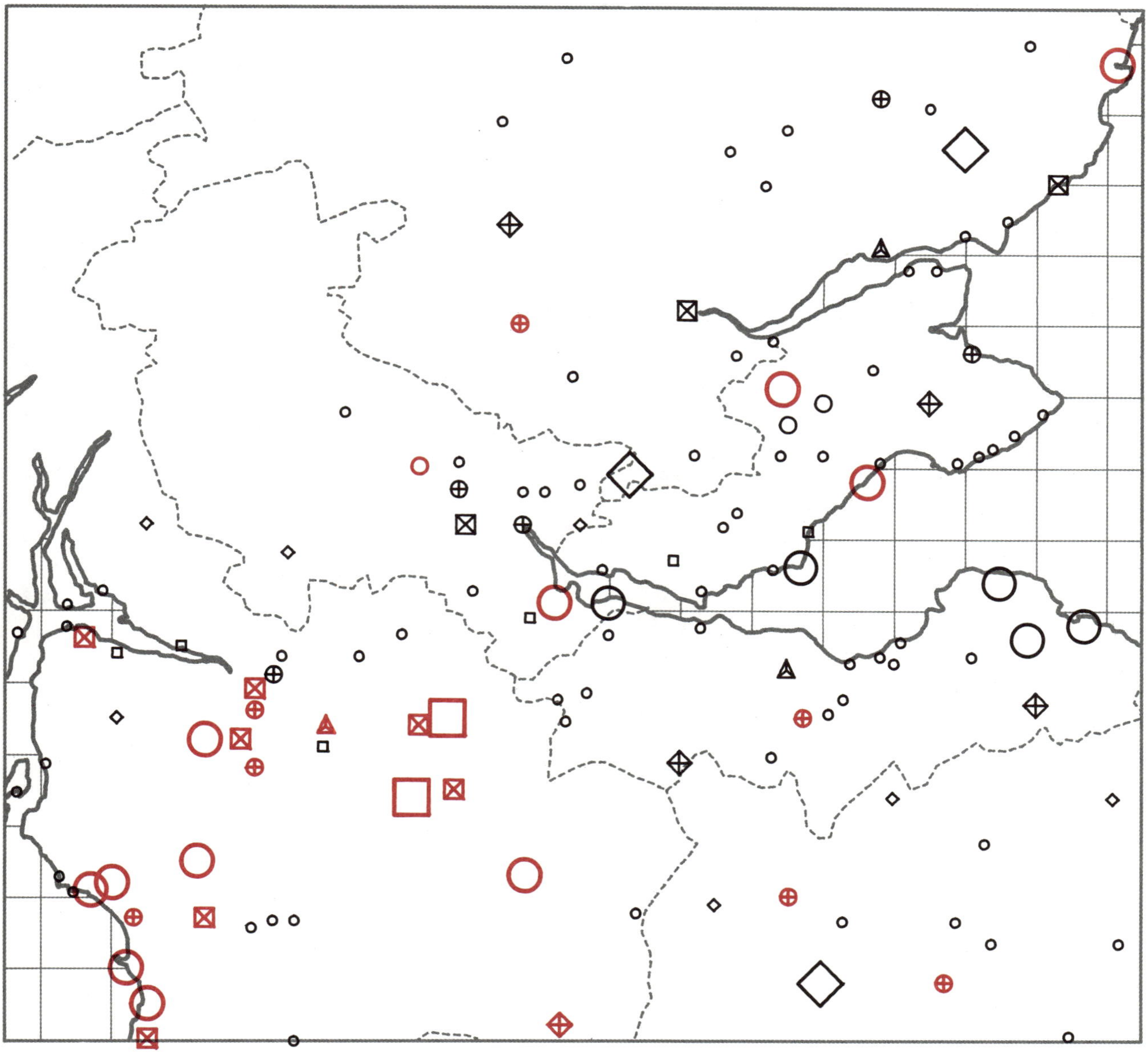

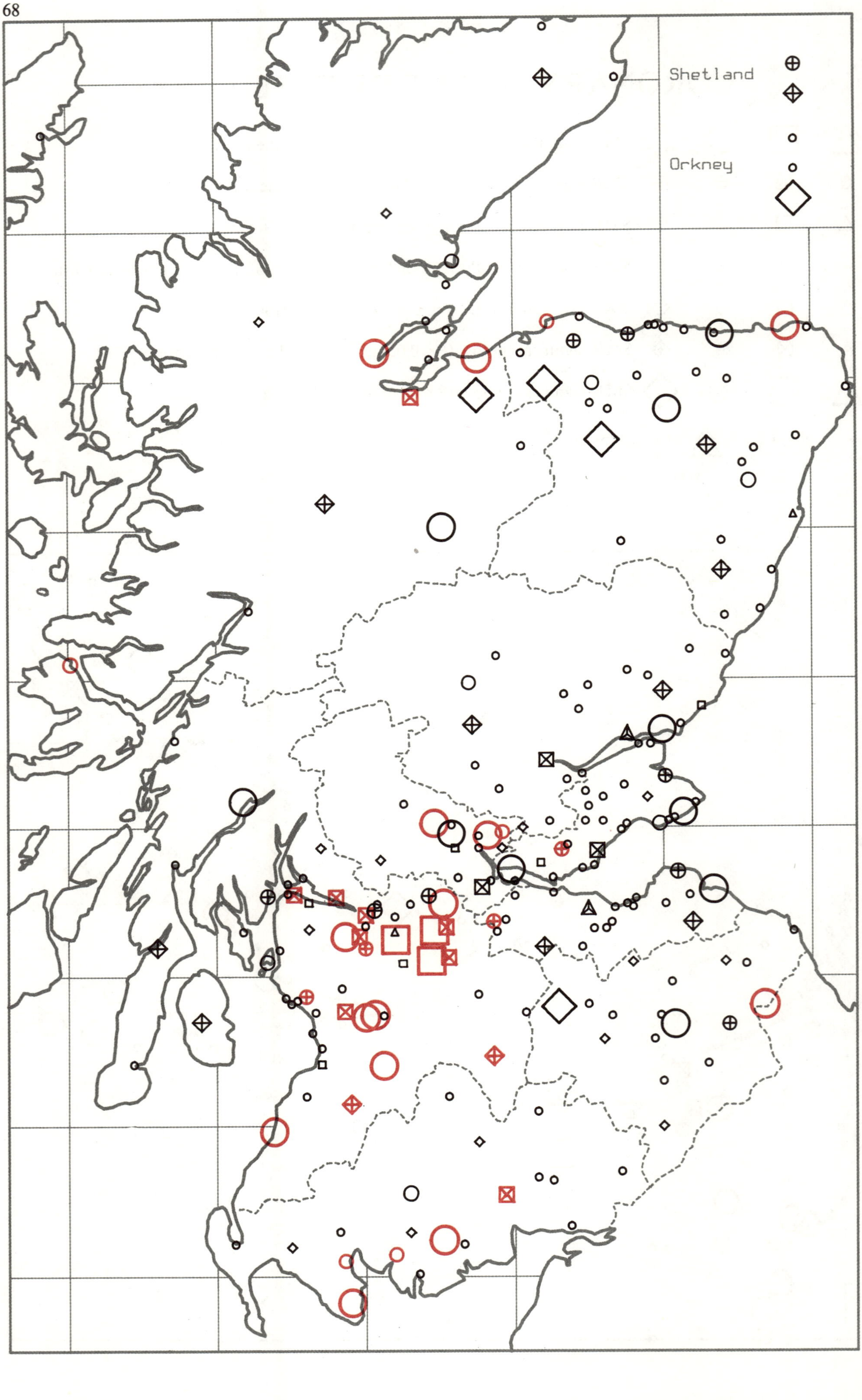
Shetland
Orkney

CORONARY HEART DISEASE 1969-73

- SMR significantly high ($p<0.05$) and within the top tenth
- SMR significantly high ($p<0.05$) not within the top tenth
- SMR not significantly high but within the top tenth
- SMR not significantly high or low and not within the top or bottom tenth
- SMR not significantly low but within the bottom tenth
- SMR significantly low ($P<0.05$) not within the bottom tenth
- SMR significantly low ($P<0.05$) and within the bottom tenth

City Large Burgh Small Burgh Landward Area

A SQUARE SYMBOL IS USED FOR THE DISTRICTS ON THE MAP OVERLEAF FOR 1979-83.

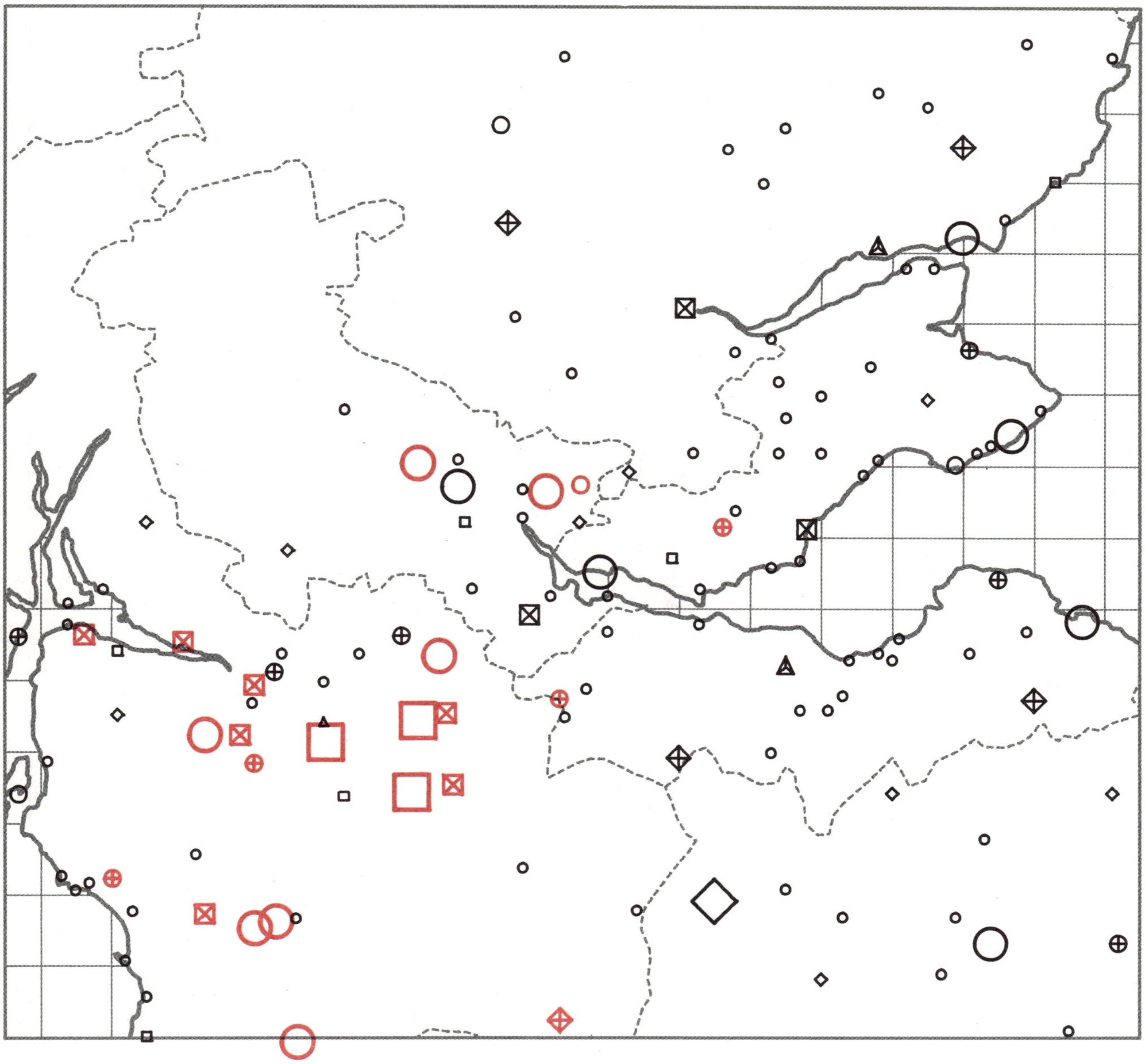

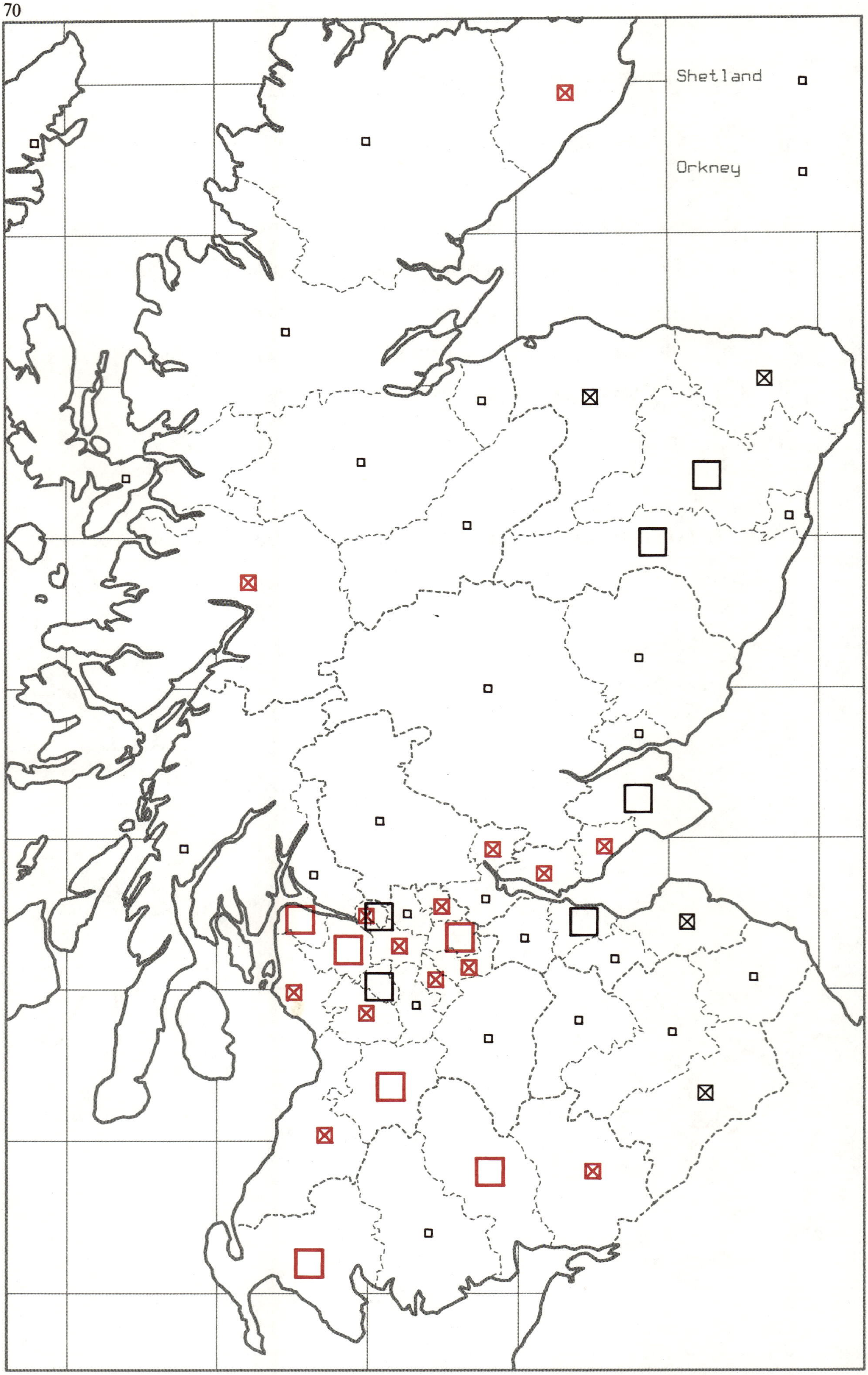
Shetland
Orkney

CORONARY AND OTHER HEART DISEASES

Although the term myocardial infarction was introduced in 1896 by Rene Marie in his paper 'L'infarctus du myocarde et ses conséquences' [39], the diagnosis of myocardial infarction is comparatively recent, as the disease was not recognized and was probably rare in the eighteenth and nineteenth centuries [40]. The upsurge in deaths seems to have begun in the 1930s, and by the 1950s this disease was the single most common cause of premature death.

The causes of Coronary Heart Disease (CHD) have not yet been fully identified, but environmental factors seem more important than genetic ones. For example, the low incidence of CHD experienced by native Japanese is not found in second generation Japanese living in the USA, who progressively adopt the rate of the Americans; in Japanese migrants who maintain their traditional lifestyles, however, there is no increased risk of CHD. The wide variations in the incidence of CHD between and within countries again indicate environmental causes.

At least eight personal factors probably contribute to an increased risk of CHD, and the effect of more than one of these factors is multiplicative. High serum cholesterol, smoking, hypertension and diabetes have been suggested as primary risk factors, whereas excess body weight, inactivity, stress and genetic endowment have been considered as secondary.

Of the primary factors, the causal connection between high serum cholesterol and an increased risk of CHD (with the exception of hypercholesterolaemia) is not clear. While some evidence suggests that the risk is linked with the consumption of saturated rather than unsaturated fats [41-43], other studies discount an aetiological role for blood cholesterol [44,45]. Nevertheless, the nutritional habits in the different parts of Scotland have not been studied sufficiently to allow dietary differences to be implicated in the geographical distribution of CHD in these maps. In the same way, ignorance about regional differences in smoking habits and in the prevalences of hypertension, diabetes, obesity, physical inactivity and stress inhibits speculation about how those factors might influence the geography of CHD.

The precise importance of genetic endowment is difficult to establish, but a positive family history of CHD is relatively frequent among patients with CHD. The variation in genetic endowment throughout the United Kingdom may be inferred in part from the unequal distribution of the various blood groups [46,47]. In Britain, the frequency of group O increases, and of group A declines, from south to north-west; and the proportions of blood groups AB and B in the central west of Scotland are uniquely high. Blood group patterns have strong statistical associations with mortality from atherosclerotic heart disease [46], and hence such genetic inequalities could play a major part in the geographical distribution of CHD.

Finally, although it is unlikely that any of the personal risk factors alone could be wholly responsible for the geographic distribution, CHD has multifactorial origins; and the possibility cannot be excluded that the central west and south west areas of Scotland have an unusually high number of these factors.

Of the environmental associations with CHD, water softness, mean daily maximum temperature, rainfall [48], and latitude and longitude [46] have been discussed frequently. Although the values for rainfall (whether expressed as rain-days or as inches) and for the parameter of sunshine hours in the central west and south west differ from the values in the north and east of Scotland [47,49], the possible causal links with CHD patterns remain obscure. The well-documented relationship between water softness and mortality from CHD is exemplified by the low mortality in the area of hard water in the south east of England, and the high mortality and concomitant soft water in Scotland. Nevertheless, the precise contribution of water quality to the geographical patterns of CHD mortality within Scotland must await more detailed information on variations of the water quality between small areas.

In western countries, cardiovascular disease has reached epidemic proportions. In Britain, it is the main cause of death of men over 35 years, accounting for 41 percent of deaths of those aged 35-44 years and 52 percent of those aged 45-54 years. The male:female ratio varies according to age. At 40 years it is 6:1 but by the age of 80 the ratio has fallen to 1:1. There is a marked social gradient at younger ages, rising from social class 1 to 5; but with increasing age this gradient diminishes.

The distribution of CHD varies both internationally and intranationally. On a global basis [18], in 1980, males in the age-group 40-69 years in Northern Ireland experienced the highest mortality (630 per 100,000 population) followed by Finland (599), Scotland (592) and England and Wales (499); while Japan (65), France (137), Yugoslavia (197) and Romania (202) showed the lowest rates. The pattern of mortality was similar for the same age-group of females, although the magnitude of the mortality was appreciably lower. Scotland had the highest mortality (208) followed by Northern Ireland (191), New Zealand (178), and Ireland (160). Japanese women experienced the lowest mortality (24) followed by France (30), Switzerland

Continued on page 77

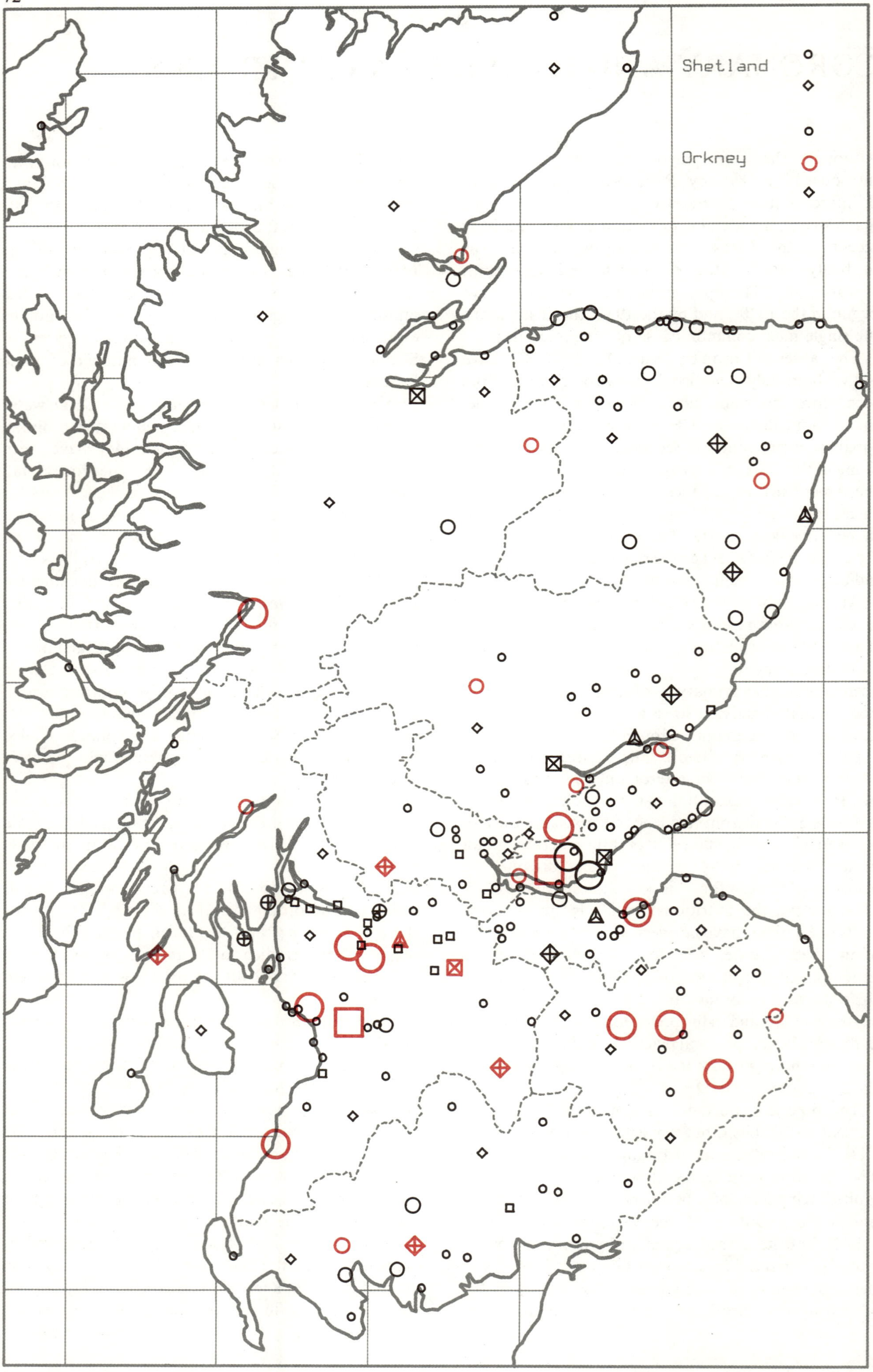
Shetland
Orkney

OTHER HEART DISEASE 1959-63

SMR significantly high $(p < 0.05)$ and within the top tenth

SMR significantly high $(p < 0.05)$ not within the top tenth

SMR not significantly high but within the top tenth

SMR not significantly high or low and not within the top or bottom tenth

SMR not significantly low but within the bottom tenth

SMR significantly low $(P < 0.05)$ not within the bottom tenth

SMR significantly low $(P < 0.05)$ and within the bottom tenth

City Large Burgh Small Burgh Landward Area

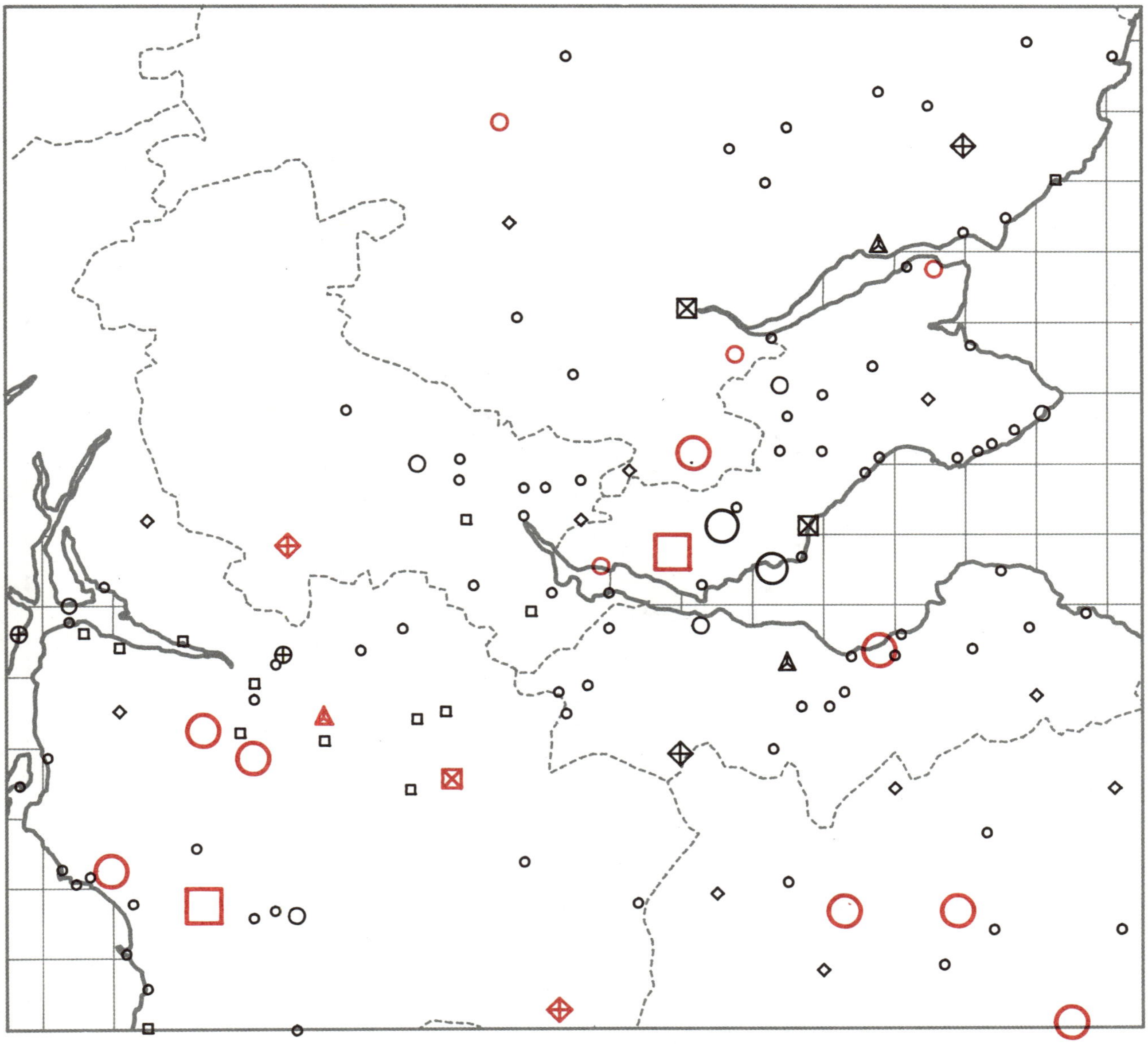

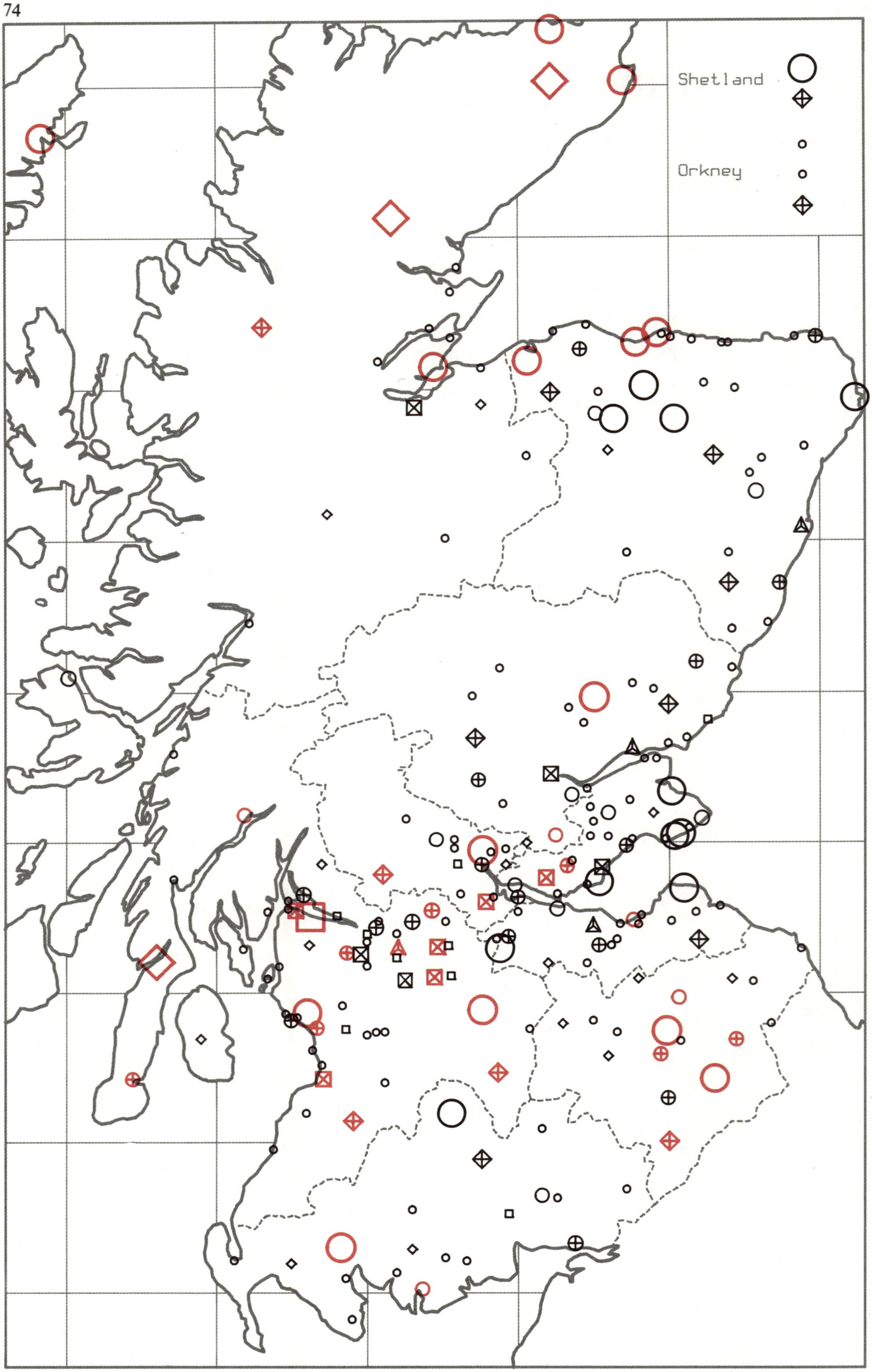
Shetland
Orkney

OTHER HEART DISEASE 1969-73

SMR significantly high ($p<0.05$) and within the top tenth

SMR significantly high ($p<0.05$) not within the top tenth

SMR not significantly high but within the top tenth

SMR not significantly high or low and not within the top or bottom tenth

SMR not significantly low but within the bottom tenth

SMR significantly low ($P<0.05$) not within the bottom tenth

SMR significantly low ($P<0.05$) and within the bottom tenth

City △ Large Burgh □ Small Burgh ○ Landward Area ◇

A SQUARE SYMBOL IS USED FOR THE DISTRICTS ON THE MAP OVERLEAF FOR 1979-83.

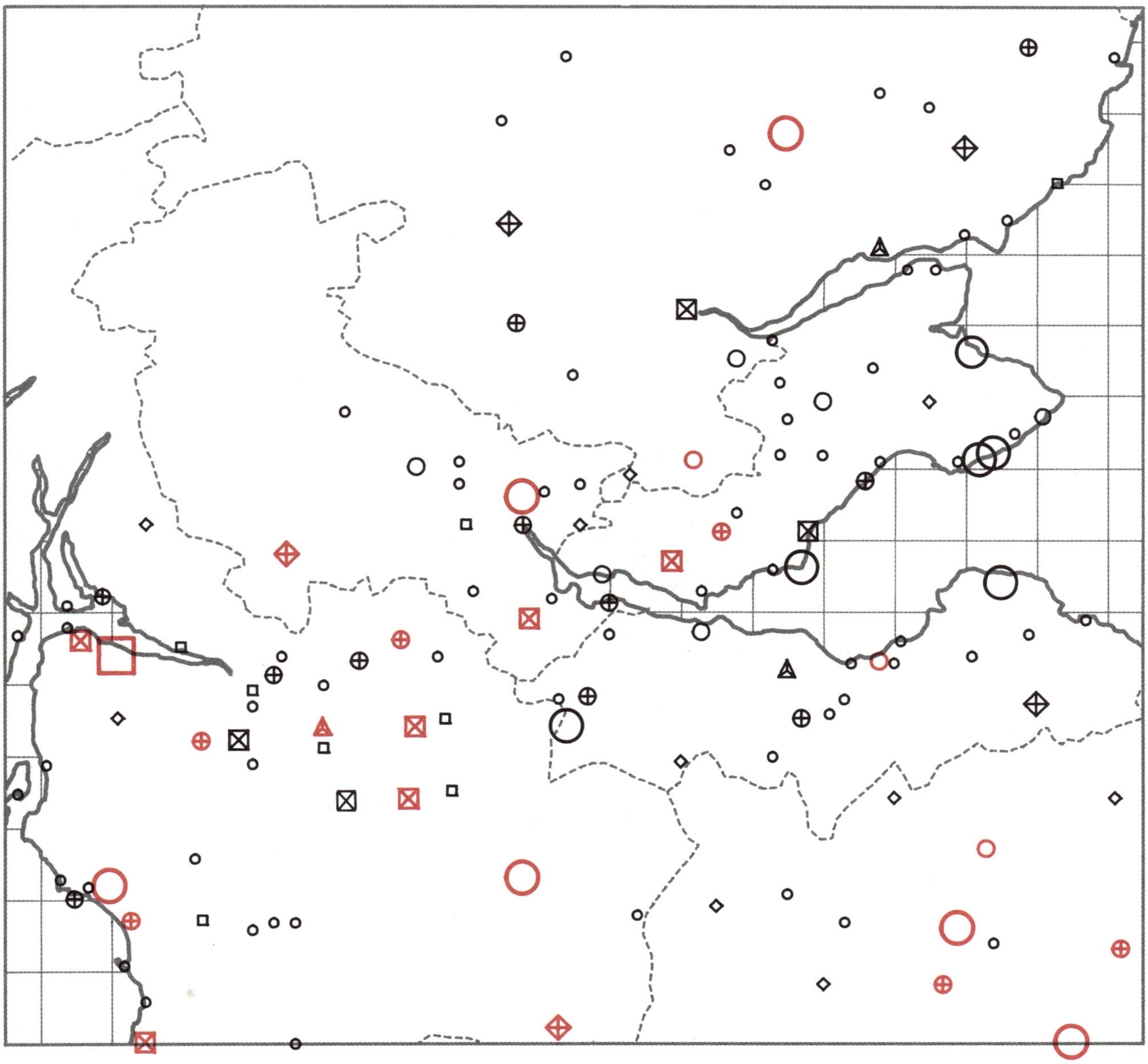

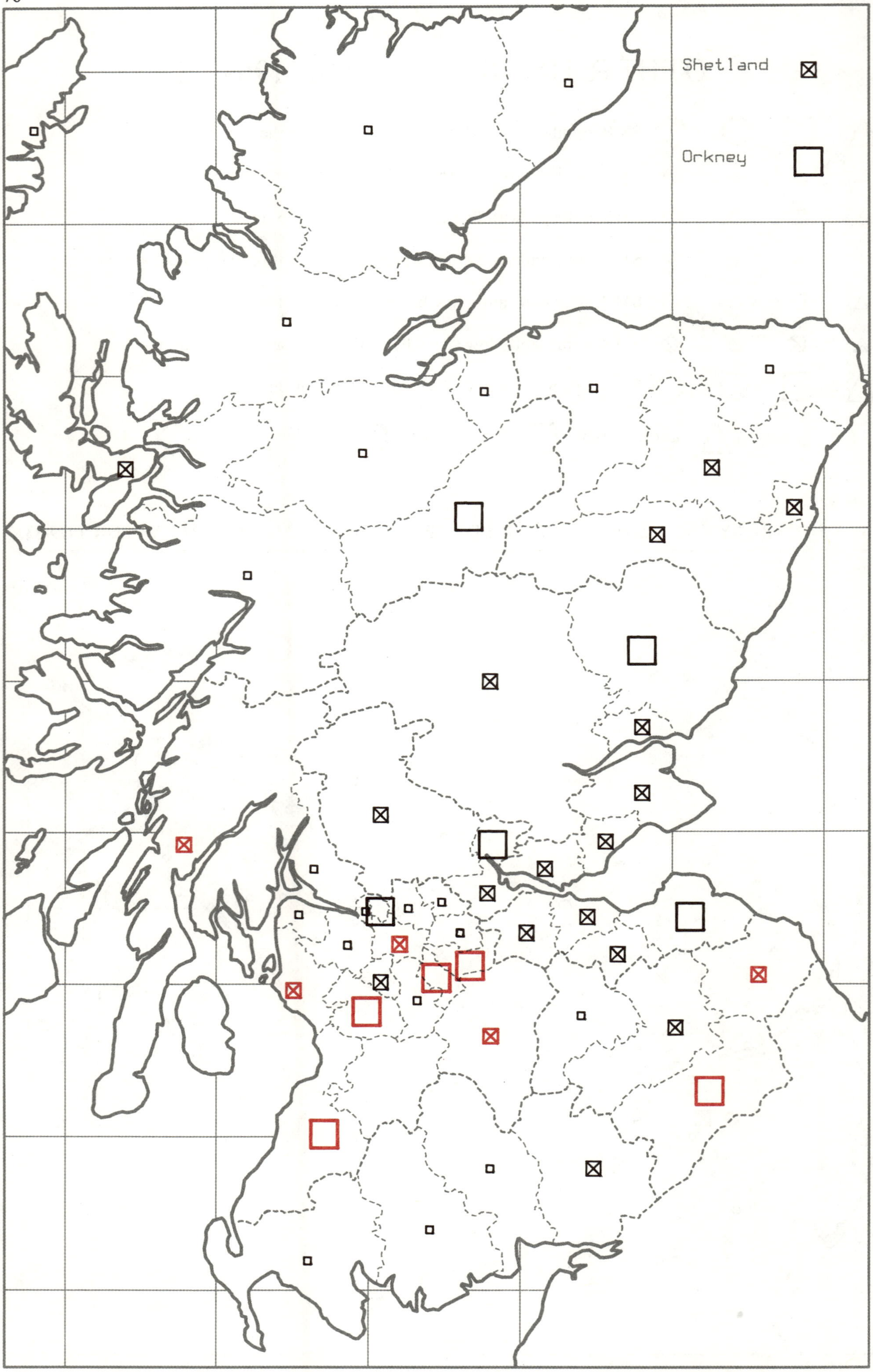
Shetland
Orkney

(47) and Italy (53). The differences between the countries are less noticeable for the females than the males, and there is a suggestion that the male:female ratio is increasing. In Europe, there is again a wide variation in the mortality rates; and an obvious gradient from north west to south east, with high attack rates for males in Helsinki, for example, and low rates in Bucharest [50]. In Britain, the gradients of mortality for both males and females decline from the high values in Scotland to the low values in East Anglia [11].

The secular trends in mortality from coronary heart disease vary considerably between countries. Between 1950 and 1978 the trends for males were generally upward, with the notable exceptions of the USA, Canada, Japan and France which showed a persistent decline. However, the trends in the female rates during the same period consistently declined [51].

In Scotland during 1959-63, high SMRs predominated in the central west and south west, especially around Glasgow, and in several Small Burghs in the south. This pattern was generally unchanged during 1969-73. Apart from four communities in each period, the communities with significantly high SMRs were situated to the south and south west of a line between the Tay estuary on the east and the Small Burgh of Lochgilphead on the west coast. The Small Burghs of Whithorn and Coldstream were in the category of the ten communities with the highest SMRs which were also significantly raised during the two earlier periods. During 1979-83 (despite the intervening boundary changes) raised SMRs were again mainly found in Districts in the central west and south west, with the exceptions of Caithness in the north and Lochaber on the west coast.

By contrast, the communities with low SMRs were found mainly in the north and east of Scotland in all three periods. The anomalies included Bearsden and Eastwood, which experienced low SMRs whilst surrounded by Districts with high mortality.

The distribution of Other Heart Disease was relevant to the interpretation of the CHD patterns because it was possible that cases of CHD had been reclassified into this category at some stage during the periods covered by the maps. As with the distribution of CHD, however, Strathclyde, Borders, and Dumfries and Galloway had the highest proportions of communities with high SMRs for Other Heart Disease. Hence, over a period of at least 26 years, mortality from cardiovascular diseases has been consistently higher in central west and south west Scotland than in other areas.

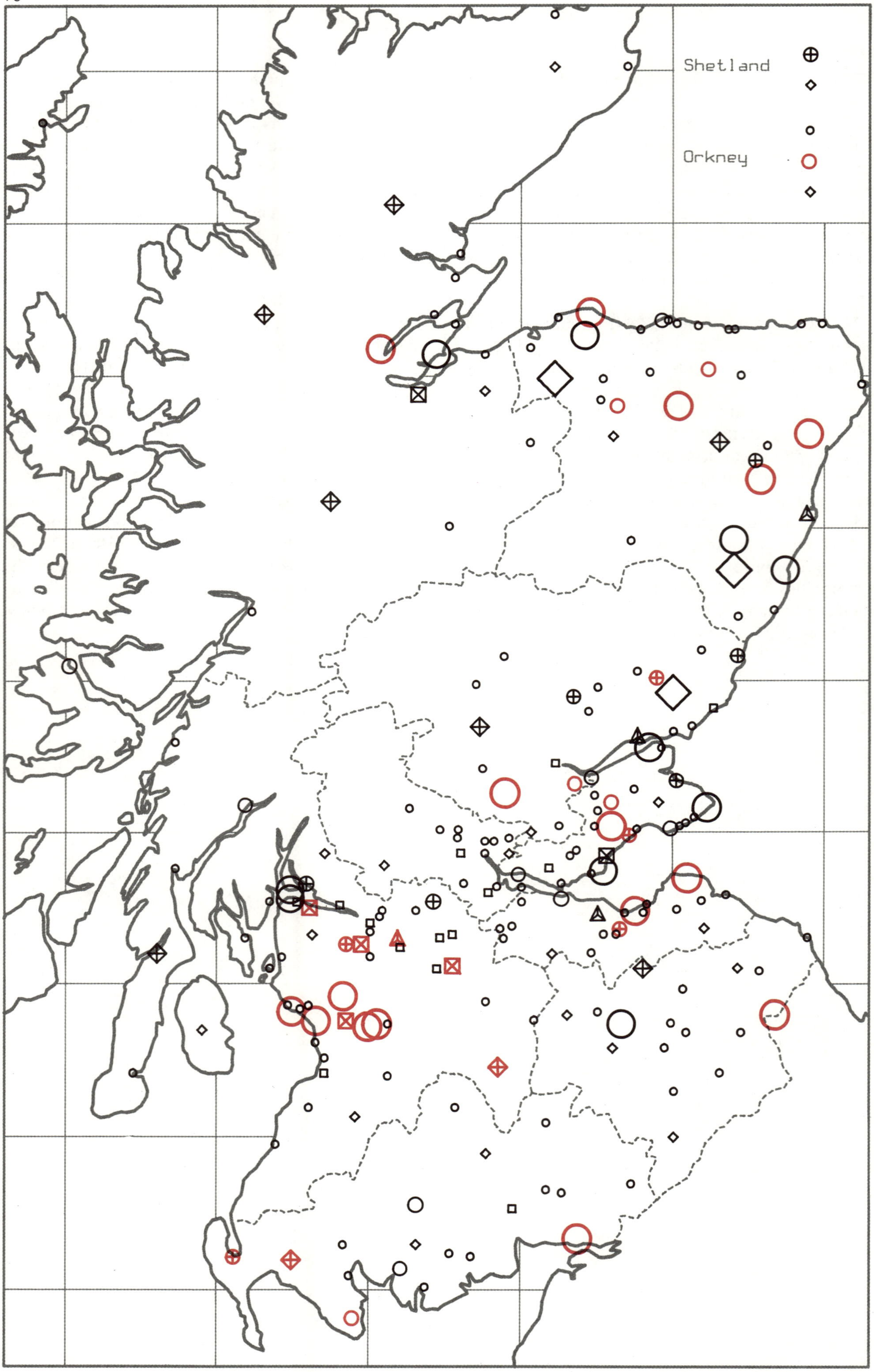
Shetland
Orkney

CEREBROVASCULAR DISEASE 1959-63

SMR significantly high ($p < 0.05$) and within the top tenth

SMR significantly high ($p < 0.05$) not within the top tenth

SMR not significantly high but within the top tenth

SMR not significantly high or low and not within the top or bottom tenth

SMR not significantly low but within the bottom tenth

SMR significantly low ($P < 0.05$) not within the bottom tenth

SMR significantly low ($P < 0.05$) and within the bottom tenth

City △ Large Burgh □ Small Burgh ○ Landward Area ◇

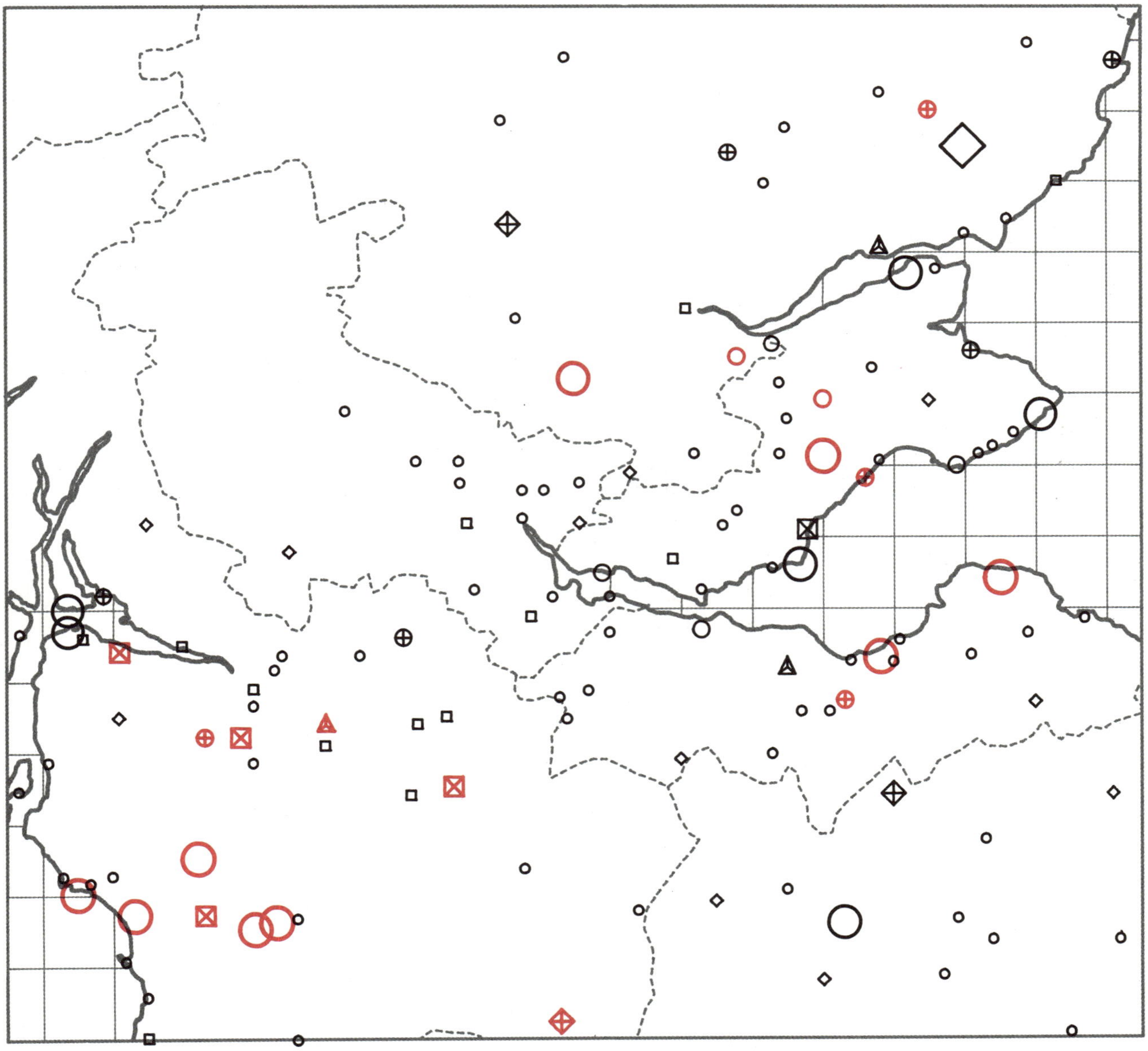

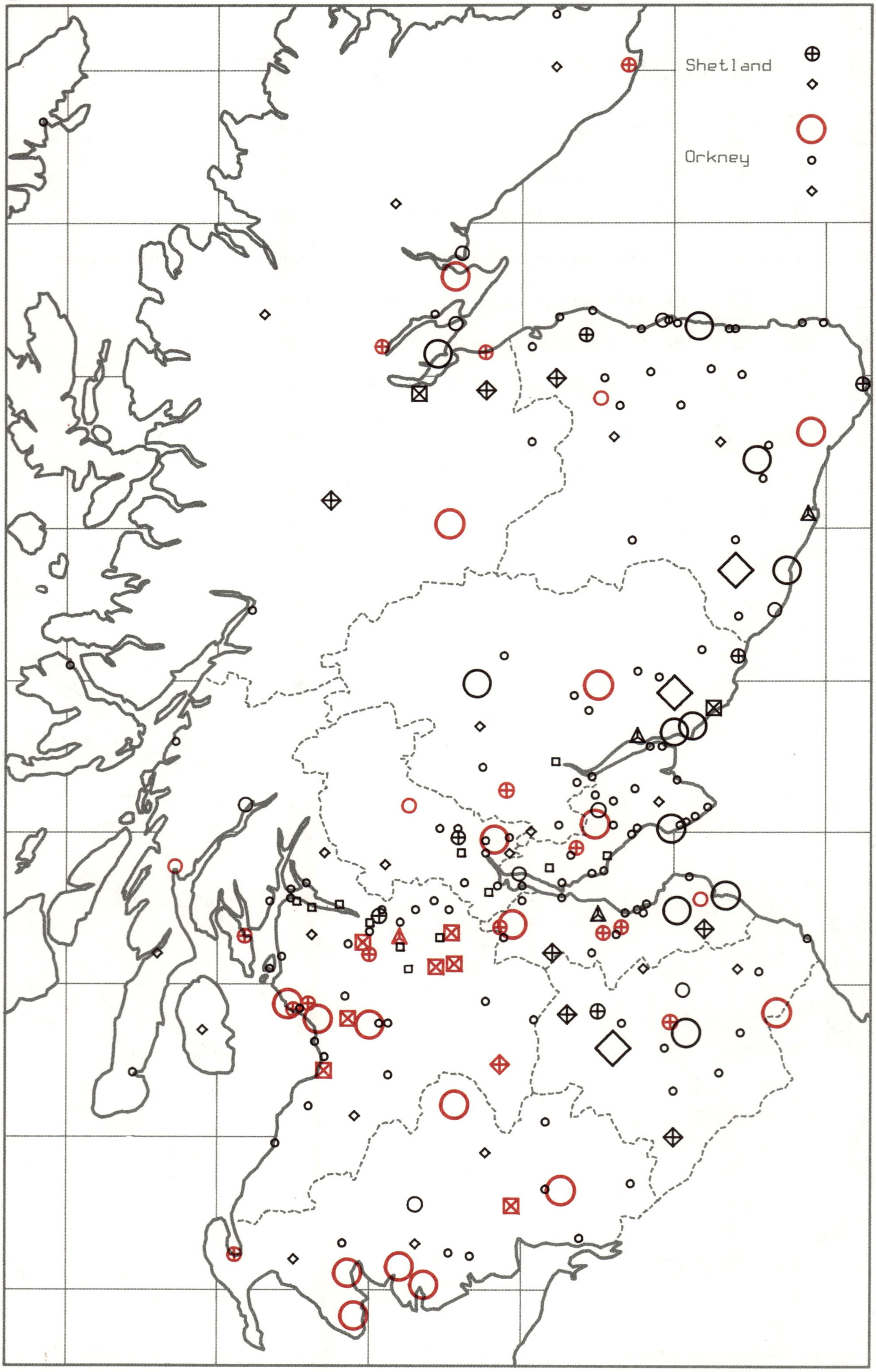
Shetland
Orkney

CEREBROVASCULAR DISEASE 1969-73

SMR significantly high ($p < 0.05$) and within the top tenth

SMR significantly high ($p < 0.05$) not within the top tenth

SMR not significantly high but within the top tenth

SMR not significantly high or low and not within the top or bottom tenth

SMR not significantly low but within the bottom tenth

SMR significantly low ($P < 0.05$) not within the bottom tenth

SMR significantly low ($P < 0.05$) and within the bottom tenth

City △ Large Burgh □ Small Burgh ○ Landward Area ◇

A SQUARE SYMBOL IS USED FOR THE DISTRICTS ON THE MAP OVERLEAF FOR 1979-83.

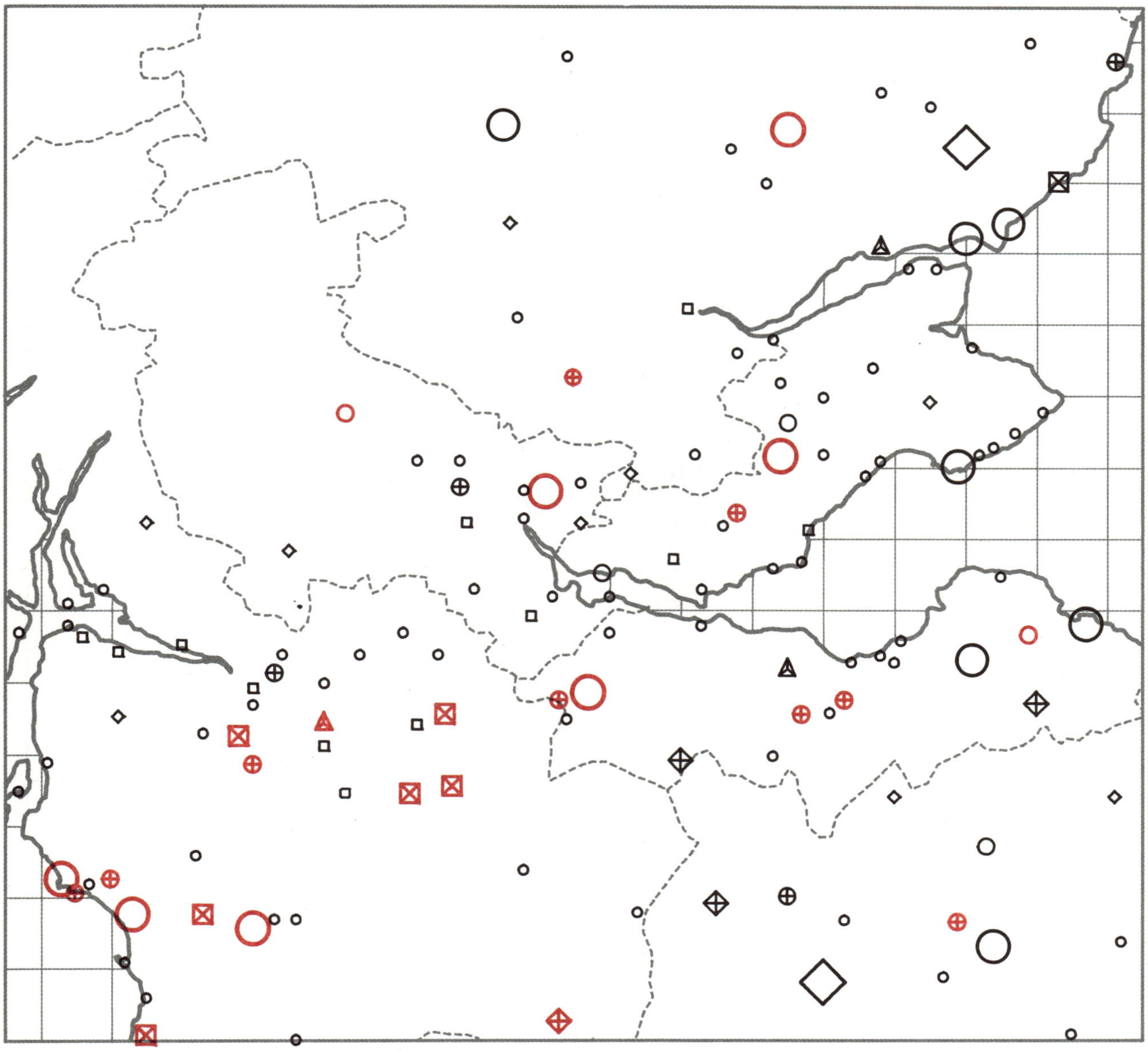

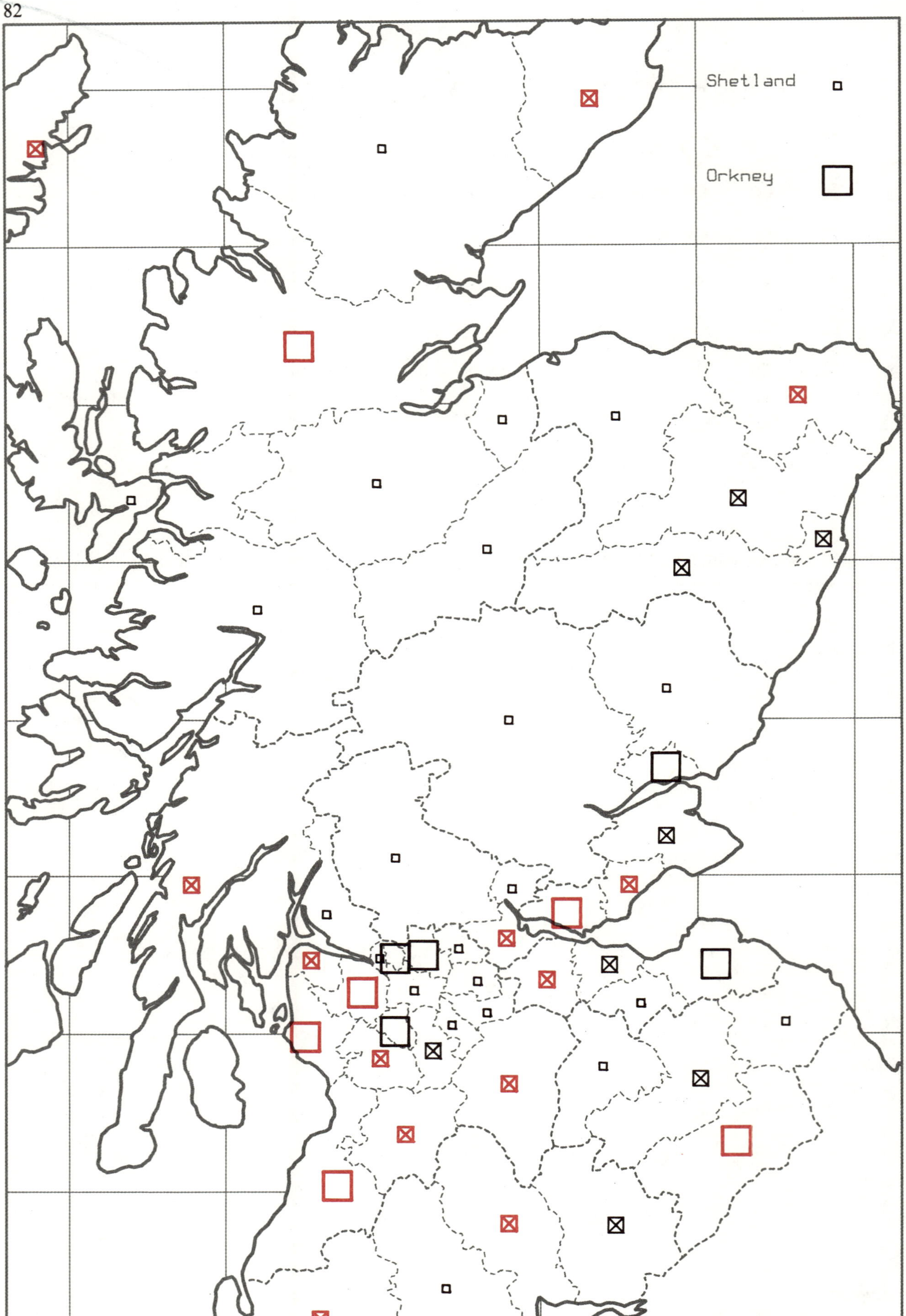
Shetland
Orkney

CEREBROVASCULAR DISEASE

'The sudden onset of a focal neurological deficit due to a local disturbance in blood supply to the brain' [52] may be followed by resolution within 24 hours (transient ischaemic attack), by more permanent symptoms or signs, or by death (stroke). Stroke includes intracerebral and subarachnoid haemorrhage and brain infarction due to atheroma, thrombosis or embolism, but distinction of these pathological entities on clinical grounds is unreliable. Comparisons of antemortem and postmortem diagnoses highlight this problem and show overdiagnosis of intracerebral haemorrhage [53]. Temporal changes in the type of stroke certified have been compared with trends in autopsy findings [54]. Even taking stroke as a single category, as many as one-third of cerebrovascular deaths may be certified as due to other causes and one-quarter of those labelled as stroke may be misclassified [53,55,56]. Comparisons of mortality rates from cerebrovascular disease should acknowledge these inaccuracies and the possible effect of temporal or spatial variation in diagnostic or coding practice.

Stroke is a major cause of death worldwide. International comparisons show high age-standardized mortality rates in Japan, Portugal and Bulgaria, and low rates in East Germany and Switzerland. In Britain, where it is the third commonest cause of death, mortality from cerebrovascular disease increases from south-east to north-west [11].

Age-standardized stroke mortality in most countries is declining. In the USA, this has been so for over 50 years, and is attributable mainly to falling incidence [57] with a smaller contribution from improved long-term survival [58]. These secular changes antedate effective antihypertensive therapy.

The incidence of stroke rises almost exponentially with age, with higher rates in males at all ages. Overall, about one-third of incident cases die within the first month, and a further third remain dependent for at least one activity of daily living. The impact of stroke on the community is seen as much in its position as a leading cause of disability and hospital bed occupancy, as in its contribution to mortality.

Much of our knowledge of personal risk factors for cerebrovascular disease is derived from prospective research designed primarily to investigate coronary heart disease, such as the Framingham study [59].

Hypertension. The dominant predisposing factor in terms of the closeness and consistency of its association with all types of stroke, it is also highly prevalent, constituting a substantial attributable risk within Western populations. The risk of stroke increases continuously with increasing blood pressure; no threshold effect is discernible. The effect does not decrease with age, and isolated systolic hypertension is important. Control of blood pressure can reduce stroke incidence and mortality in middle-aged and elderly persons with diastolic blood pressures above 90mmHg [60-65]. However, because most strokes occur in persons with only mild elevation of blood pressure, a small downward shift of blood pressure in the whole population could, on theoretical grounds, have as much impact on stroke incidence as the pharmacological treatment of hypertensive individuals [66].

Blood Lipids. In contrast to coronary disease, the association of stroke with blood cholesterol is weak and inconsistent. Recent results suggest that low levels of cholesterol, LDL-cholesterol and HDL-cholesterol are all associated with higher rates of atherothrombotic brain infarction.

Diabetes. Independent of other factors, glucose intolerance increases the risk of stroke two-fold in both sexes. Control of blood sugar levels does not affect outcome.

Obesity. A weak positive association is probably accounted for by the effect of body weight on blood pressure and carbohydrate tolerance.

Haematocrit. A positive association persists after controlling for the association of packed cell volume with blood pressure.

Cardiac Disease. Even after adjustment for the effect of blood pressure, coronary heart disease increases the risk of stroke threefold, or fivefold if congestive failure or ECG evidence of left ventricular hypertrophy are present. Atrial fibrillation and rheumatic heart disease are important and independent risk factors, particularly for embolic stroke.

Much less is known about aetiological influences underlying these clinical and pathophysiological risk factors. Within families, there is some inherited predisposition to hypertension and diabetes. American blacks have a high prevalence of hypertension and a higher stroke mortality than whites, but recently these racial differences have been decreasing.

The following features of lifestyle and the environment have been associated with cerebrovascular disease :

Cigarette Smoking. This is only weakly associated with stroke, mainly men under 65 [59].

Alcohol. A positive association with stroke incidence [59] is consistent with other evidence implicating alcohol as an aetiological factor in hypertension. There may be an acute effect from alcohol intoxication [67].

Water. In some nationwide studies, cardiovascular mortality (including stroke) is higher in areas with soft

Continued on page 89

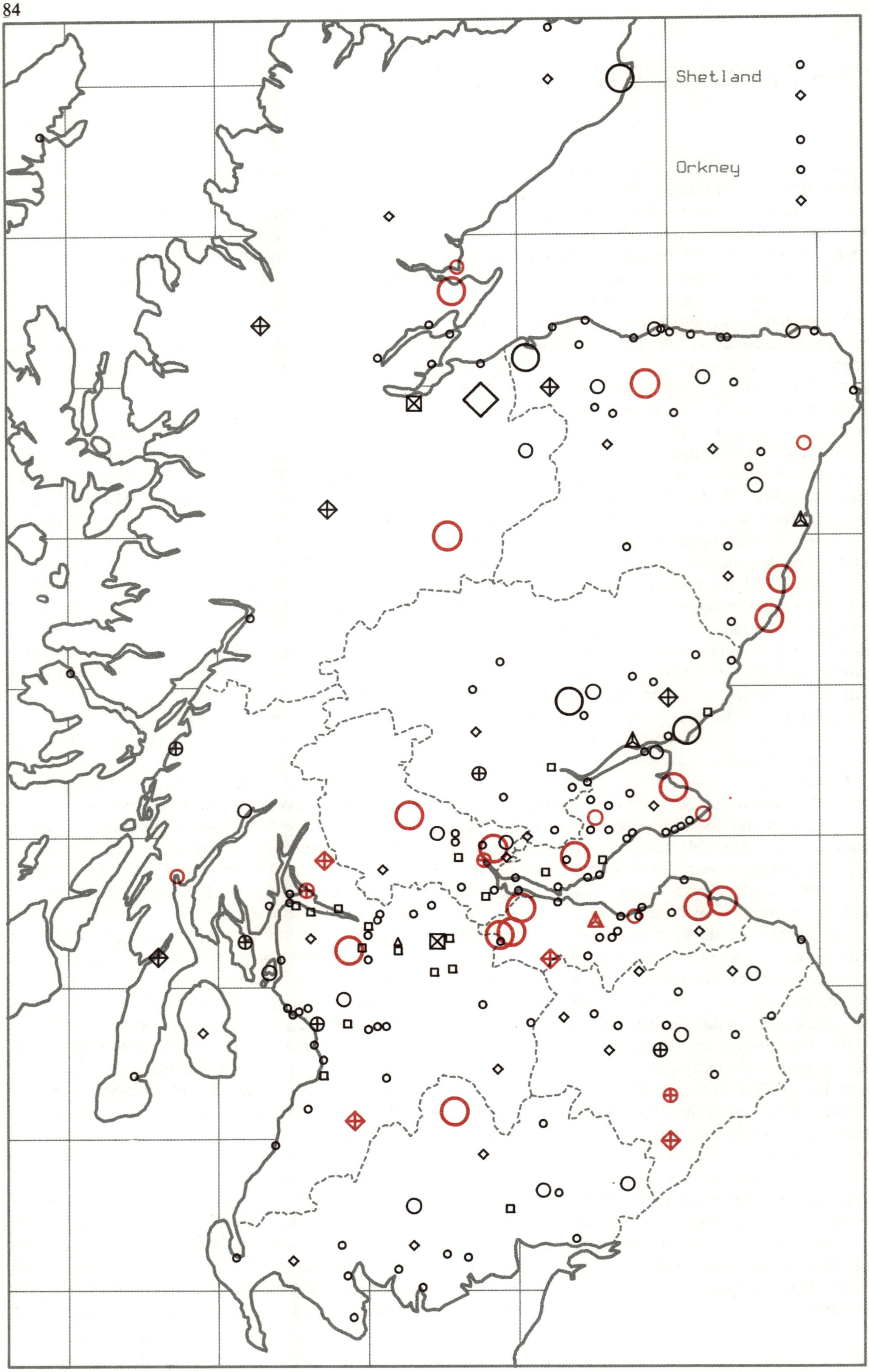
Shetland
Orkney

OTHER CIRCULATORY DISEASE 1959-63

SMR significantly high ($p < 0.05$) and within the top tenth

SMR significantly high ($p < 0.05$) not within the top tenth

SMR not significantly high but within the top tenth

SMR not significantly high or low and not within the top or bottom tenth

SMR not significantly low but within the bottom tenth

SMR significantly low ($P < 0.05$) not within the bottom tenth

SMR significantly low ($P < 0.05$) and within the bottom tenth

City Large Burgh Small Burgh Landward Area

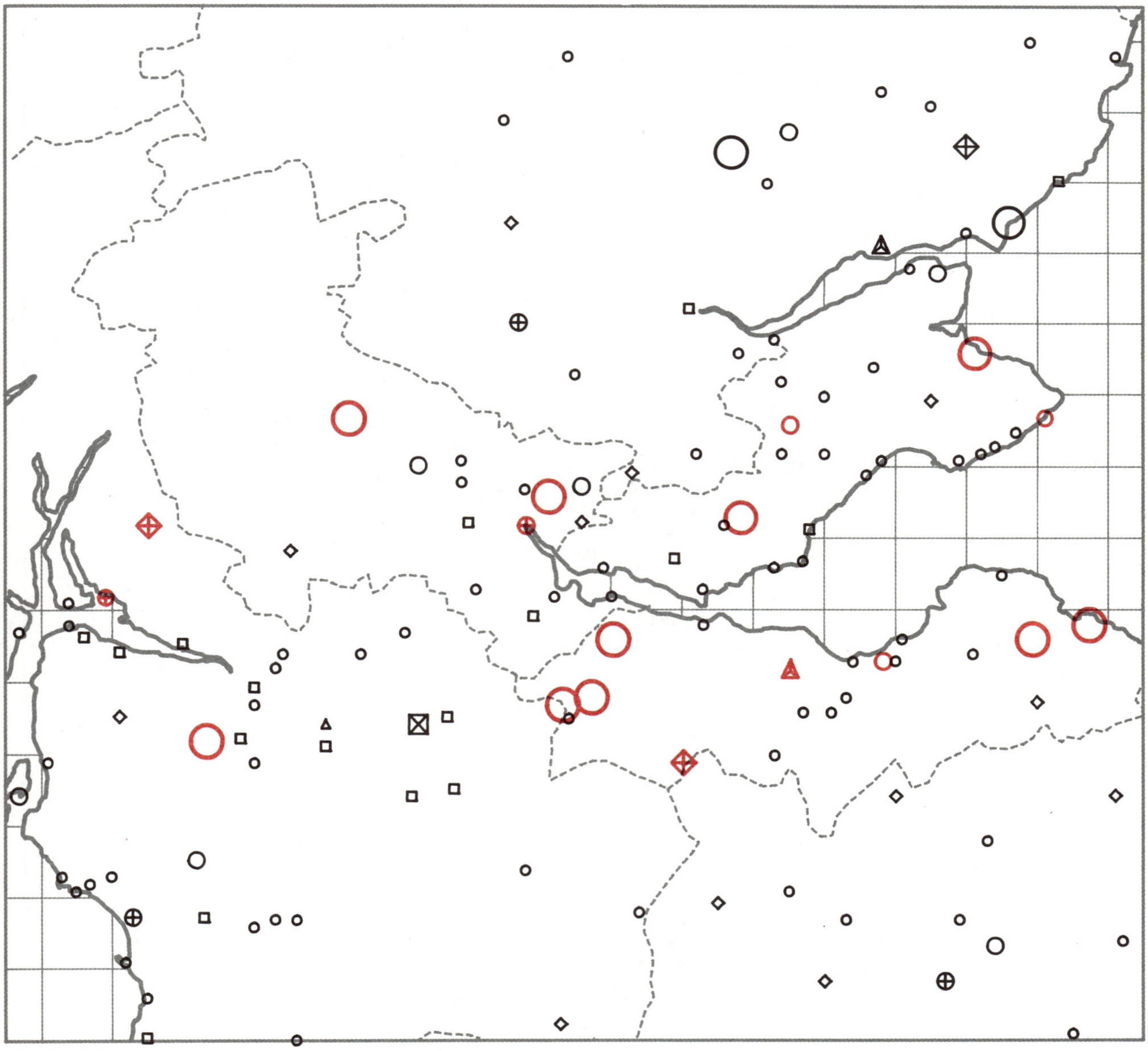

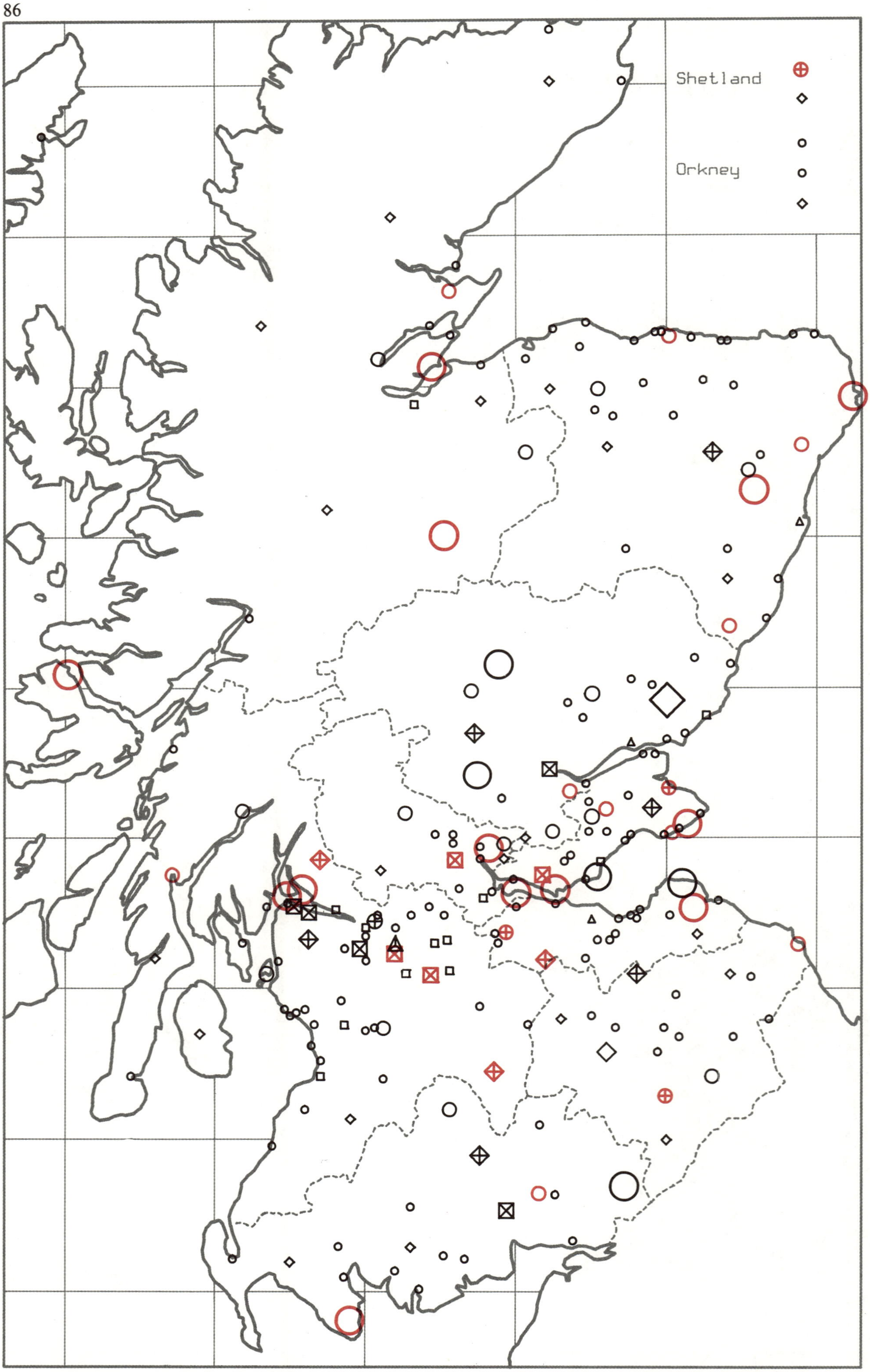
Shetland
Orkney

OTHER CIRCULATORY DISEASE 1969-73

City	Large Burgh	Small Burgh	Landward Area	
△	□	○	◇	SMR significantly high ($p < 0.05$) and within the top tenth
◬	⊠	⊕	◈	SMR significantly high ($p < 0.05$) not within the top tenth
△	□	○	◇	SMR not significantly high but within the top tenth
▵	▫	∘	⋄	SMR not significantly high or low and not within the top or bottom tenth
△	□	○	◇	SMR not significantly low but within the bottom tenth
◬	⊠	⊕	◈	SMR significantly low ($P < 0.05$) not within the bottom tenth
△	□	○	◇	SMR significantly low ($P < 0.05$) and within the bottom tenth

City △ Large Burgh □ Small Burgh ○ Landward Area ◇

A SQUARE SYMBOL IS USED FOR THE DISTRICTS ON THE MAP OVERLEAF FOR 1979-83.

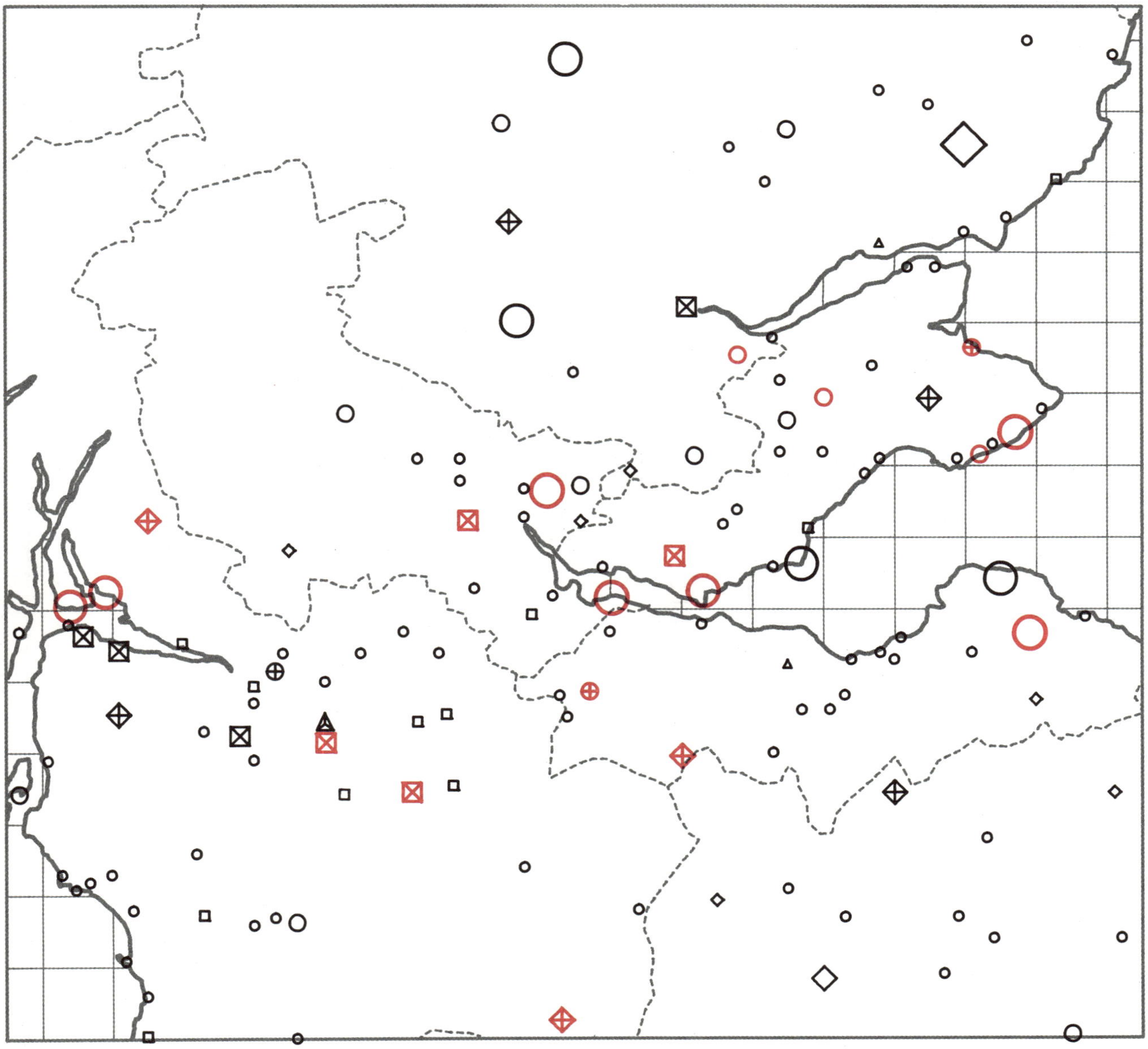

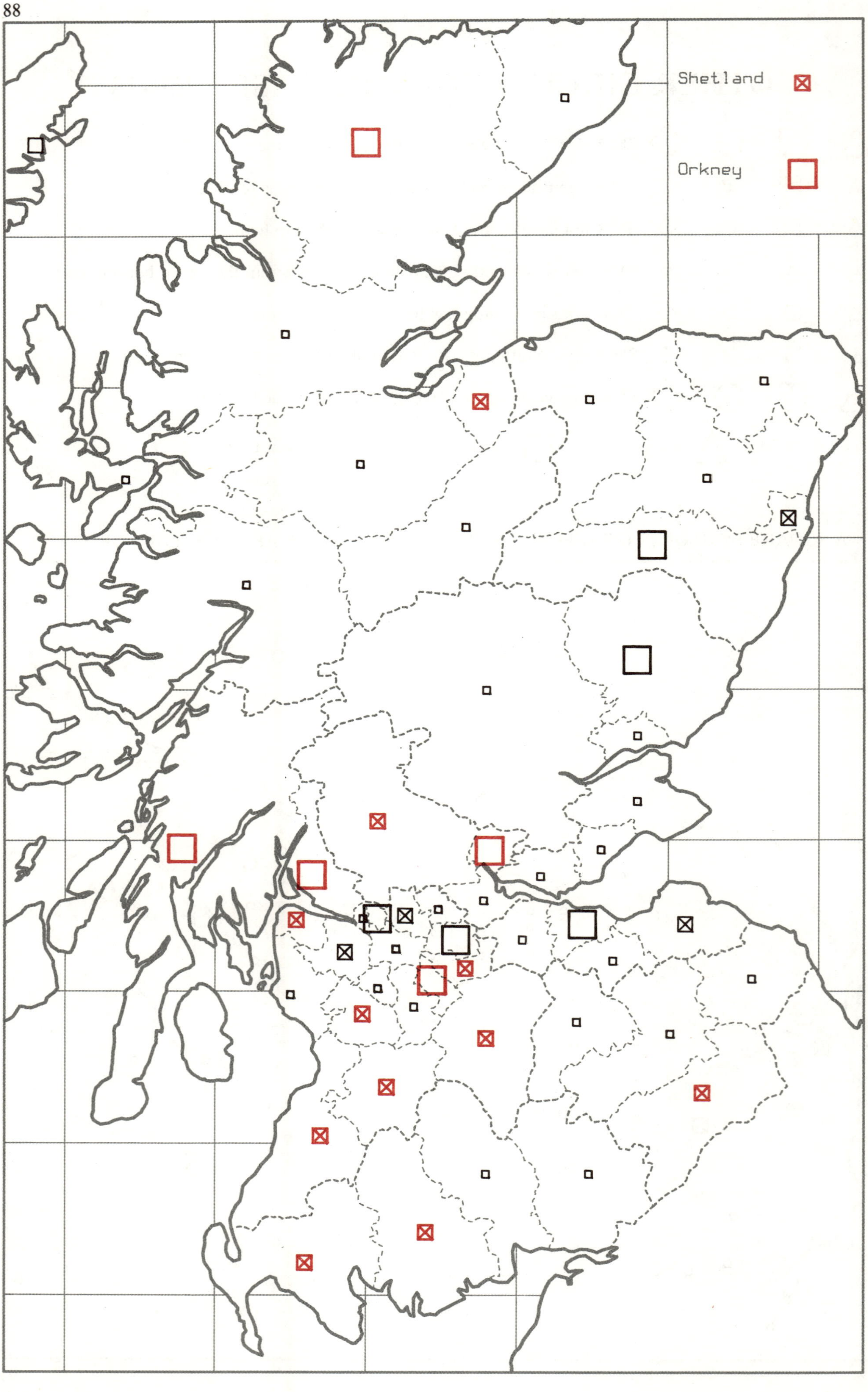
Shetland
Orkney

water. This is not confirmed in more local comparisons, and may reflect regional variation in other risk factors [68].

Diet. Few studies have examined the link between diet and stroke directly, but a recent British survey reported an inverse association with fresh fruit and vegetable consumption. More evidence exists on possible links between diet and intermediate risk factors, particularly hypertension and blood lipids. However, the interpretation of these data remains uncertain. The following dietary constituents have been proposed as aetiological determinants of blood pressure: sodium, potassium, calcium, magnesium, fat, fibre and alcohol [69].

Oral Contraceptives. Combined oestrogen-progestogen pills increase the risk of cerebrovascular events among users ninefold [70]. Cigarette smoking increases the risk. However, because incidence of stroke during the reproductive years is so low, the absolute risk is small, and the contribution to overall incidence is insignificant.

Social Class. Mortality from stroke is higher among the lower social classes in the UK. It is not known to what extent this reflects differential exposure to aetiological factors, or variations in the uptake of preventive services, notably the detection and treatment of hypertension.

Climate. Mortality from all cardiovascular diseases is lower during the summer months in temperate climates, perhaps due to small seasonal changes in blood pressure which are themselves unexplained.

The geographical patterns of mortality due to Cerebrovascular Disease shown here include a cluster of high SMRs to the south west of Glasgow during 1959-63 and 1969-73, and a small cluster of high SMRs on the southern coastline during 1969-73. Communities with high SMRs in both periods included: the City of Glasgow; the Large Burghs of Paisley, Motherwell and Kilmarnock; the Small Burghs of Ellon, Auchterarder, Dalkeith, Galston Irvine, Saltcoats, Coldstream and Stranraer; and the Landward Area of Lanark. During 1979-83, the Districts to the south west of Glasgow again showed high values, and the whole south west quarter of Scotland appeared to have a large proportion of high values. For low SMRs, the converse distribution was found in all periods, with the eastern half of Scotland showing a relatively high proportion of low values.

High values were rarely seen for both Cerebrovascular Disease and for Other Circulatory Disease simultaneously, indicating that local variations in diagnostic fashion might have helped to generate the abnormal values in some communities. In 1959-63, high values in the two categories were found only for the Small Burghs of Ellon, Prestonpans and Johnstone. In 1969-73, the comparable communities were: the Large Burgh of Hamilton; the Small Burghs of Tain, Ellon again, Kingussie, Lochgilphead, Tillicoutry, East Linton, Bathgate and Whithorn; and the Landward Area of Lanark. For 1979-83, the pattern of Other Circulatory Disease resembled that of Cerebrovascular Disease in showing Districts with high SMRs mainly in the south west quarter of Scotland, but with the low SMRs more evenly balanced between east and west.

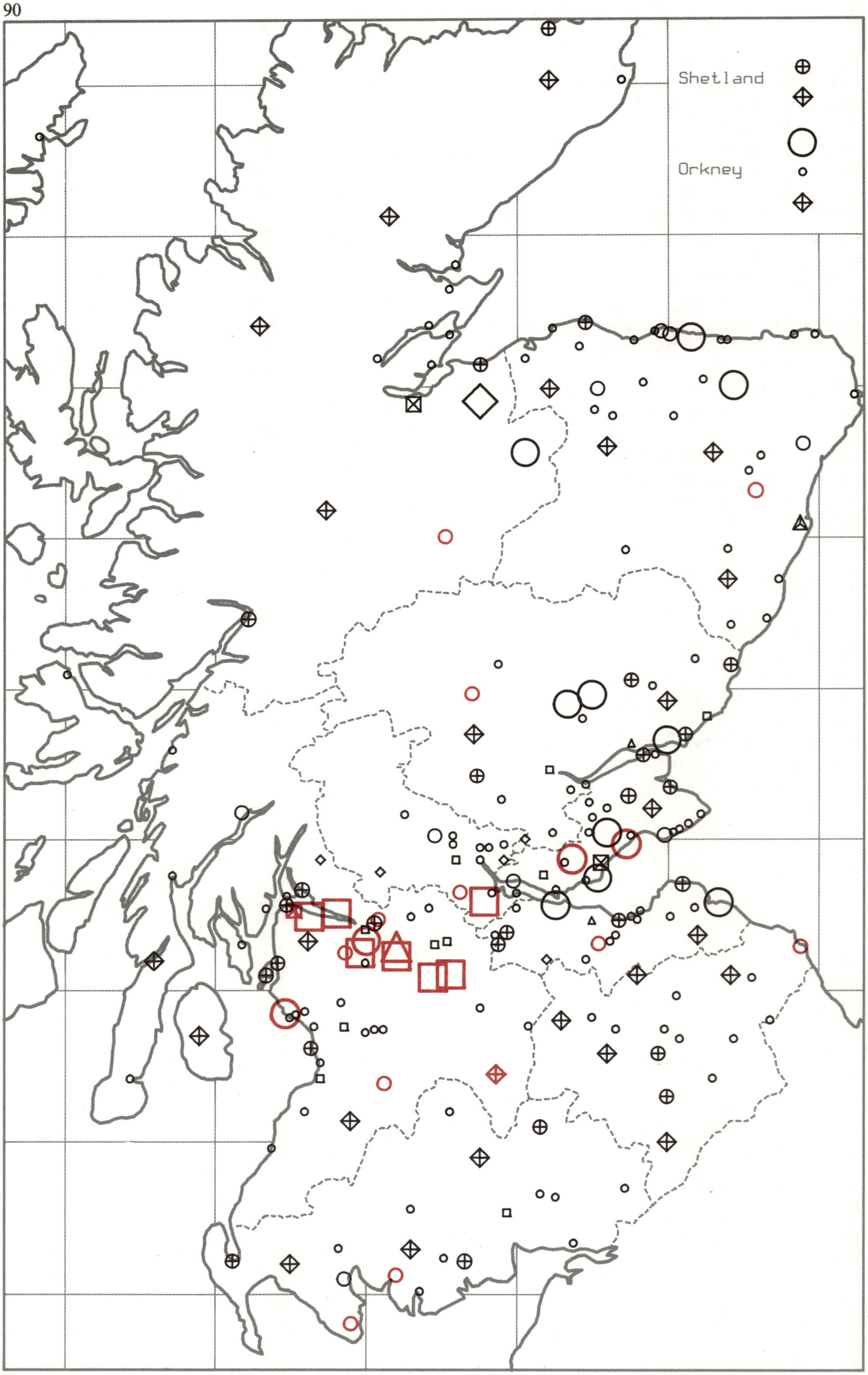
Shetland
Orkney

BRONCHITIS 1959-63

- SMR significantly high ($p < 0.05$) and within the top tenth
- SMR significantly high ($p < 0.05$) not within the top tenth
- SMR not significantly high but within the top tenth
- SMR not significantly high or low and not within the top or bottom tenth
- SMR not significantly low but within the bottom tenth
- SMR significantly low ($P < 0.05$) not within the bottom tenth
- SMR significantly low ($P < 0.05$) and within the bottom tenth

City △ Large Burgh □ Small Burgh ○ Landward Area ◇

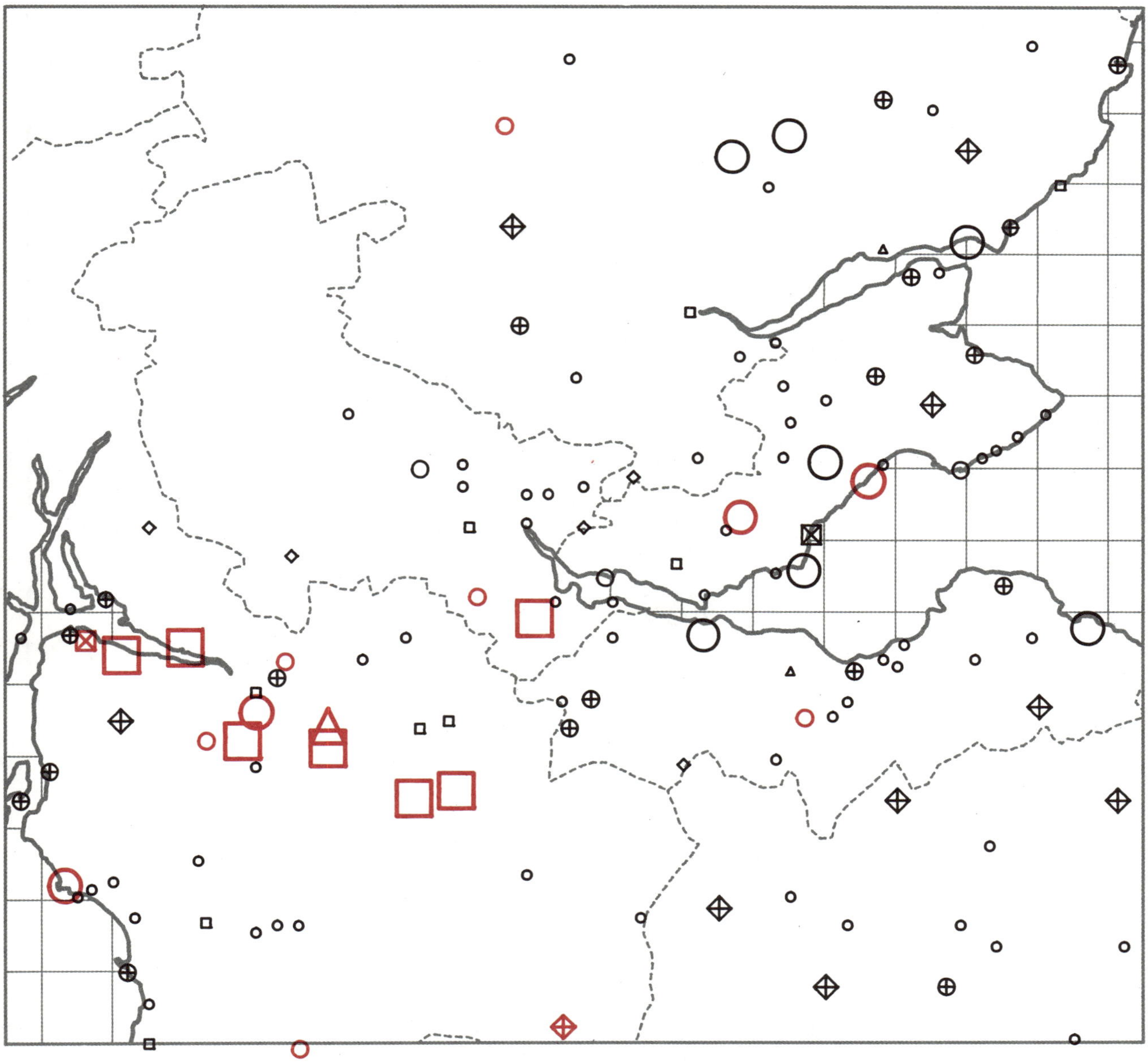

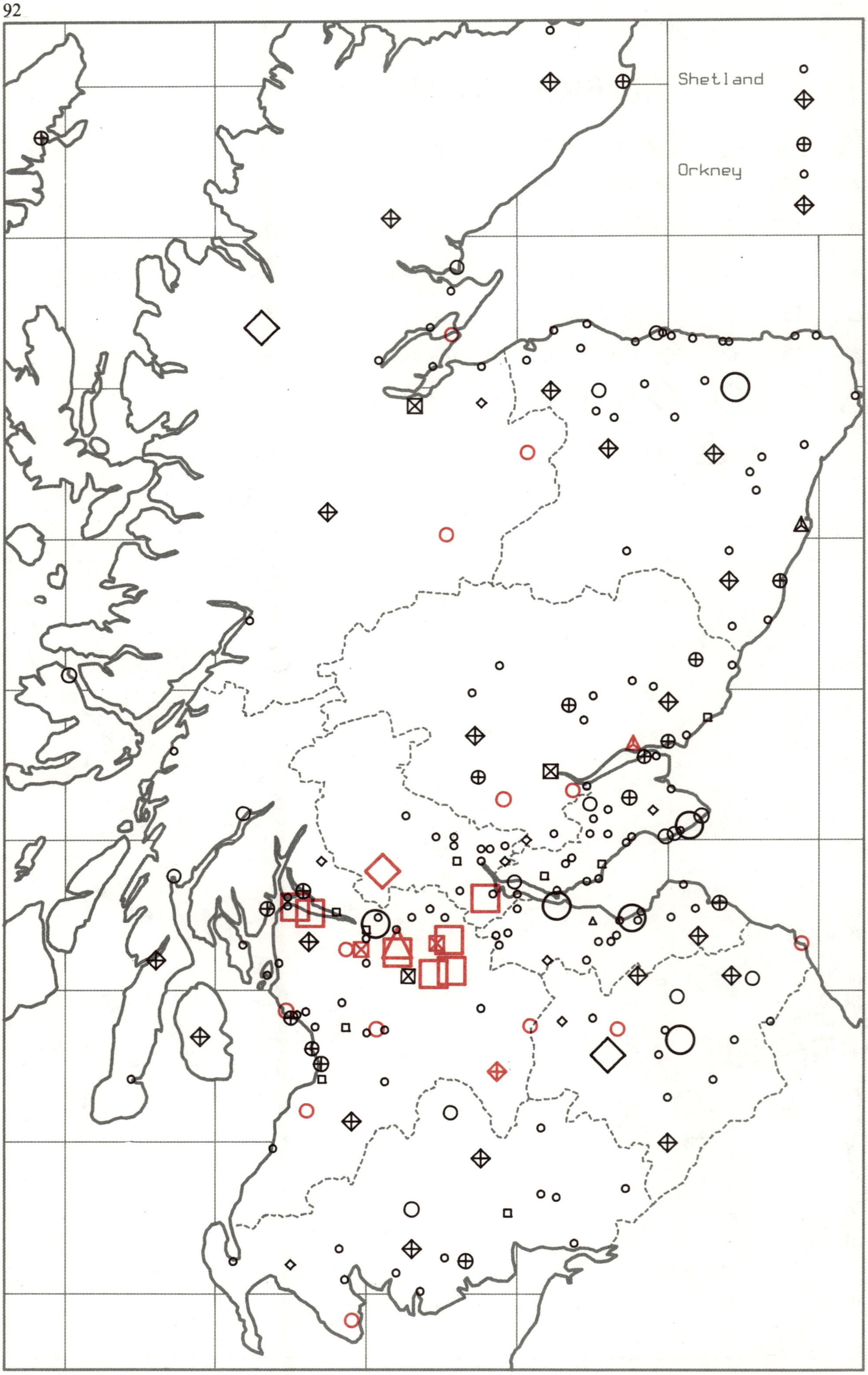
Shetland
Orkney

BRONCHITIS, EMPHYSEMA AND ASTHMA 1969-73

SMR significantly high ($p < 0.05$) and within the top tenth

SMR significantly high ($p < 0.05$) not within the top tenth

SMR not significantly high but within the top tenth

SMR not significantly high or low and not within the top or bottom tenth

SMR not significantly low but within the bottom tenth

SMR significantly low ($P < 0.05$) not within the bottom tenth

SMR significantly low ($P < 0.05$) and within the bottom tenth

City △ Large Burgh □ Small Burgh ○ Landward Area ◇

A SQUARE SYMBOL IS USED FOR THE DISTRICTS ON THE MAP OVERLEAF FOR 1979-83.

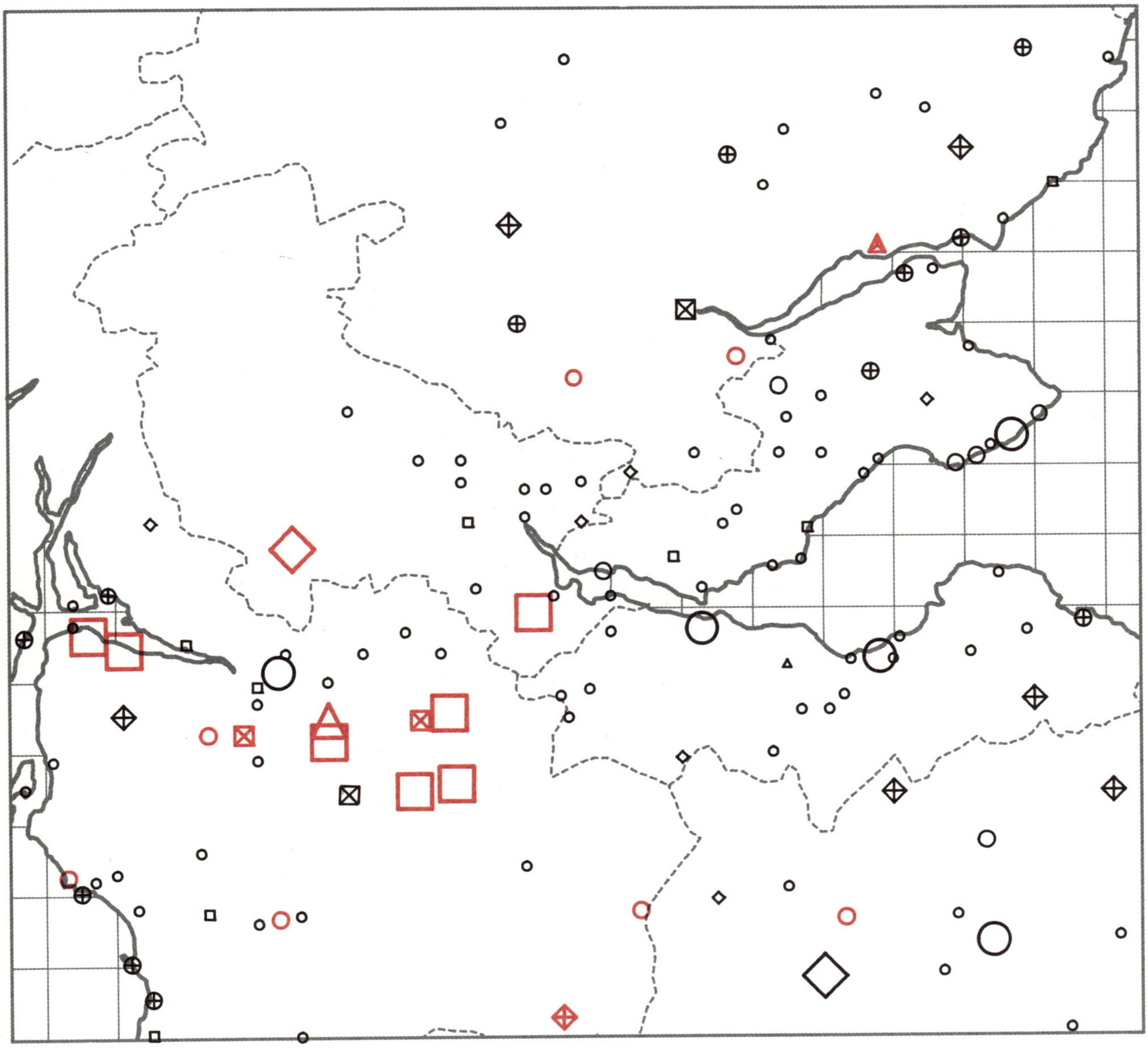

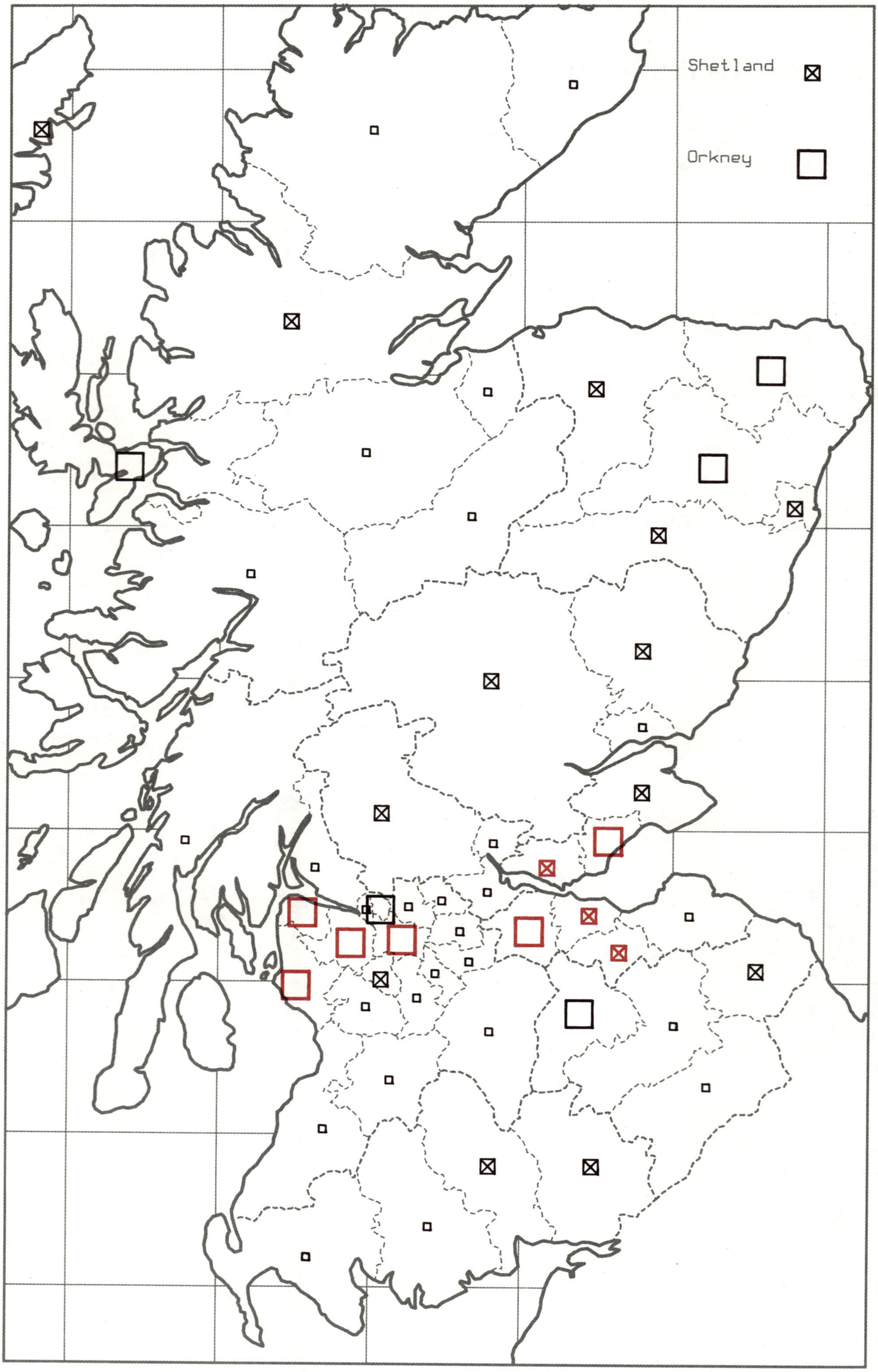
Shetland
Orkney

BRONCHITIS, EMPHYSEMA AND ASTHMA

Chronic bronchitis can be defined as a chronic or recurrent increase in the volume of mucoid bronchial secretion sufficient to cause expectoration. Emphysema is sometimes used as an alternative diagnosis to chronic bronchitis, so for the purposes of mortality analysis they should be considered together. Emphysema is recorded as an underlying cause of death in Scotland in about five percent of deaths in the ICD-9:490-493. Asthma is defined clinically by its symptoms and response to therapy and may not be recognized in its milder forms [71,72]. Since only five percent of mortality due to bronchitis, emphysema and asthma is ascribed to asthma, variation in asthma mortality is unlikely to have an important effect on area ranking. This diagnosis is therefore not considered further.

The uncertainty of the diagnosis of chronic bronchitis is an important factor in mortality data since some 80 percent of deaths do not have diagnostic verification by autopsy. Studies of pre- and post-mortem diagnoses have shown that clinicians underdiagnose the condition by between 15 and 30 percent [53,73]. Among the risk factors for chronic bronchitis, the smoking of tobacco is the most important [74]. For example, in the study of British doctors [75], the standardized mortality rate from chronic bronchitis in smokers consuming 25 or more cigarettes per day was 21 times as great as for non-smokers.

Air pollution is probably the next most important factor, at least when outdoor values of particulate matter are continuously high. Variation in daily ambient smoke and sulphur dioxide values in London were shown to be positively correlated with changes in bronchitics' symptoms [76]. Furthermore, the symptoms of bronchitis are more common among adults living in areas of high compared with low pollution [77,78]. A clear relation has been demonstrated between bronchitis mortality and air pollution in two studies from England and Wales covering the periods 1948-54 and 1959-63 [79,80]. These relations were not detectable in a similar analysis for data from 1969-73 [81] due possibly to the marked decline over the previous decade in pollution values in almost all urban areas. Exacerbations of, and mortality from, chronic bronchitis are also related inversely to outdoor temperature [82], which presents difficulties when analyzing the effects of pollution since values vary inversely with temperature.

Other factors are probably of less general importance. However, the risk of bronchitis may be increased by occupational environments such as mines, iron foundries and cotton mills. Bronchitis is also associated with lower social class, which may in part be a reflection of smoking habits and adverse domestic environments as well as occupation [83,84]. Early childhood respiratory illnesses are associated with bronchitic symptoms in adulthood [85,86]. Bronchitis increases with age and is more common in men than women, probably a reflection of smoking habits.

The maps fit partially with the known risk factors. High SMRs are seen in the Glasgow region for all three periods. Falkirk, situated in an industrial area, had significantly high mortality for the two earlier periods, but not in 1979-83. Of the Cities, Dundee had an elevated SMR in 1969-73 but was otherwise average, Edinburgh, despite its size, had average SMRs until 1979-83 when several of the Lothian Districts had SMRs among the top ten. Somewhat surprisingly, Aberdeen has had consistently low SMRs. There is some correspondence between patterns for bronchitis and lung cancer (qv): in all periods, high SMRs for both diseases were present in, and to the west of, Glasgow.

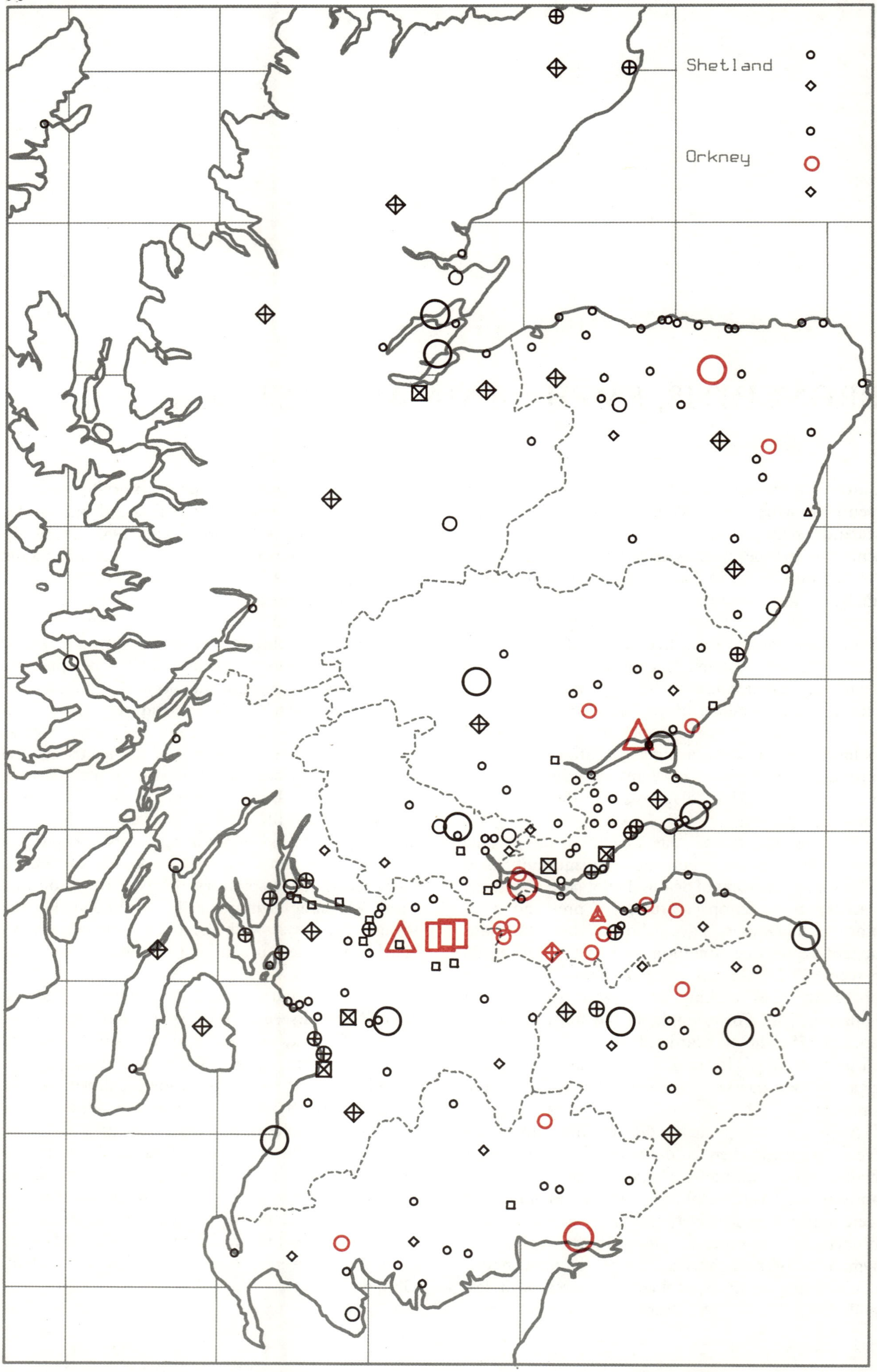
Shetland
Orkney

PNEUMONIA 1959-63

- SMR significantly high ($p<0.05$) and within the top tenth
- SMR significantly high ($p<0.05$) not within the top tenth
- SMR not significantly high but within the top tenth
- SMR not significantly high or low and not within the top or bottom tenth
- SMR not significantly low but within the bottom tenth
- SMR significantly low ($P<0.05$) not within the bottom tenth
- SMR significantly low ($P<0.05$) and within the bottom tenth

City △ Large Burgh □ Small Burgh ○ Landward Area ◇

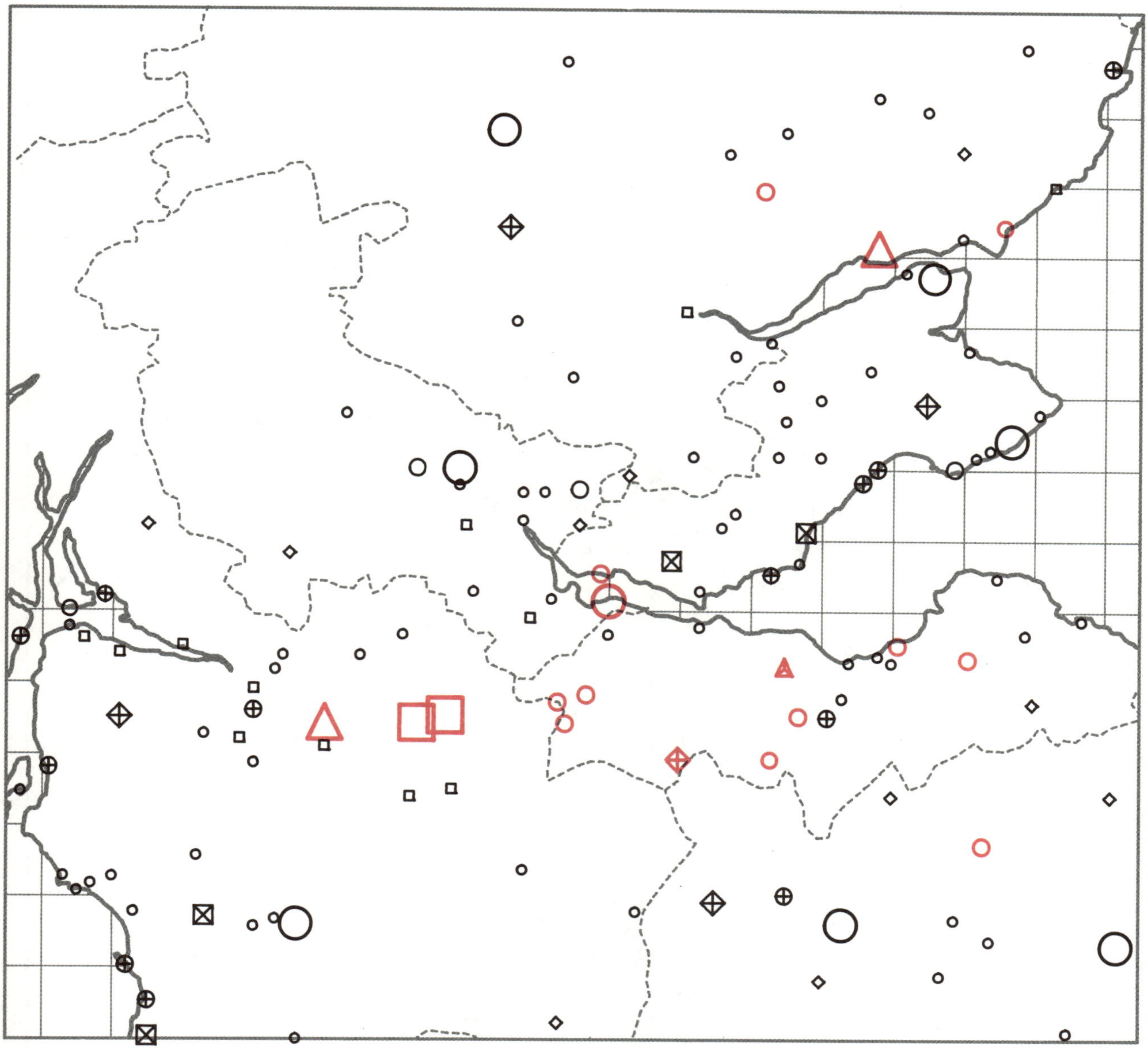

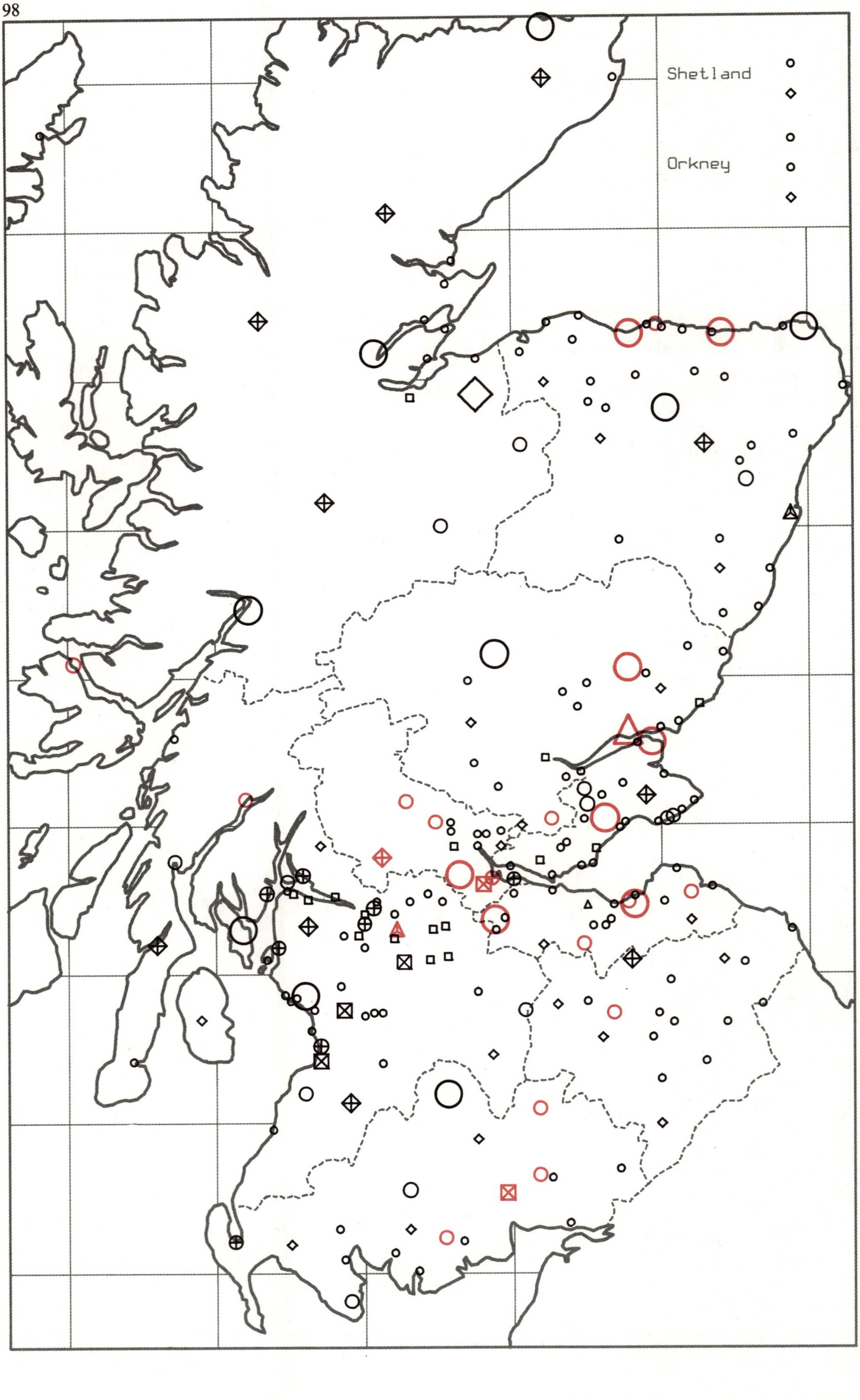
Shetland
Orkney

PNEUMONIA 1969-73

SMR significantly high ($p<0.05$) and within the top tenth

SMR significantly high ($p<0.05$) not within the top tenth

SMR not significantly high but within the top tenth

SMR not significantly high or low and not within the top or bottom tenth

SMR not significantly low but within the bottom tenth

SMR significantly low ($P<0.05$) not within the bottom tenth

SMR significantly low ($P<0.05$) and within the bottom tenth

City △ Large Burgh □ Small Burgh ○ Landward Area ◇

A SQUARE SYMBOL IS USED FOR THE DISTRICTS ON THE MAP OVERLEAF FOR 1979-83.

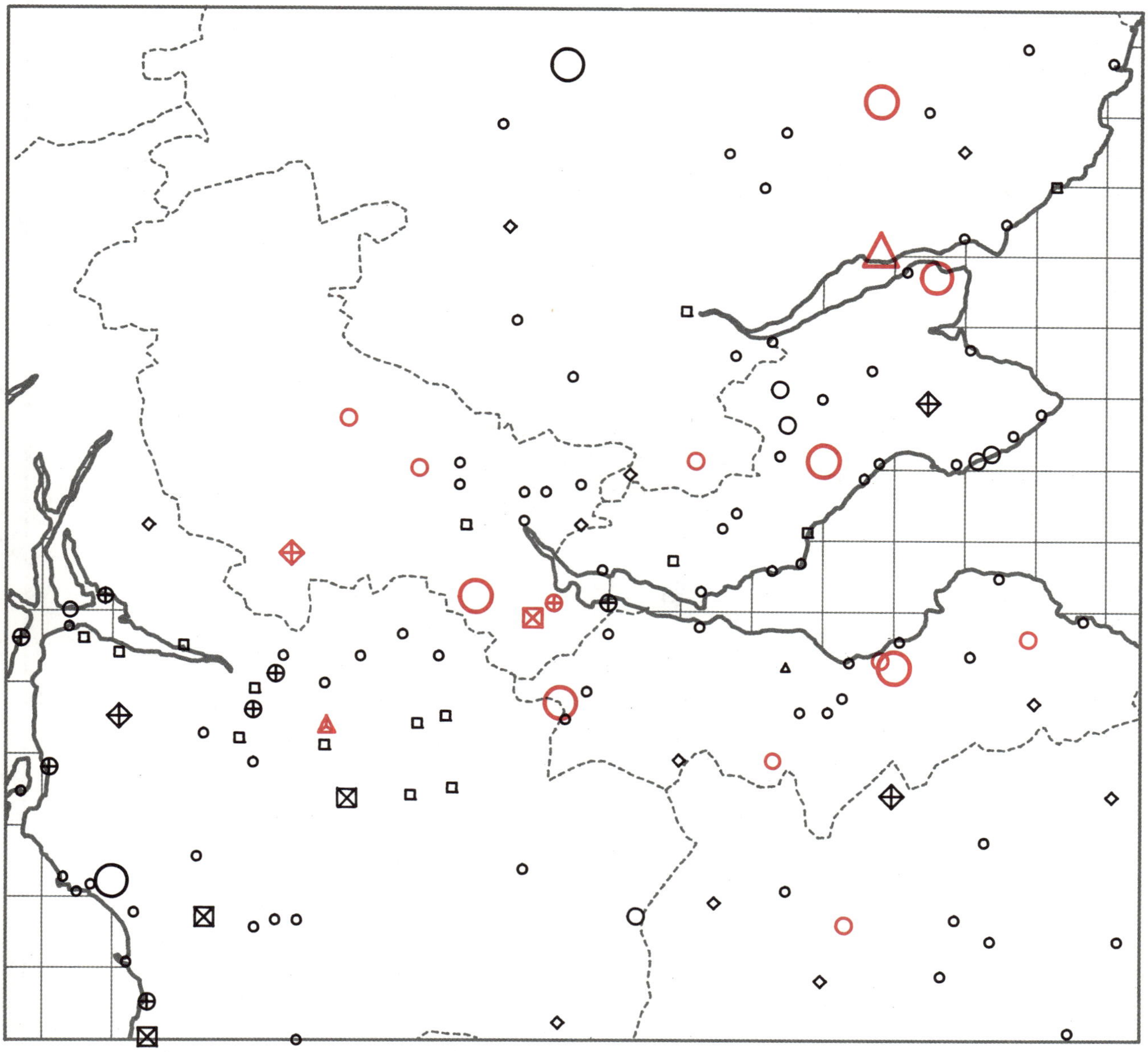

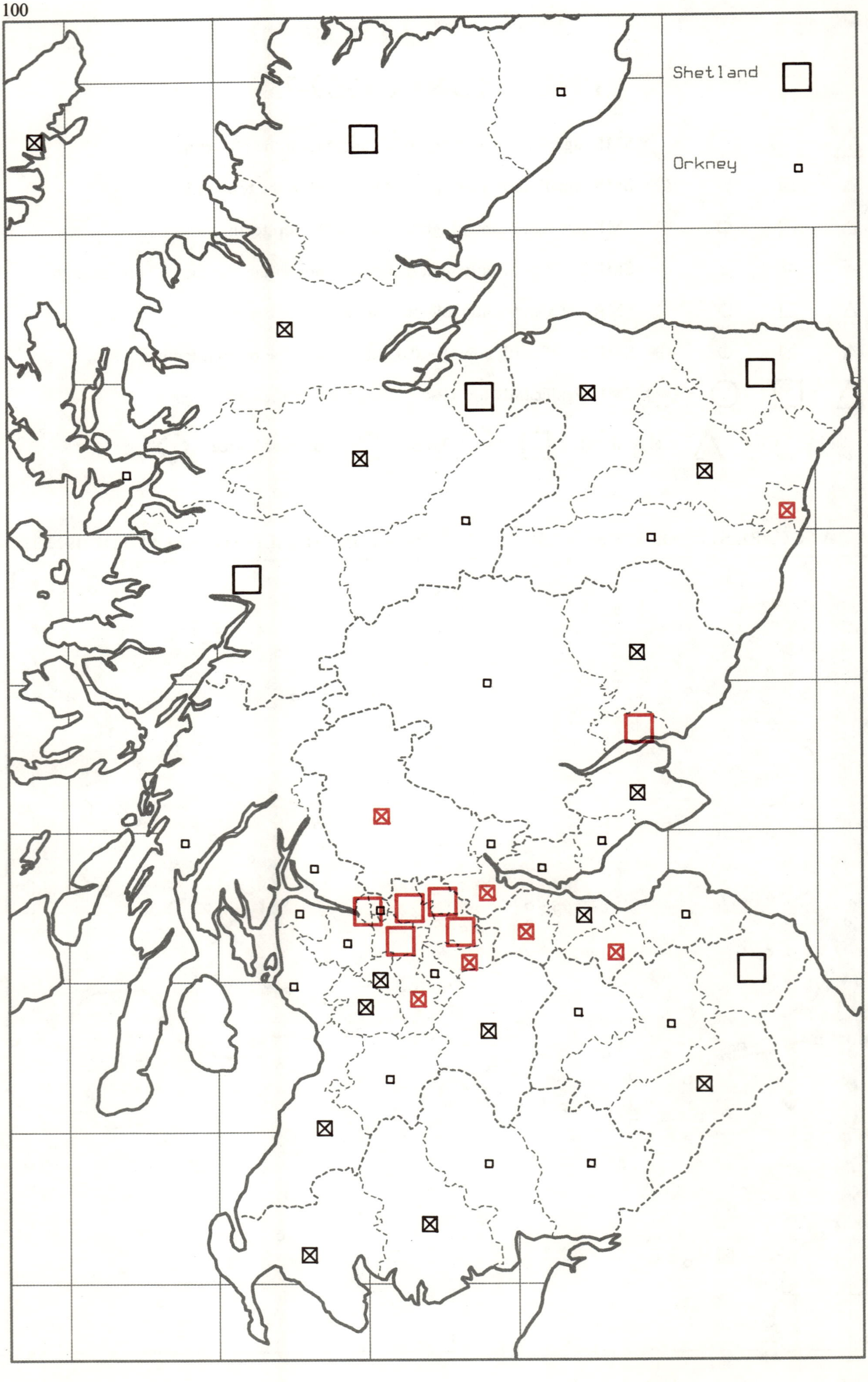
Shetland
Orkney

ACUTE RESPIRATORY INFECTION: INFLUENZA AND PNEUMONIA

Over 90 percent of acute respiratory infections are caused or initiated by viruses; bacteria are usually secondary invaders [87]. In Scotland, as elsewhere in the United Kingdom, epidemic respiratory infection is dominated by two viruses - influenza and respiratory syncytial virus - although other viruses (eg rhinovirus, para-influenza virus and adenovirus) play a considerable role in producing respiratory problems for the community.

Influenza is a disease of great antiquity. An epidemic with influenza like symptoms was described in 412 BC by Hippocrates, and the earliest description of the disease in the United Kingdom appeared in the Chronicle of Melrose in 1173. In Scotland, increased prevalence of infection happens nearly every year. At much longer intervals, spectacular epidemics occur due to a major change ('antigenic shift') in the structure of the influenza virus. Perhaps the most devastating of these epidemics was at the end of the First World War, when over twenty million people were estimated to have died of influenza [88].

Three influenza viruses have so far been identified - types A, B and C - and they have different epidemiological characteristics. Outbreaks due to type A are usually annual events; those caused by type B are at intervals of one to five years; those due to type C are sporadic, producing only minor respiratory illness. More than one virus type can appear in the same year, as in 1982, 1984 and 1985. Outbreaks characteristically make most impact during the winter months, with illness extending into the spring. When caused by a single virus type, the epidemic normally lasts about two months. Elevations in the numbers of deaths from pneumonia usually coincide with increasing laboratory evidence of influenza type A and with deaths diagnosed as due to influenza.

Respiratory syncytial virus classically causes bronchiolitis in young children, but it is increasingly being recognized as causing respiratory problems in the elderly. Sharp outbreaks of this infection occur almost annually in Scotland, starting in December and lasting for about two months. Children from the poorer urban areas are chiefly affected.

Whatever the causal organism, respiratory infections are a major cause of morbidity and mortality throughout the world [89], despite the advent of antimicrobial therapy. In the United Kingdom, illness from respiratory infection accounts for about one third of absences from work and from school, and this proportion increases during those years when influenza appears in epidemic form [90]. Respiratory and allied disorders are responsible for about one quarter of general practitioners' consultations, and they result in about half of the patient-doctor contact with children [91].

Some years ago, it was shown that over 60 percent of infections in children under five years are respiratory [92]. As regards mortality, respiratory disease accounts for about seven percent of all deaths in the developed world [93], affecting particularly the very young and the elderly. As with other infections, respiratory infection is the resultant of the virulence of the germ responsible, the susceptibility of the host and the ability of the environment to facilitate the spread of infection. Factors involved in the spread of influenza principally include the appearance of a new strain of the virus, the number of susceptible individuals in the local population and the opportunity for contact with infected persons. In Scotland, a feature of the epidemiology of the disease in recent years has been the presence of communities which, despite their remoteness, have the opportunity to experience significant epidemics due to special circumstances of contact with the virus. Perhaps the most spectacular of these outbreaks occurred during the winter of 1969-70 when the population of Stornoway in the Isle of Lewis was exposed to the then novel variant of influenza A virus ('Hong Kong Flu') before anywhere else in north western Europe. Surveillance studies had shown that this new variant had spread across Asia from Hong Kong and into southern Europe during 1968 and early 1969, but there had been no evidence of spread into northern Europe. However, the presence of large shoals of herring in the Minch (the strait between the Western Isles, the mainland and Skye) attracted numerous fishing boats from many European countries, including San Sebastian in Spain where influenza due to this virus was prevalent. Vessels from San Sebastian with sick fishermen aboard came to Stornoway just before the influenza epidemic broke out in the local population. Hence the source of the subsequent outbreak affecting 27 percent of persons surveyed in Stornoway [94] was probably infected fishermen on the Spanish boats. Not surprisingly, outbreaks were later reported from Peterhead, Fraserburgh and Aberdeen, as many of the boats in Stornoway at the time of the illness had come from the north-east of Scotland. Further, the large number of Norwegian boats fishing at that time off Stornoway probably accounted for the epidemic reported soon after in Norway [95]. Thus, the fishing

Continued on page 107

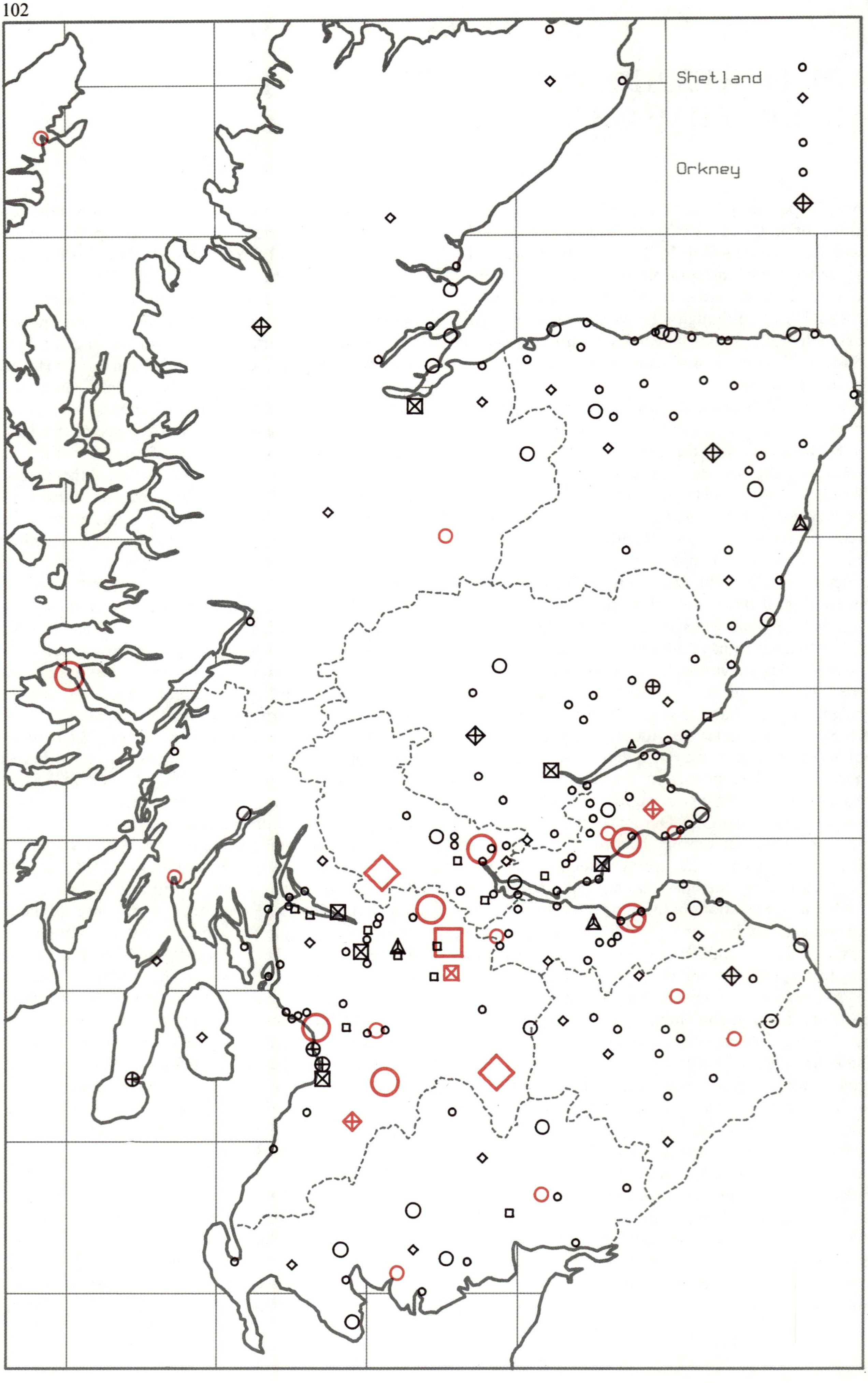
Shetland
Orkney

OTHER RESPIRATORY DISEASE 1959-63

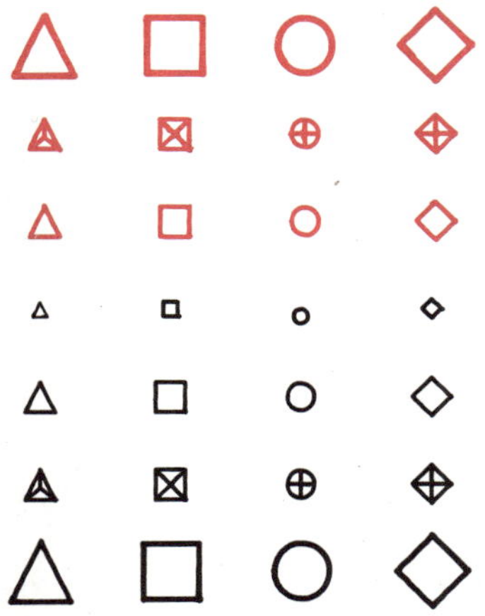

SMR significantly high ($p<0.05$) and within the top tenth

SMR significantly high ($p<0.05$) not within the top tenth

SMR not significantly high but within the top tenth

SMR not significantly high or low and not within the top or bottom tenth

SMR not significantly low but within the bottom tenth

SMR significantly low ($P<0.05$) not within the bottom tenth

SMR significantly low ($P<0.05$) and within the bottom tenth

City △ Large Burgh □ Small Burgh ○ Landward Area ◇

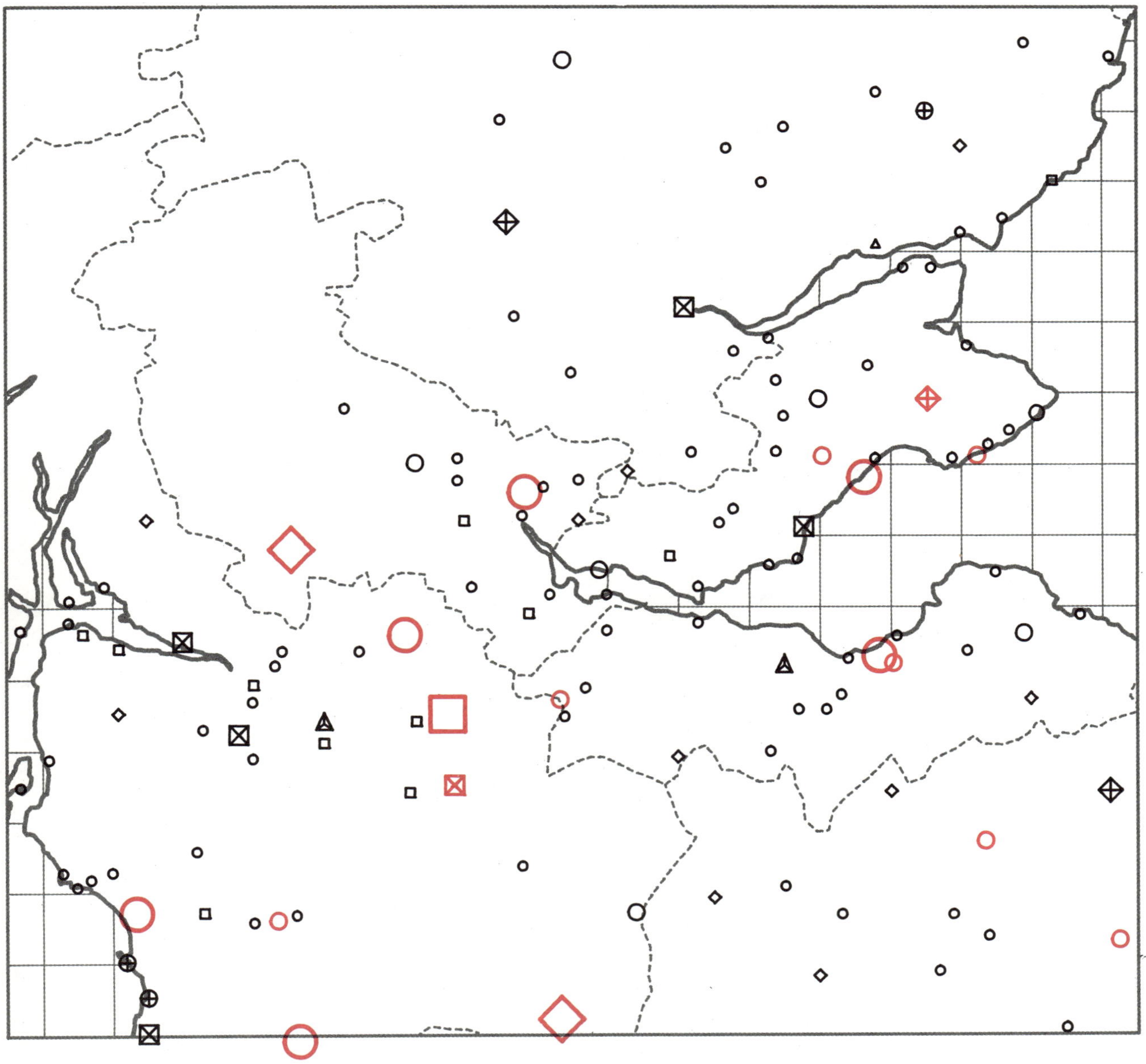

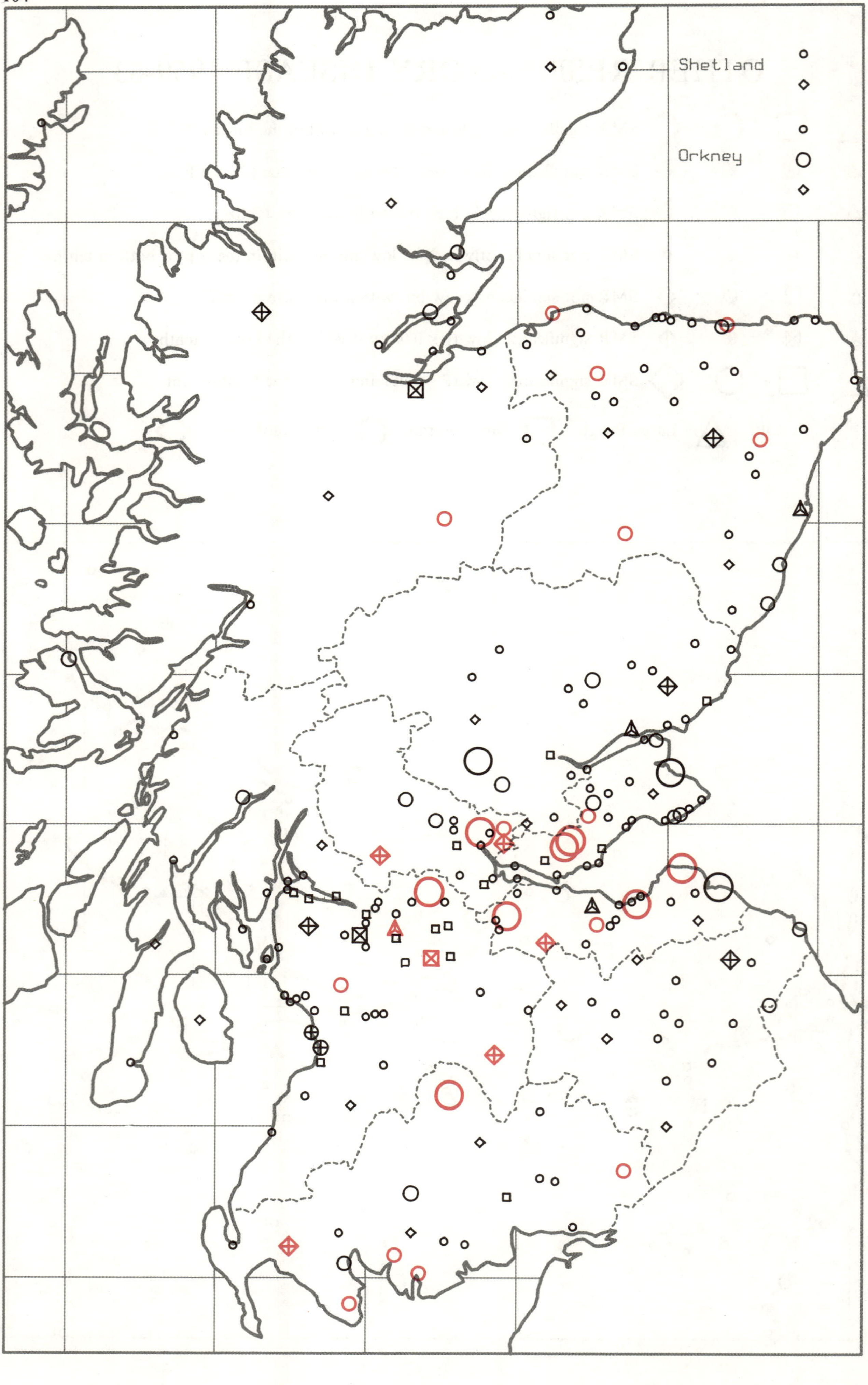
Shetland
Orkney

OTHER RESPIRATORY DISEASE 1969-73

SMR significantly high ($p < 0.05$) and within the top tenth

SMR significantly high ($p < 0.05$) not within the top tenth

SMR not significantly high but within the top tenth

SMR not significantly high or low and not within the top or bottom tenth

SMR not significantly low but within the bottom tenth

SMR significantly low ($P < 0.05$) not within the bottom tenth

SMR significantly low ($P < 0.05$) and within the bottom tenth

City △ Large Burgh □ Small Burgh ○ Landward Area ◇

A SQUARE SYMBOL IS USED FOR THE DISTRICTS ON THE MAP OVERLEAF FOR 1979-83.

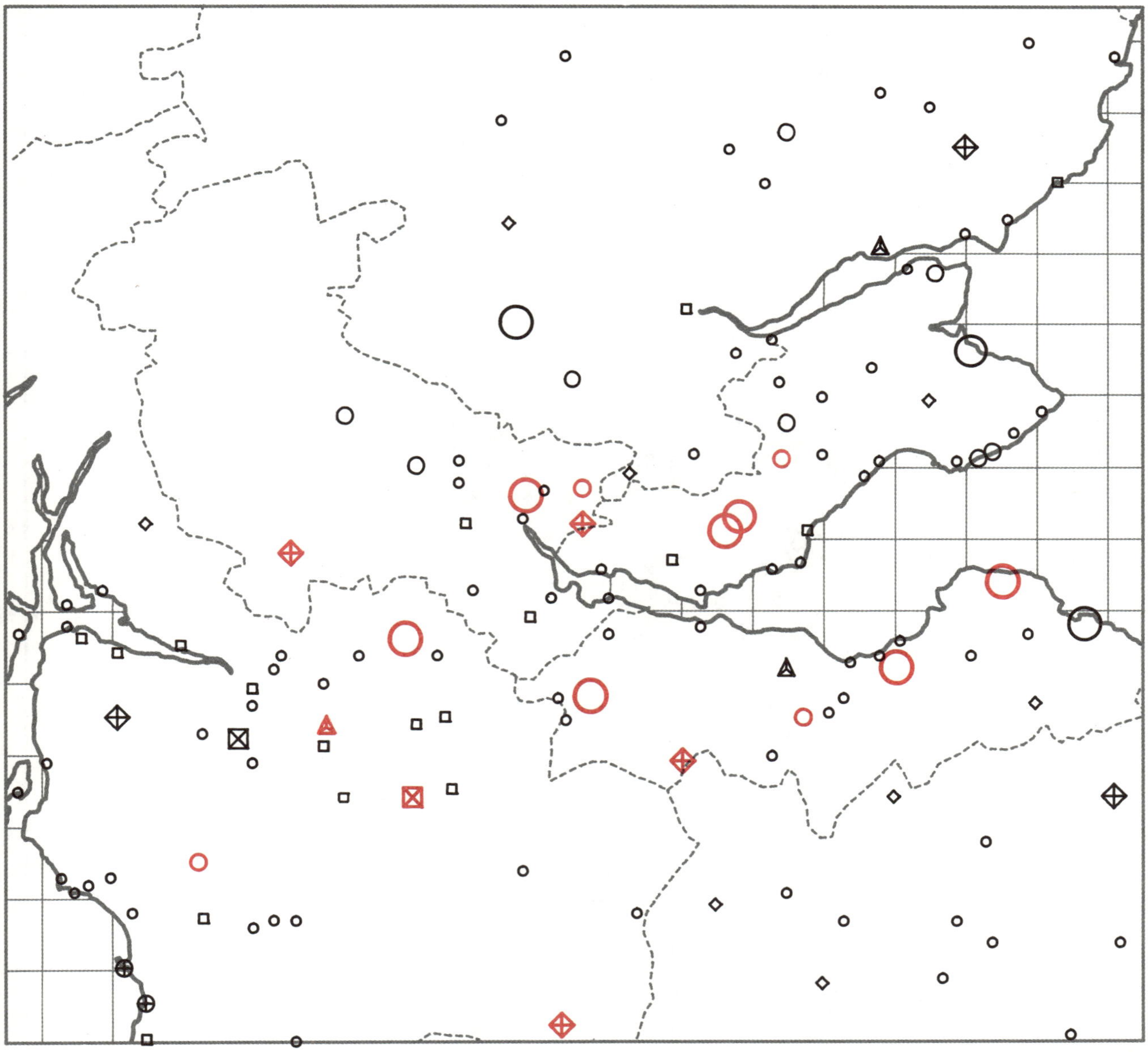

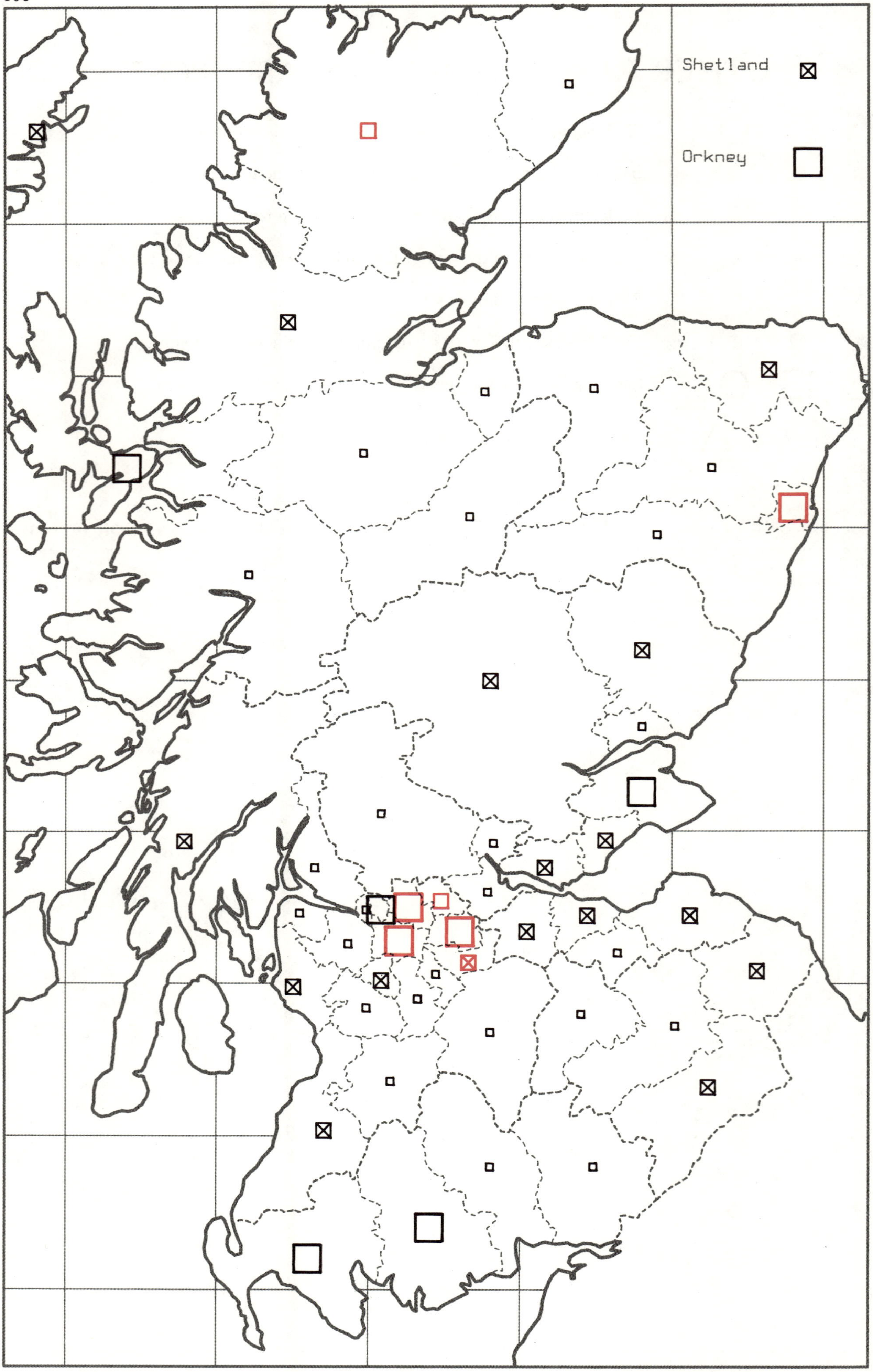
Shetland
Orkney

boat proved not only the likely importer of infection but also the distributor and exporter. Since then, early outbreaks of influenza have been in the ports of Gairloch, Lerwick and Eyemouth, providing possible further evidence that the crowded quarters of a fishing vessel can be a suitable 'medium' in which viruses can propagate as effectively as in the densely-populated urban areas.

Surveillance of influenzal activity in Scotland involves the recording of various complementary indices, such as information from 'spotter' general practitioners, consultation rates for influenza-like illnesses, school absenteeism, sickness benefit claims (now ceased) and evidence of influenza obtained from virus laboratories. In addition to morbidity, mortality increases substantially in a year when influenza is prevalent, and this is the case whether the index used is 'influenza mortality', 'pneumonia mortality' or even 'total mortality'. Influenza exerts its most lethal effect on the elderly, and outbreaks associated with high mortality rates in geriatric and eventide homes are relatively common.

Although influenza virus may gain entry to Scotland whenever there is movement of population, the main impact, so far as mortality is concerned, is in areas where persons (especially the elderly) with pre- existing respiratory disease are concentrated. Of particular importance are those with chronic bronchitis who subsequently may develop influenzal pneumonia. Because of the number of persons compromised by bronchitis who live in the industrialized areas of Scotland, the SMR for pneumonia is higher in parts of Strathclyde (Glasgow City, Strathkelvin, Monklands, Cumbernauld and Kilsyth) and Dundee City than elsewhere in the country. Significantly high ratios are also found in the Districts of Stirling, Falkirk, West Lothian, Midlothian, Motherwell, East Kilbride and Aberdeen City.

Mortality from respiratory infection may also be expressed by recording clinical entities other than pneumonia (eg exacerbations of chronic bronchitis, pulmonary oedema and lung abscess), as the maps of Other Respiratory Diseases show. As with mortality ascribed to pneumonia, those most affected live in Strathclyde (Glasgow City, Monklands and Strathkelvin, with Motherwell also significantly high).

Scotland is very much a patchwork quilt so far as risk factors for respiratory infections are involved. As well as the many open spaces where overcrowding does not need to be taken into consideration, there are still areas where the populations are concentrated - often for social, economic and historical reasons; and, being already affected by pre-existing respiratory damage, the impact of respiratory viruses can be severe. An understanding of the relevant environmental and geographical factors is important so that successful preventive measures can be undertaken.

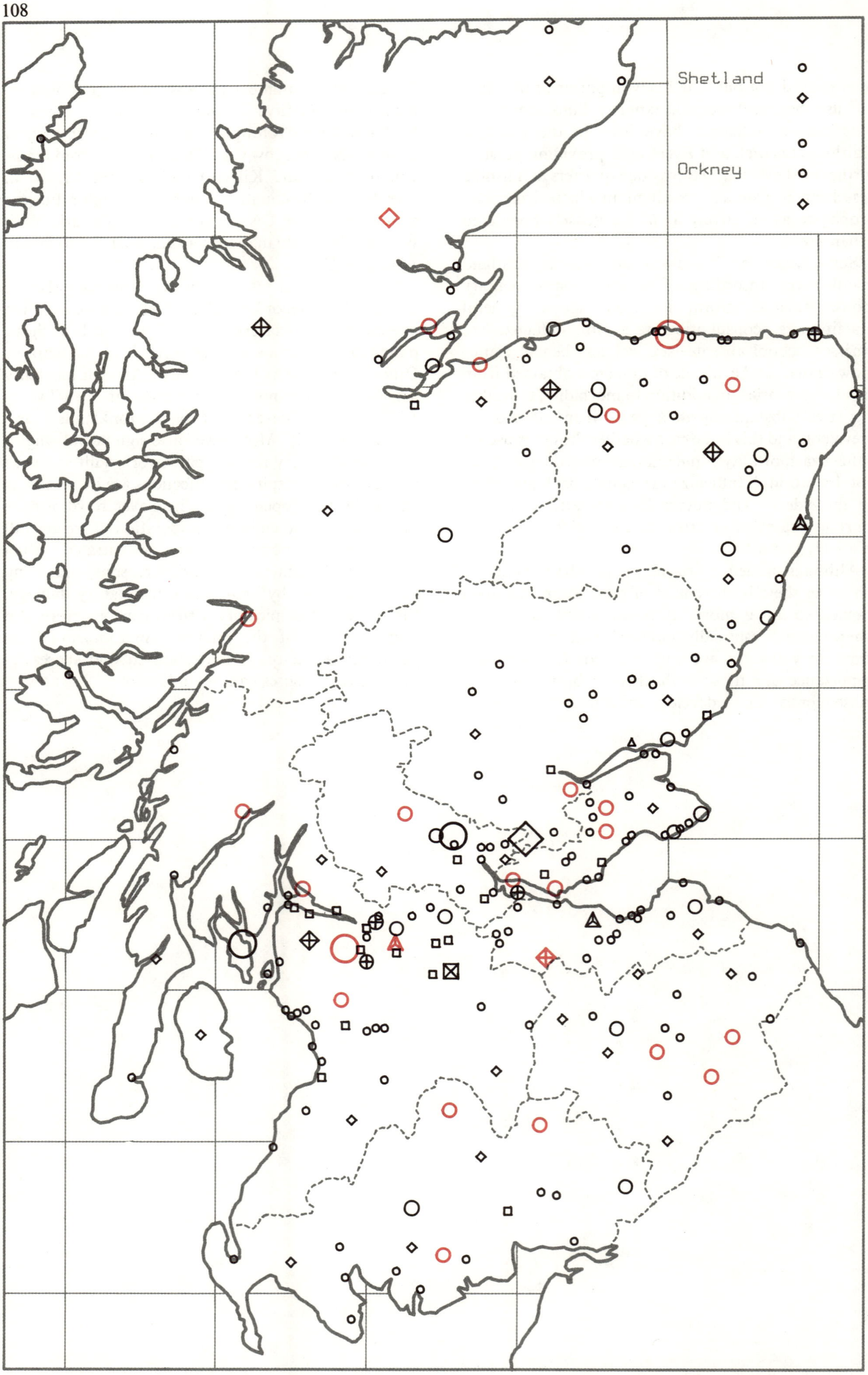
Shetland
Orkney

STILLBIRTHS 1959-63

SMR significantly high ($p < 0.05$) and within the top tenth

SMR significantly high ($p < 0.05$) not within the top tenth

SMR not significantly high but within the top tenth

SMR not significantly high or low and not within the top or bottom tenth

SMR not significantly low but within the bottom tenth

SMR significantly low ($P < 0.05$) not within the bottom tenth

SMR significantly low ($P < 0.05$) and within the bottom tenth

City △ Large Burgh □ Small Burgh ○ Landward Area ◇

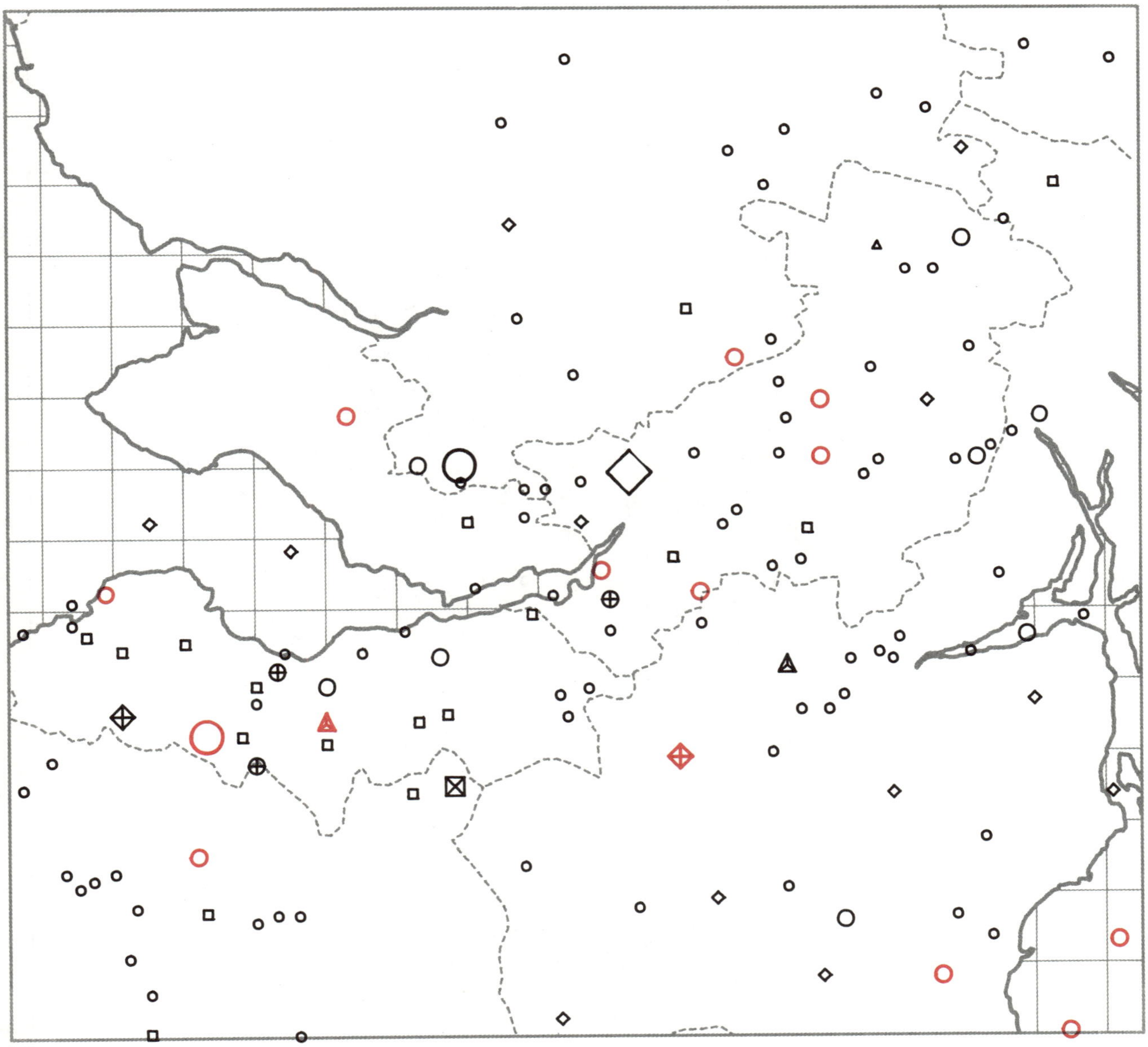

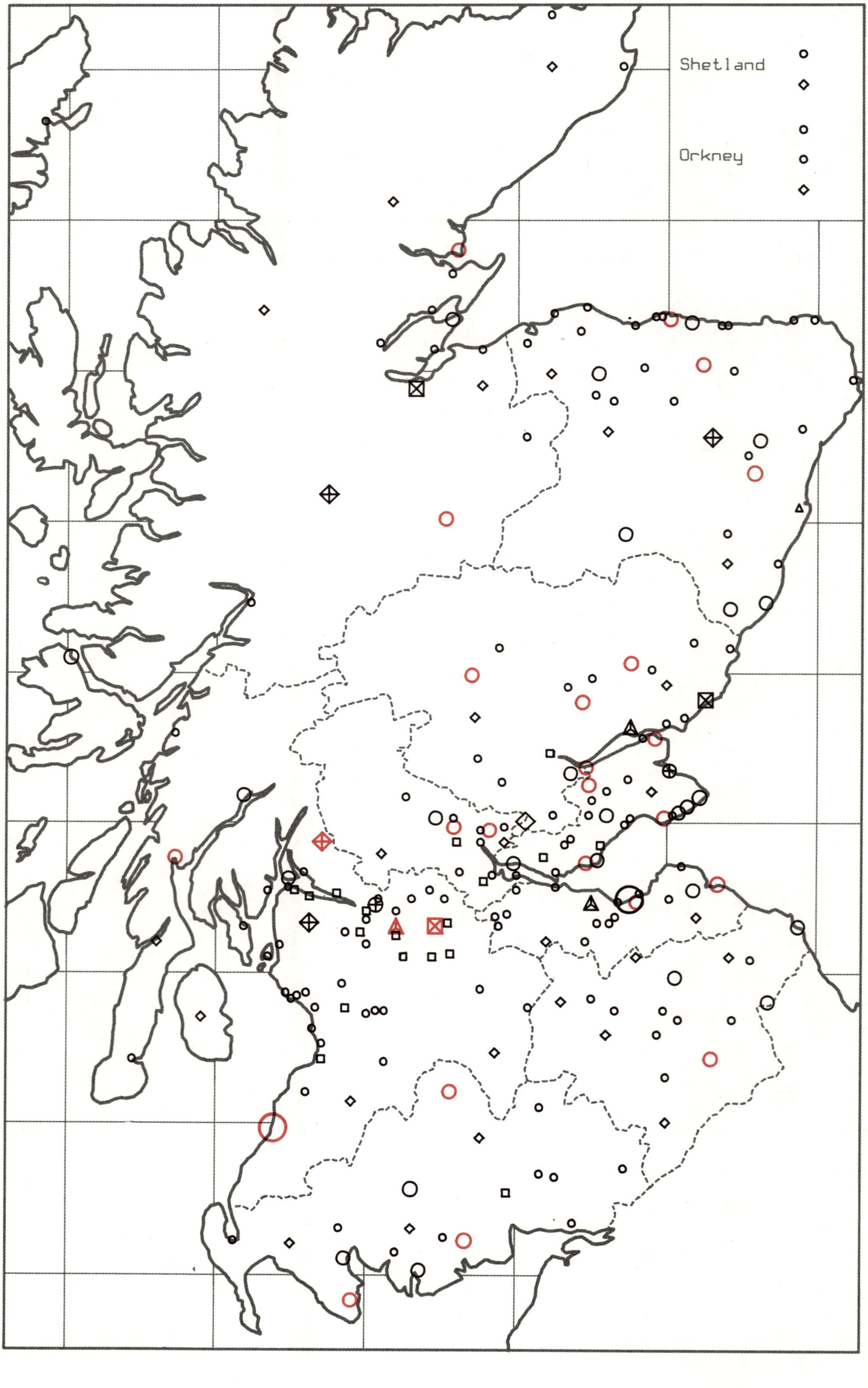
Shetland
Orkney

STILLBIRTHS 1969-73

- SMR significantly high ($p < 0.05$) and within the top tenth
- SMR significantly high ($p < 0.05$) not within the top tenth
- SMR not significantly high but within the top tenth
- SMR not significantly high or low and not within the top or bottom tenth
- SMR not significantly low but within the bottom tenth
- SMR significantly low ($P < 0.05$) not within the bottom tenth
- SMR significantly low ($P < 0.05$) and within the bottom tenth

City △ Large Burgh □ Small Burgh ○ Landward Area ◇

A SQUARE SYMBOL IS USED FOR THE DISTRICTS ON THE MAP OVERLEAF FOR 1979-83.

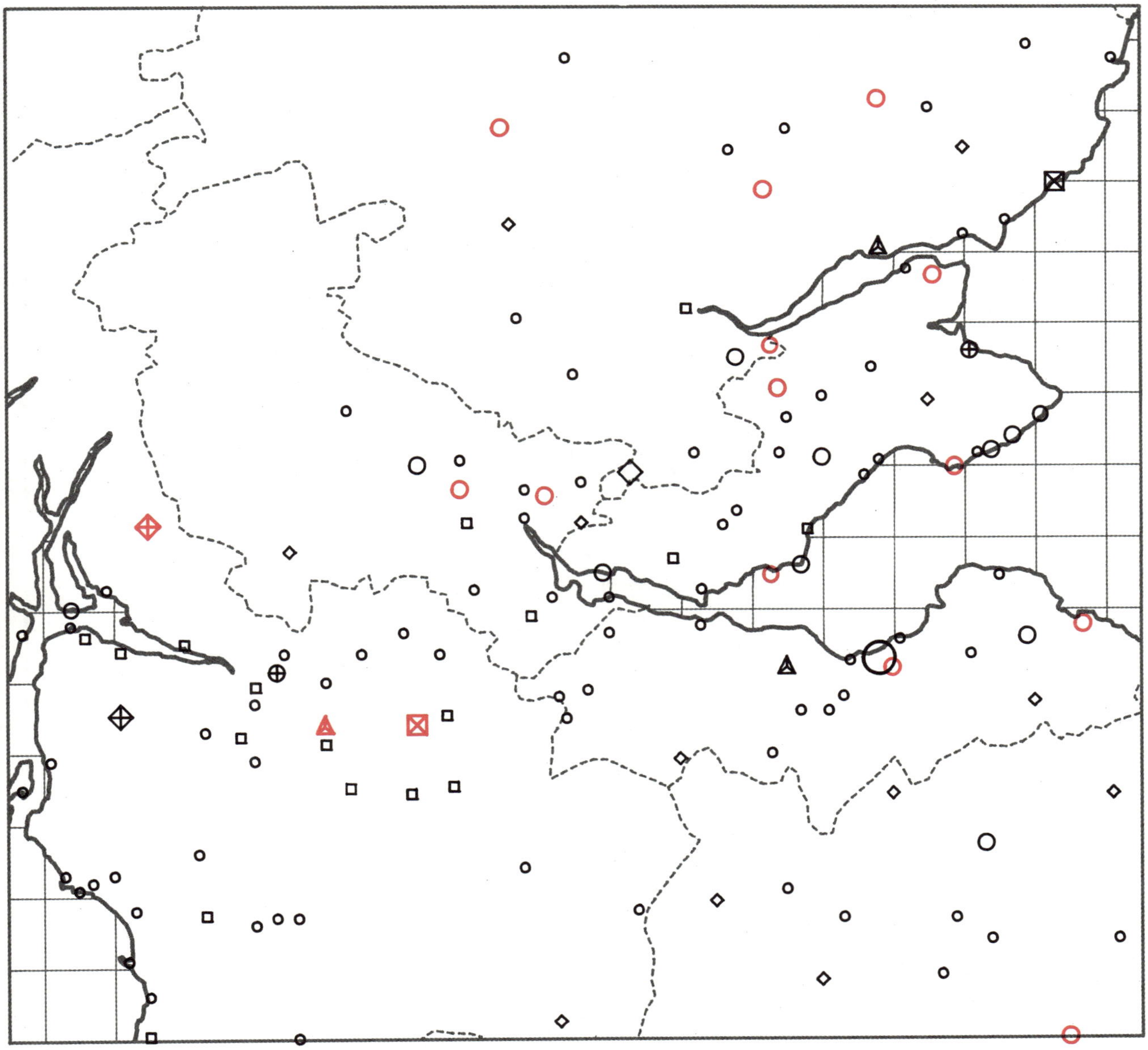

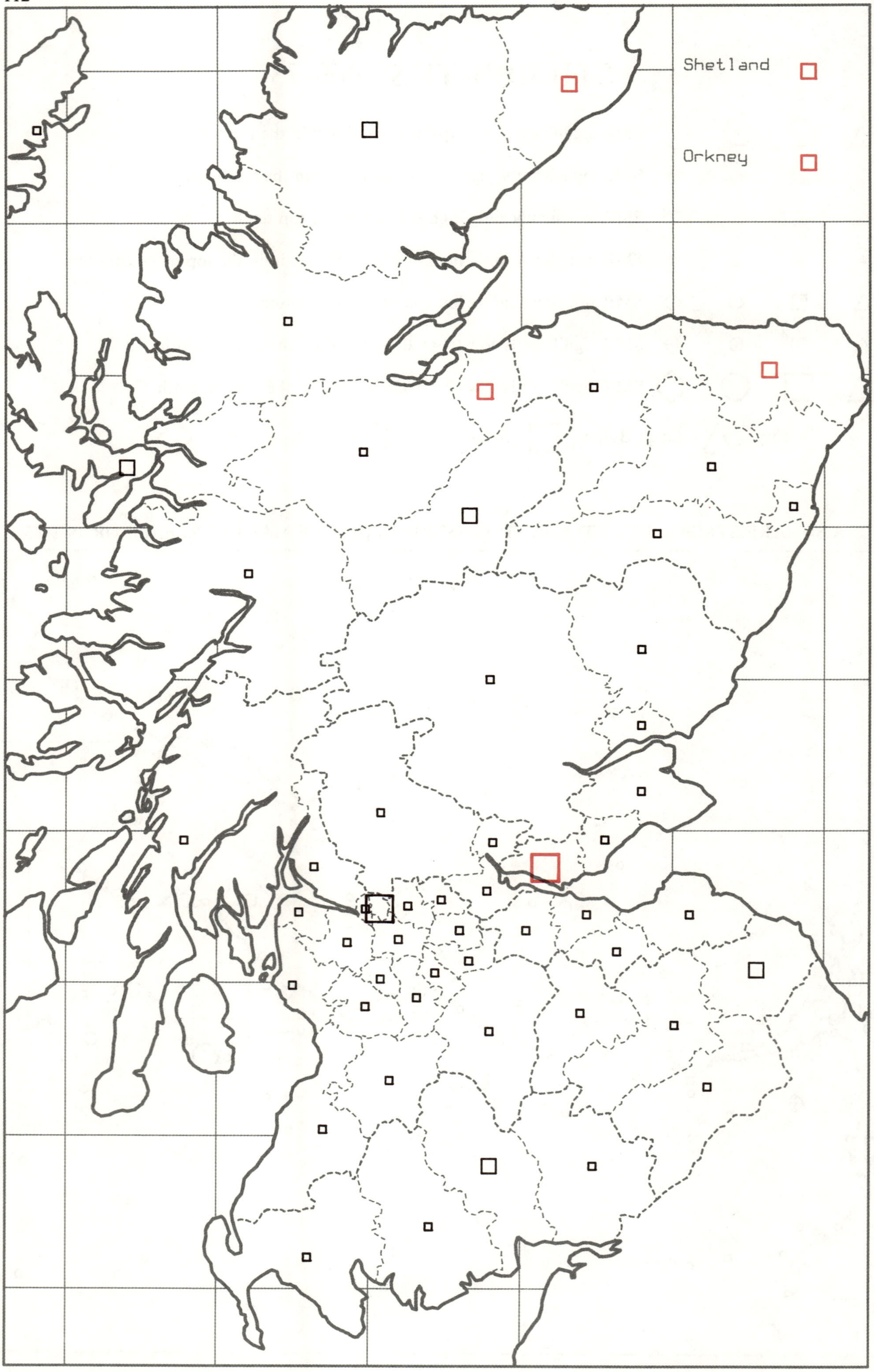
Shetland
Orkney

MORTALITY AT EARLY AGES

Awareness of the excessive vulnerability of children dates back as far as the mid 1660s [96], but regular recording and study of perinatal death nationally began only after the turn of this century. Obstetricians and paediatricians have been, to a large extent, the pioneers of medical self-audit because they have had relatively easy access to mortality data conveniently divisible into the antepartum, interpartum and neonatal periods. There has been a gratifying fall in all of these mortality rates in the 'developed' parts of the world in the last half century, and similar trends are now being seen in third world countries.

The improvement in perinatal mortality has been most manifest in the last 25 years, due no doubt to a combination of factors including improved health of the mother, coincident with a better socio-economic environment, advances in obstetric skill and more recently a revolution in technology which has provided full intensive care and life support measures for the newborn baby. Hence, there is now a 'swings and roundabouts' situation with respect to stillbirths and first week deaths. As the stillbirth rate falls there may well be an increase in first week death rates so that as a measure of progress these must be taken into account together. While this has served adequately until the present time, it is now becoming clear that, with modern therapy, the newborn is being supported well past the first week of life; so it becomes necessary to include deaths up to the end of the first month if a true measure of obstetric and paediatric success is to be obtained. Indeed, it is probably not until the child is at school and into the second decade that the outcome of pregnancy and the perinatal period can be said with confidence to be successfully 'normal'.

Infant mortality has also shown a steady downward trend since the turn of the century and especially since the 1940s, and this no doubt has been associated with improved socio-economic conditions in combination with improved surveillance and care during infancy and the availability of antimicrobials. Death from preventable illness in the UK today is now relatively unusual, and almost half of the post perinatal deaths are due to the enigmatic Sudden Infant Death Syndrome (Cot Death).

Improvement in mortality rates is becoming much harder to achieve since deaths are now due either to extreme immaturity (at times with the long-term complications of pulmonary and central nervous system pathology), to severe congenital defect, and to unexpected (and often unexplained) fetal asphyxia during late pregnancy or delivery. The first of these conditions requires further efforts to determine the causes and prevention of preterm labour, the second requires attention to factors operating in early pregnancy and even preconception, and the third requires an entirely new and as yet undiscovered method of predicting which fetus is vulnerable. The cause of death is often multifactorial, and it is hard to identify the factor or factors which play the most significant role.

As mortality rates have fallen they have lost some of their value as measures of the successful provision of medical and social services, and attempts are now being made to assess the latter by studying morbidity rates. Nevertheless there is much which can still be learned from mortality data, and the mapping technique reveals the changes that occur as time passes. It tells us where the need is greatest and where to concentrate the limited resources which are available. Mapping, even down to the level of the Small Burgh, is however only a beginning since, even within small communities, mortality and morbidity vary from district to district. A study recently published describing infant mortality and morbidity in the Tayside area of Scotland [97] revealed noticeable differences in the structure of the population from town to town with, as might be expected, differences in mortality rates. Even within a single city such as Dundee, mapping of the addresses of infants attending hospital Accident and Emergency Departments or suffering from Sudden Infant Death Syndrome reveals striking clustering and identifies areas requiring the most medical and social support.

Study of the accompanying mapping confirms the findings of what was reputedly the first mapping of this nature [1], namely that it is not always the densely populated urban areas that have the highest mortality rates. Some rural areas may go through 'bad patches' and some cities do relatively well, thus indicating that mortality rates are not 'static statistics'. Likewise, while infant (birth to one year) mortality rates are of general interest as indicators of trends, a breakdown into neonatal and post-neonatal rates, such as that illustrated by Heady and Heasman [98] as long ago as 1958, is required if managers are to be able to determine which aspects of child health care deserve priority. Mapping these rates separately illustrates more clearly the age group in which the need is greatest. Small Burghs which are closely related geographically have surprisingly different rates, a factor entirely missed by the provision of a general District rate only. Therefore if health authorities are going to be successful in meeting the needs of populations, regular reviews in considerable detail are (unfortunately) necessary. It is regretted, therefore, that the central authorities have seen fit, since District

Continued on page 117

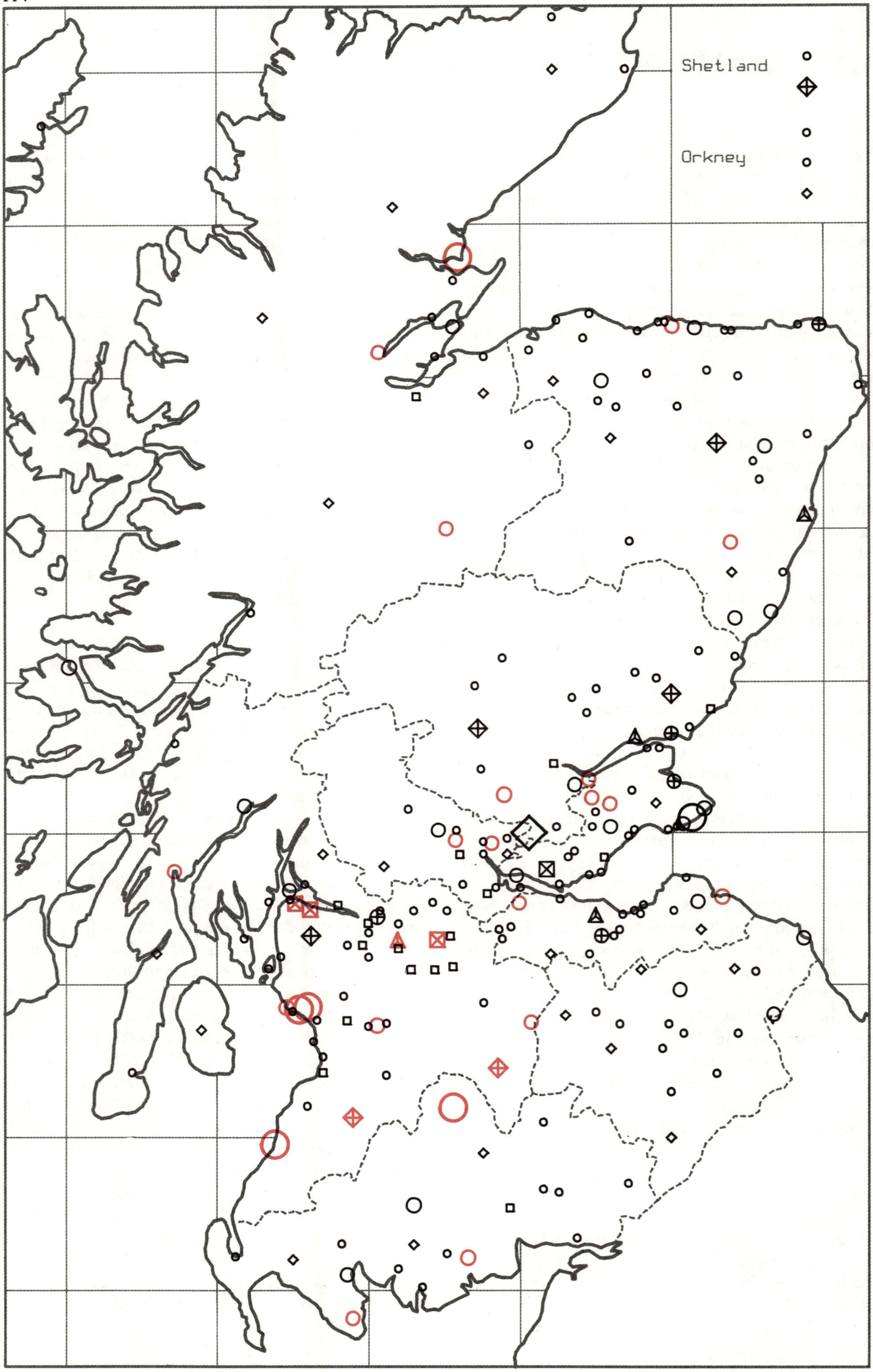
Shetland
Orkney

PERINATAL MORTALITY 1969-73

- SMR significantly high ($p < 0.05$) and within the top tenth
- SMR significantly high ($p < 0.05$) not within the top tenth
- SMR not significantly high but within the top tenth
- SMR not significantly high or low and not within the top or bottom tenth
- SMR not significantly low but within the bottom tenth
- SMR significantly low ($P < 0.05$) not within the bottom tenth
- SMR significantly low ($P < 0.05$) and within the bottom tenth

City △ Large Burgh □ Small Burgh ○ Landward Area ◇

A SQUARE SYMBOL IS USED FOR THE DISTRICTS ON THE MAP OVERLEAF FOR 1979-83.

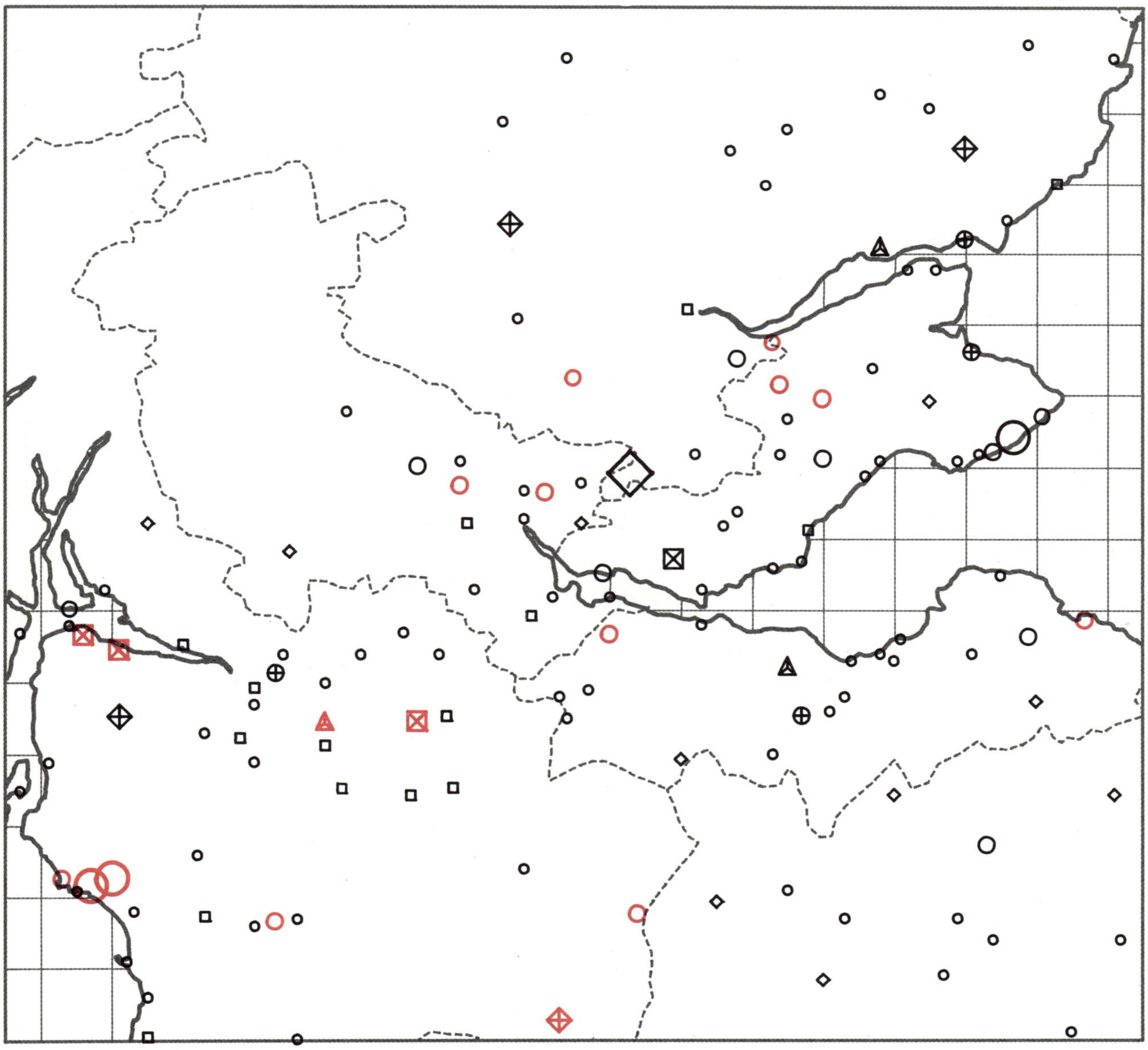

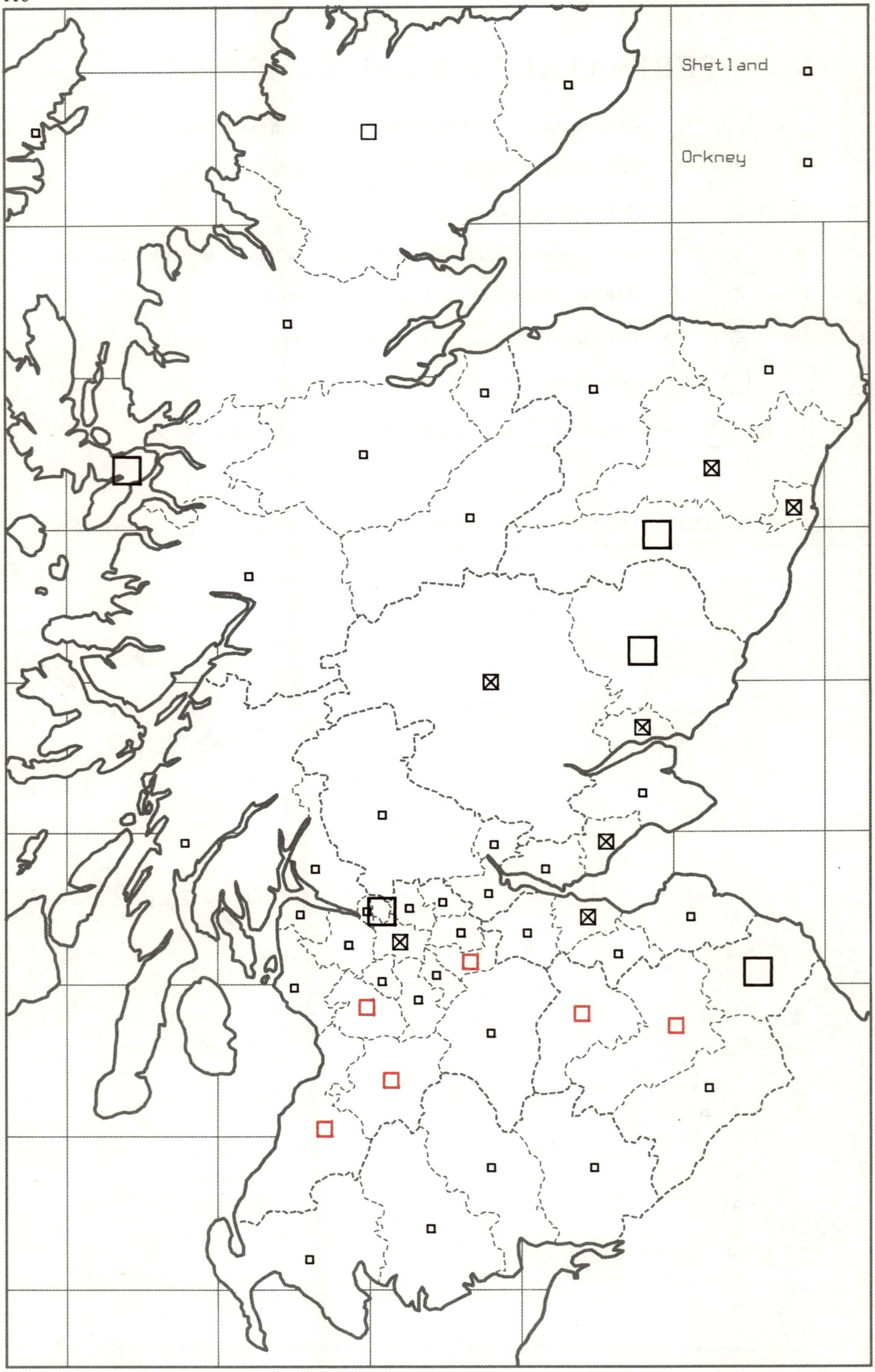
Shetland
Orkney

boundaries were changed in 1974, to limit the publication of mortality data to relatively large geographical areas. This makes detailed comparison with previous years difficult if not impossible and, while this flags broad areas in need of help, a great deal of additional work must be undertaken by epidemiologists if they are to identify successfully the local 'bad spots' needing investigation and additional medical and social assistance. It is hoped that the information available from the increased use of computers for data capture and analysis within the NHS will facilitate the routine preparation of the type of information illustrated here. The NHS National Child Health Computer System [99] is capable of providing this type of data routinely and was designed not only to improve provision of health surveillance and care but also to help managers and health authorities make the most appropriate use of resources.

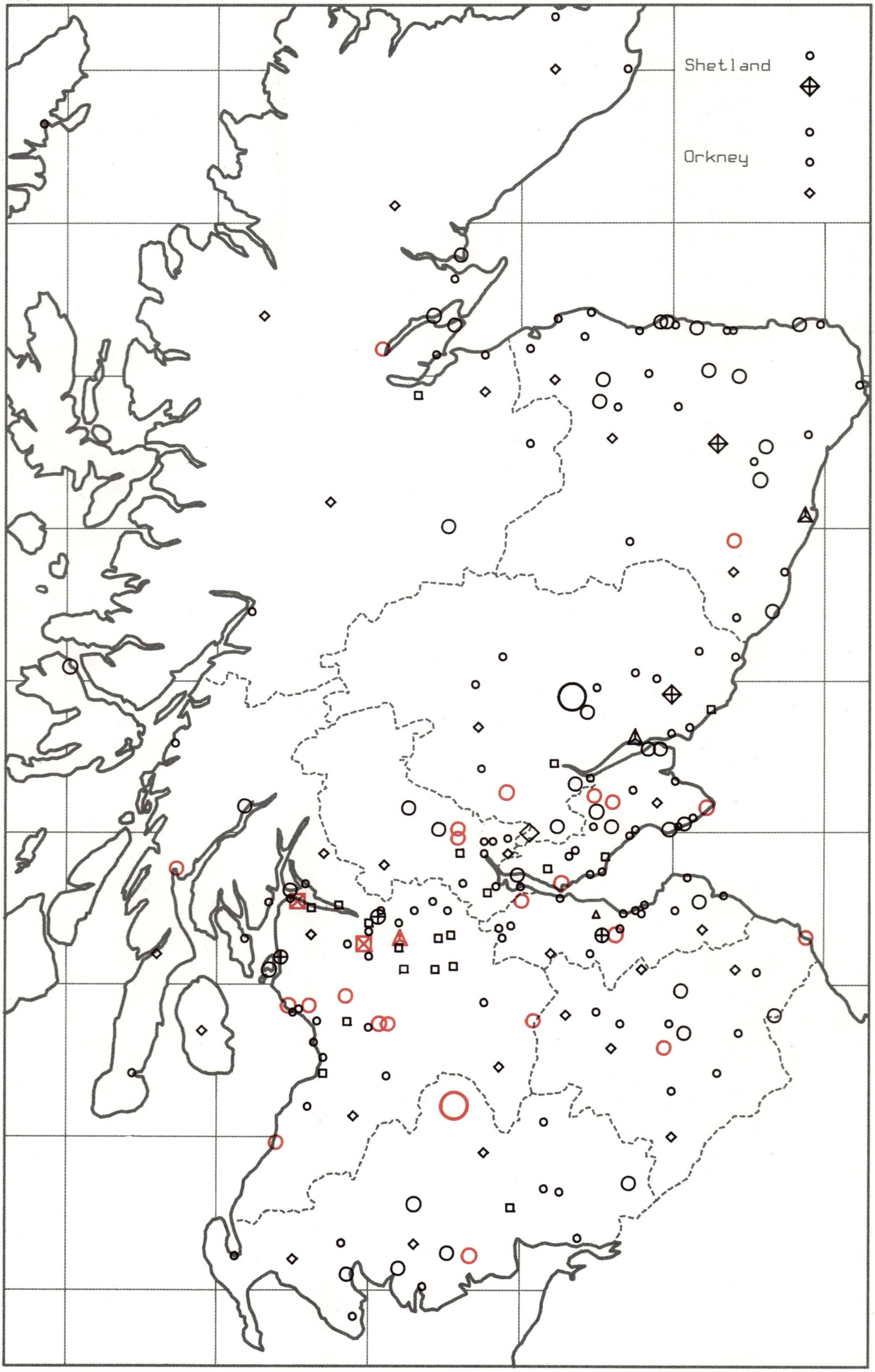
Shetland
Orkney

NEONATAL MORTALITY 1969-73

- SMR significantly high ($p < 0.05$) and within the top tenth
- SMR significantly high ($p < 0.05$) not within the top tenth
- SMR not significantly high but within the top tenth
- SMR not significantly high or low and not within the top or bottom tenth
- SMR not significantly low but within the bottom tenth
- SMR significantly low ($P < 0.05$) not within the bottom tenth
- SMR significantly low ($P < 0.05$) and within the bottom tenth

City △ Large Burgh □ Small Burgh ○ Landward Area ◇

A SQUARE SYMBOL IS USED FOR THE DISTRICTS ON THE MAP OVERLEAF FOR 1979-83.

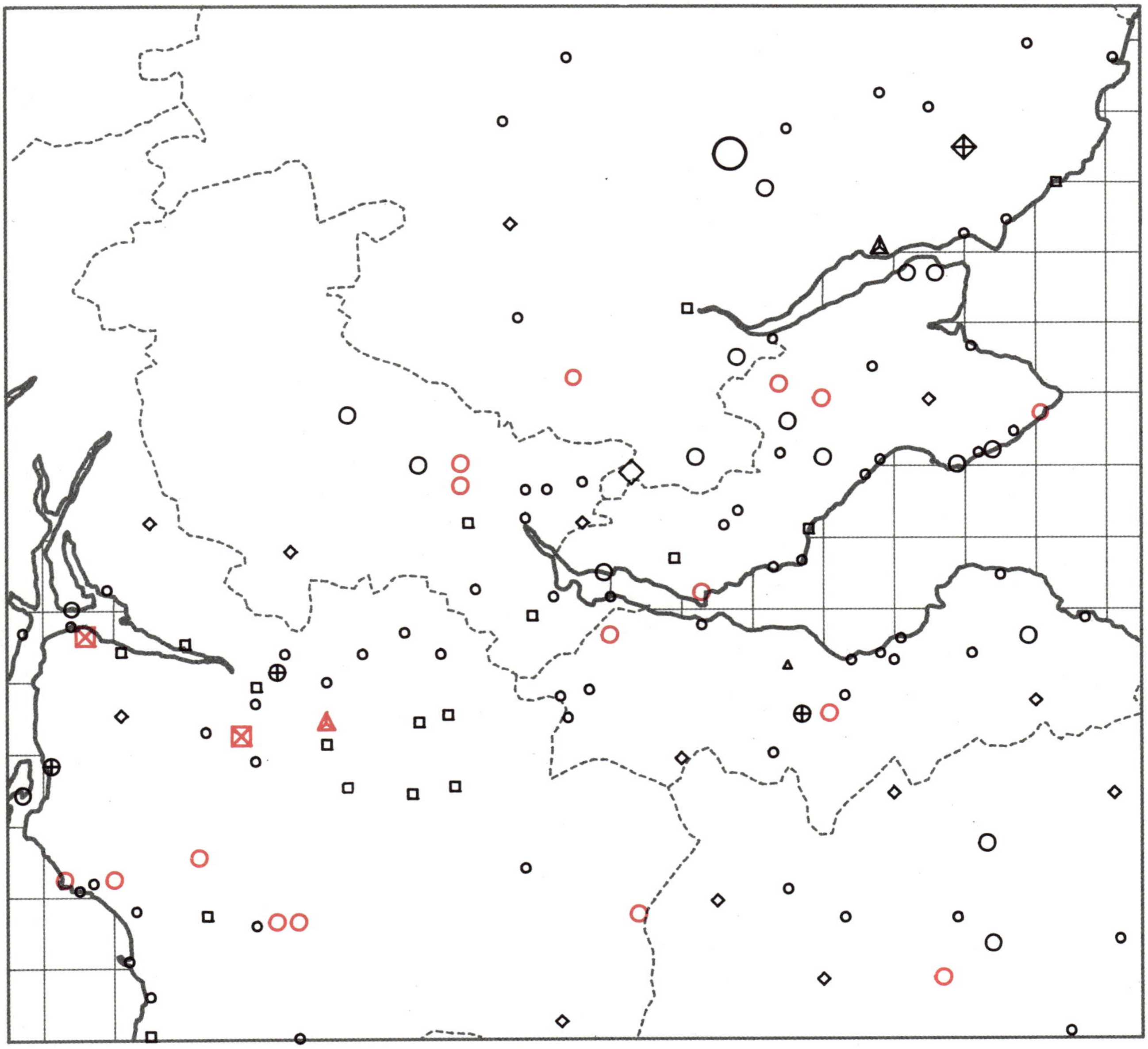

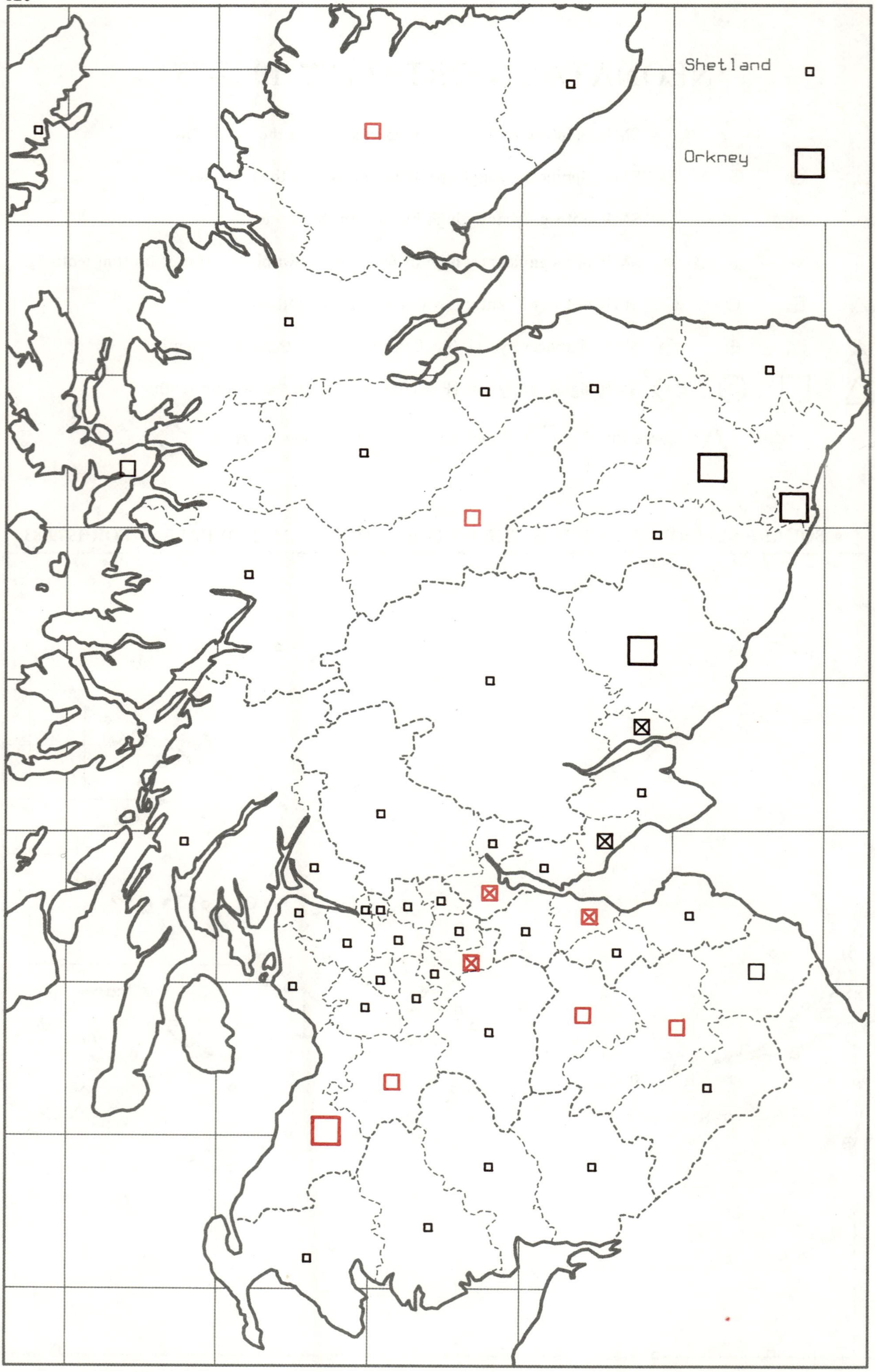

Shetland
Orkney

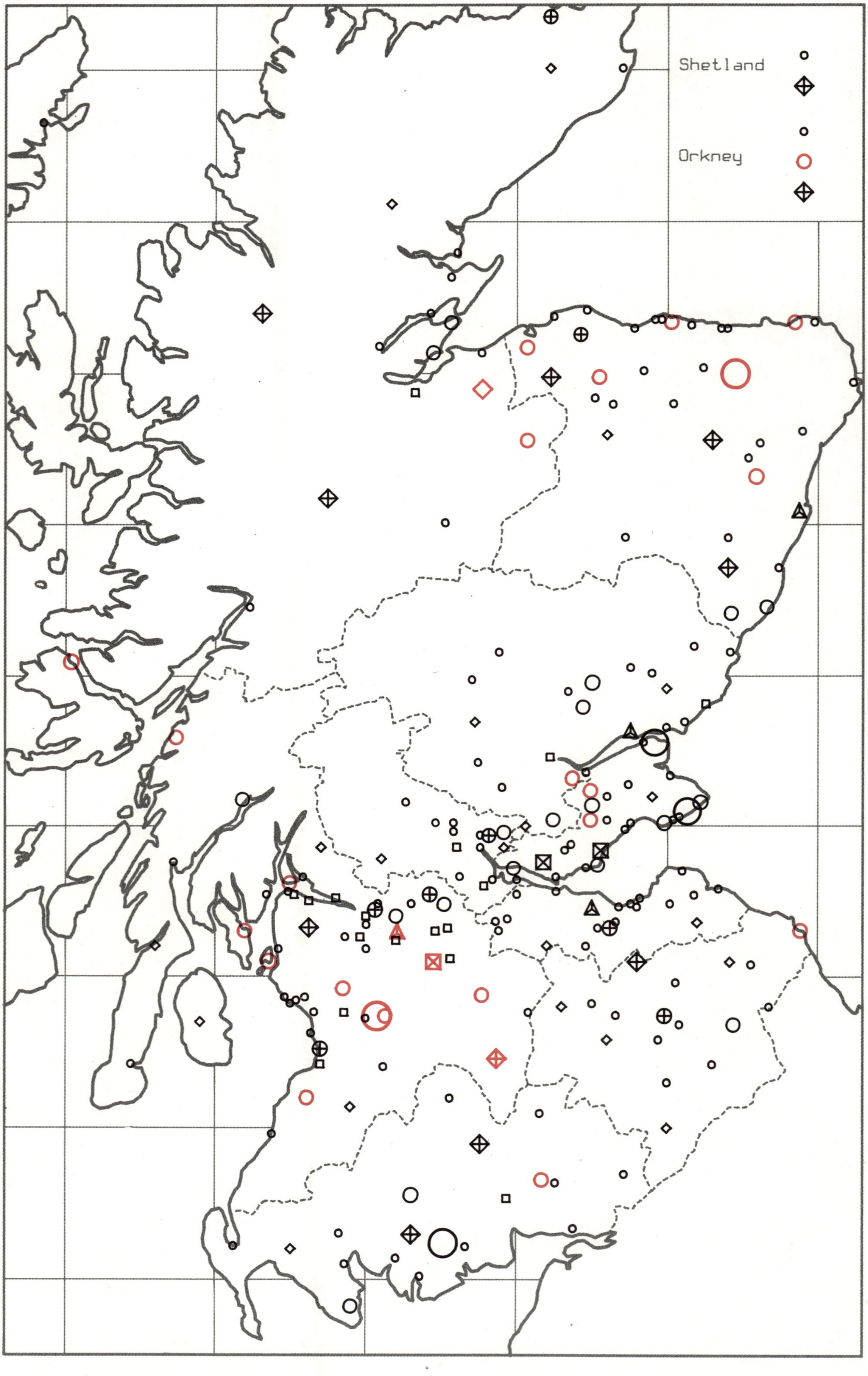
Shetland
Orkney

INFANT MORTALITY 1959-63

SMR significantly high ($p<0.05$) and within the top tenth

SMR significantly high ($p<0.05$) not within the top tenth

SMR not significantly high but within the top tenth

SMR not significantly high or low and not within the top or bottom tenth

SMR not significantly low but within the bottom tenth

SMR significantly low ($P<0.05$) not within the bottom tenth

SMR significantly low ($P<0.05$) and within the bottom tenth

City △ Large Burgh □ Small Burgh ○ Landward Area ◇

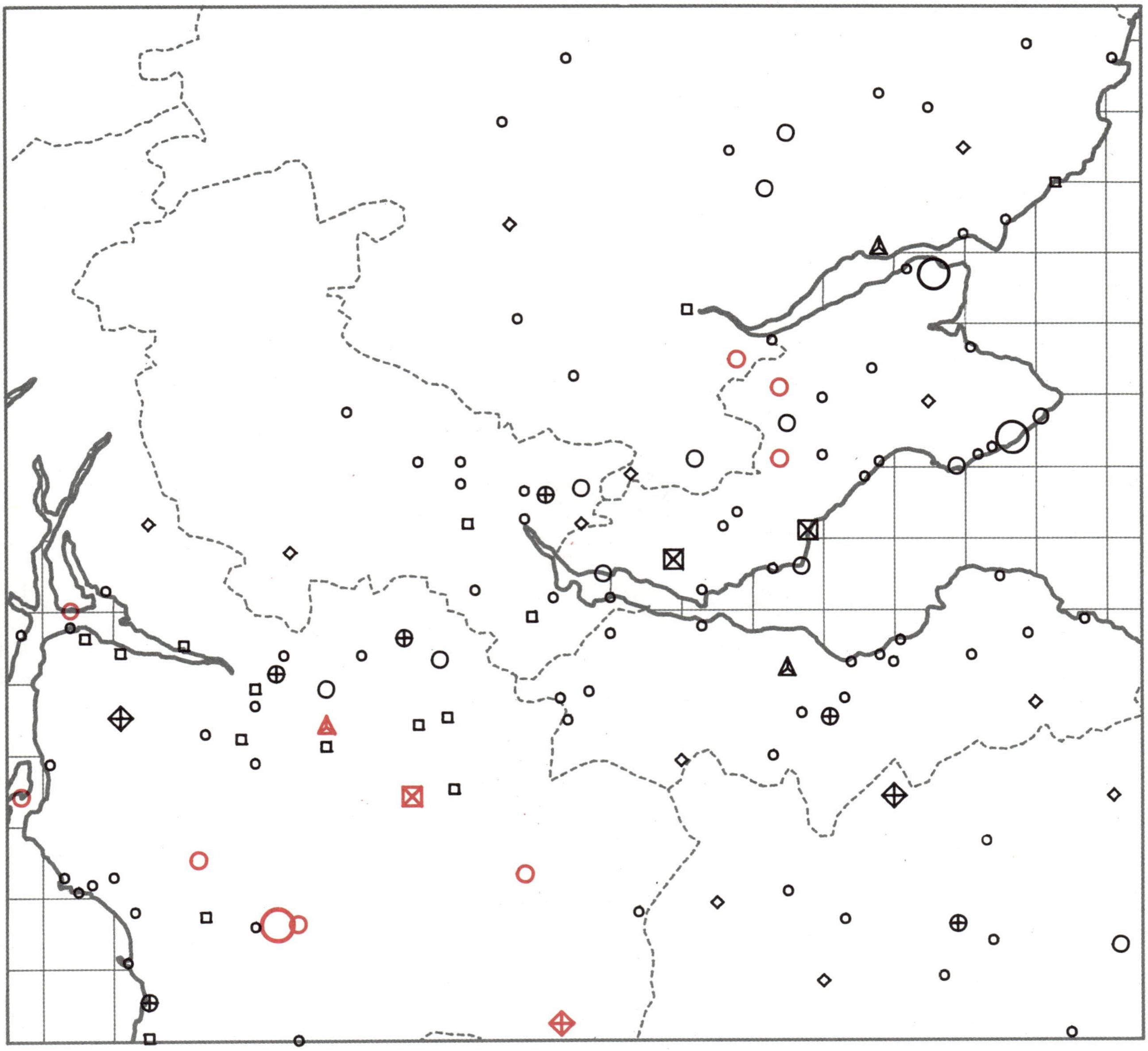

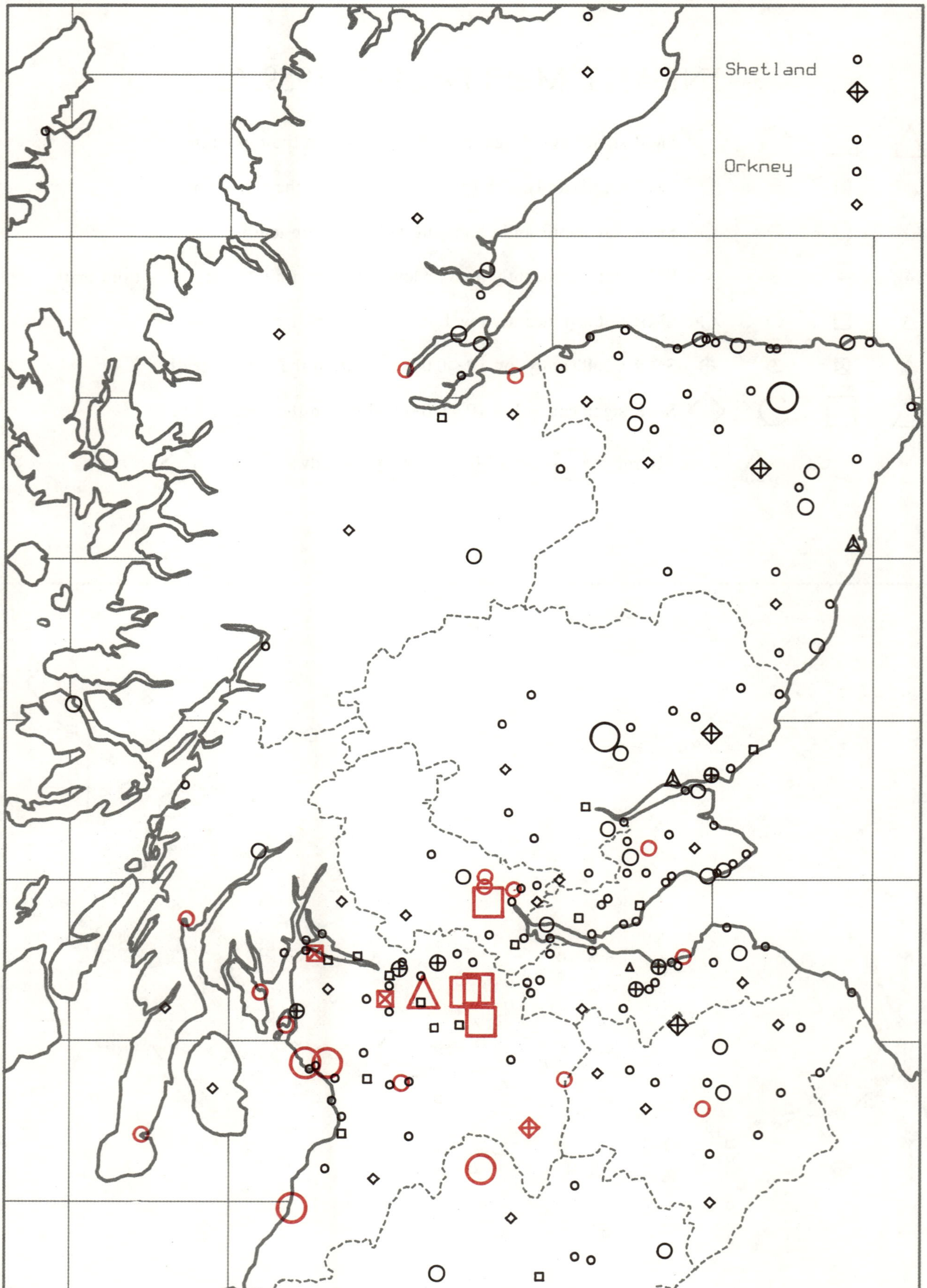
Shetland
Orkney

INFANT MORTALITY 1969-73

- SMR significantly high ($p<0.05$) and within the top tenth
- SMR significantly high ($p<0.05$) not within the top tenth
- SMR not significantly high but within the top tenth
- SMR not significantly high or low and not within the top or bottom tenth
- SMR not significantly low but within the bottom tenth
- SMR significantly low ($P<0.05$) not within the bottom tenth
- SMR significantly low ($P<0.05$) and within the bottom tenth

City Large Burgh Small Burgh Landward Area

A SQUARE SYMBOL IS USED FOR THE DISTRICTS ON THE MAP OVERLEAF FOR 1979-83.

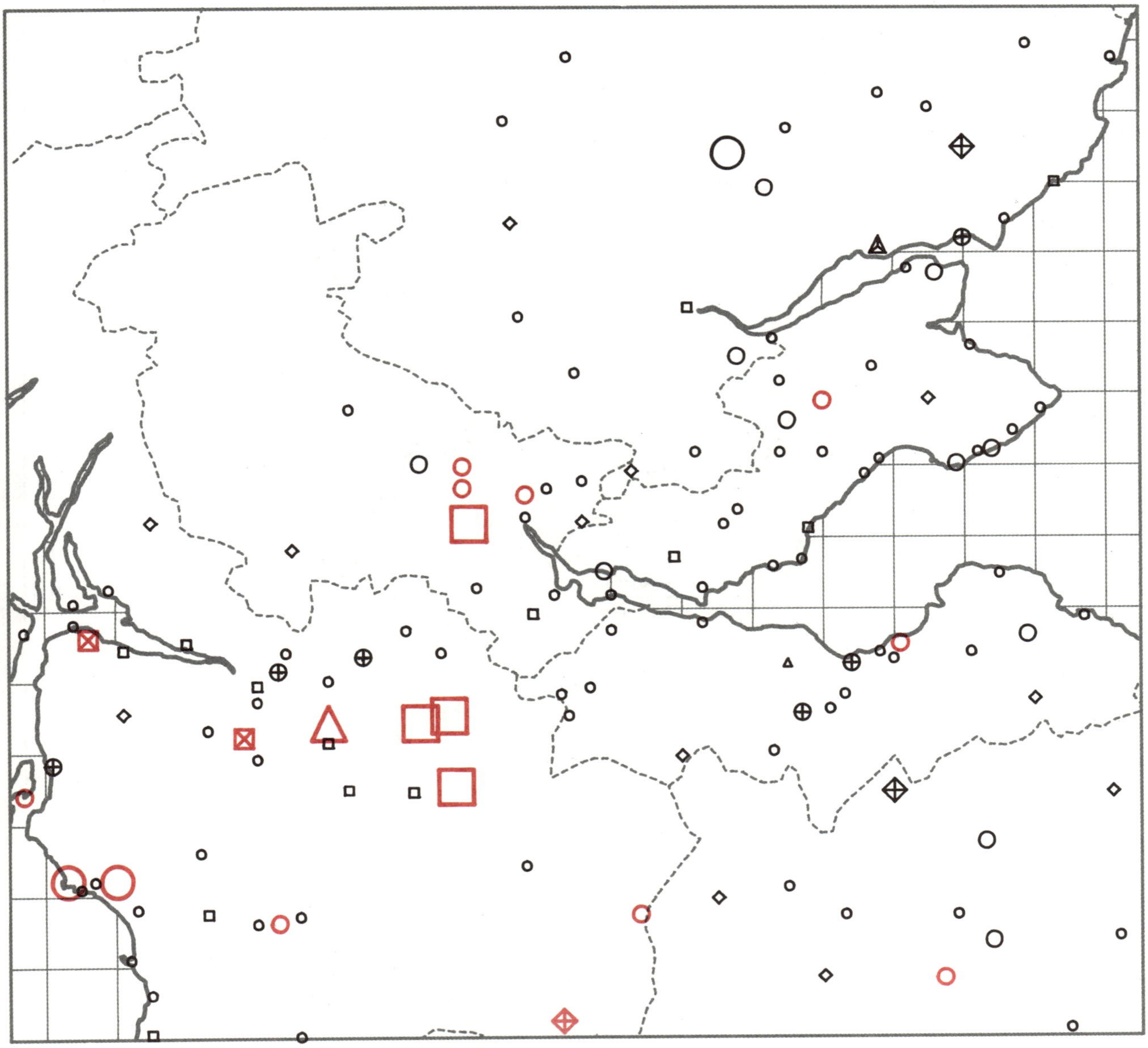

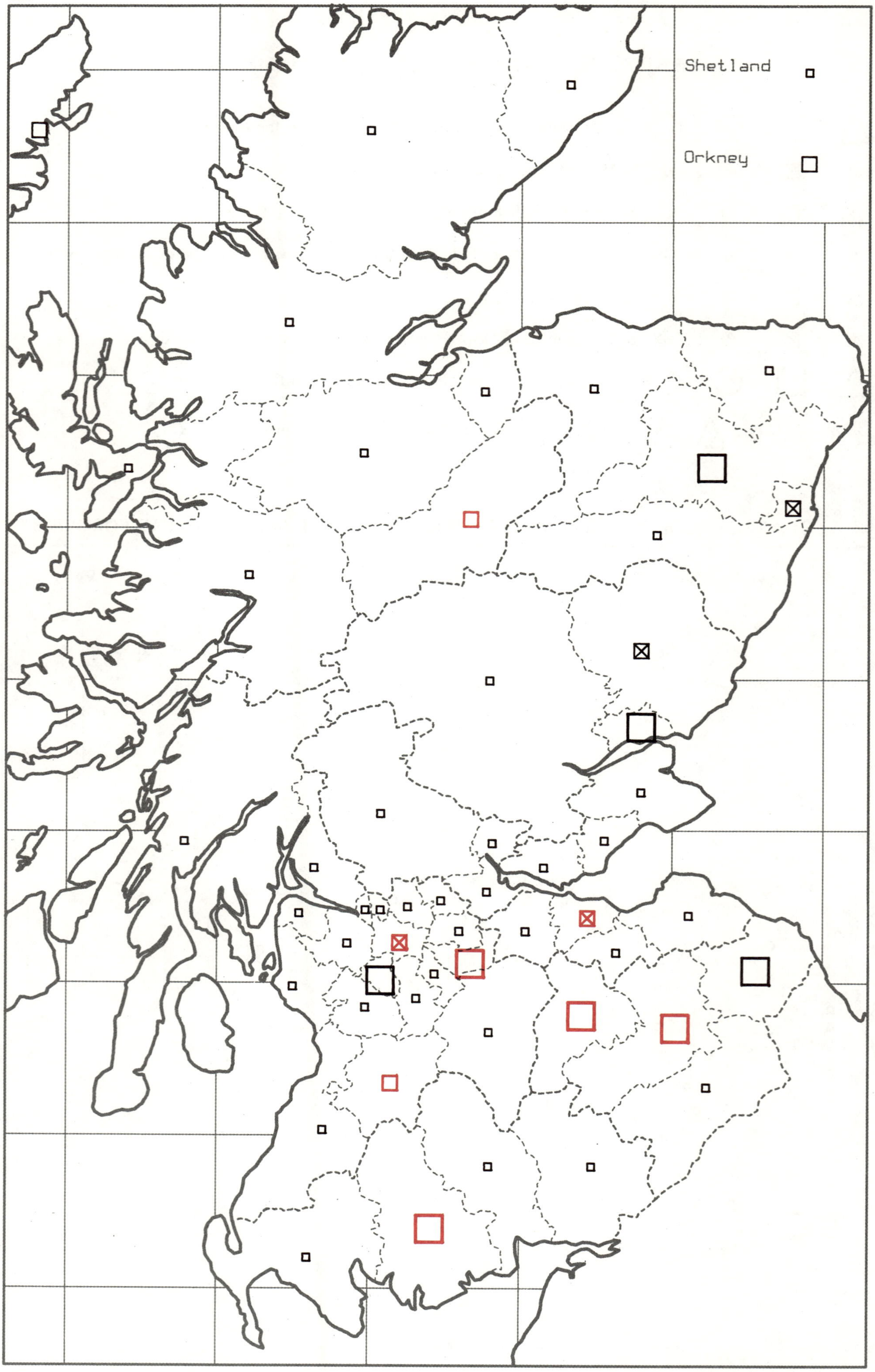
Shetland
Orkney

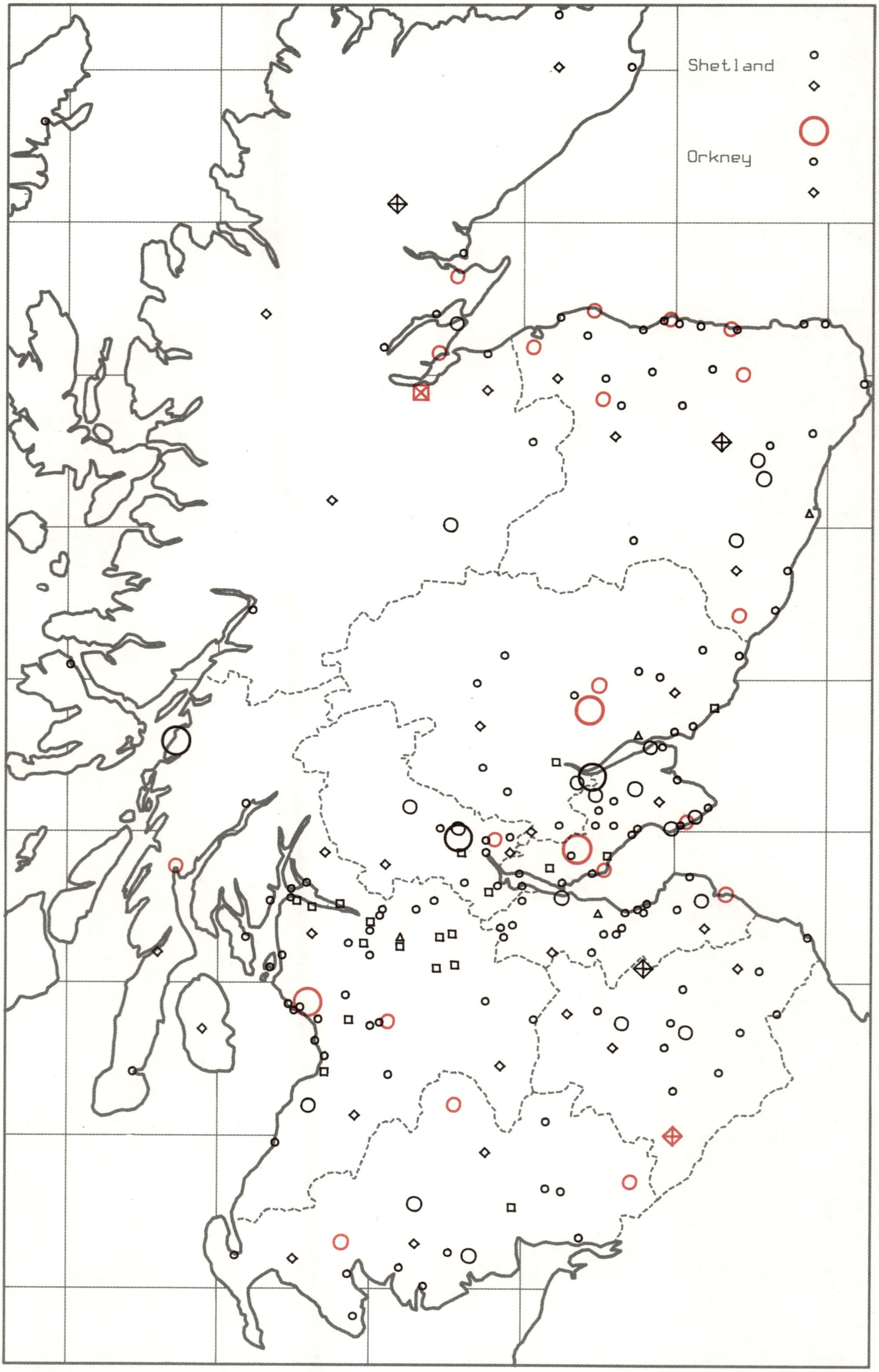
Shetland
Orkney

SEX RATIOS OF BIRTHS 1959-63

- SMR significantly high ($p < 0.05$) and within the top tenth
- SMR significantly high ($p < 0.05$) not within the top tenth
- SMR not significantly high but within the top tenth
- SMR not significantly high or low and not within the top or bottom tenth
- SMR not significantly low but within the bottom tenth
- SMR significantly low ($P < 0.05$) not within the bottom tenth
- SMR significantly low ($P < 0.05$) and within the bottom tenth

City △ Large Burgh □ Small Burgh ○ Landward Area ◇

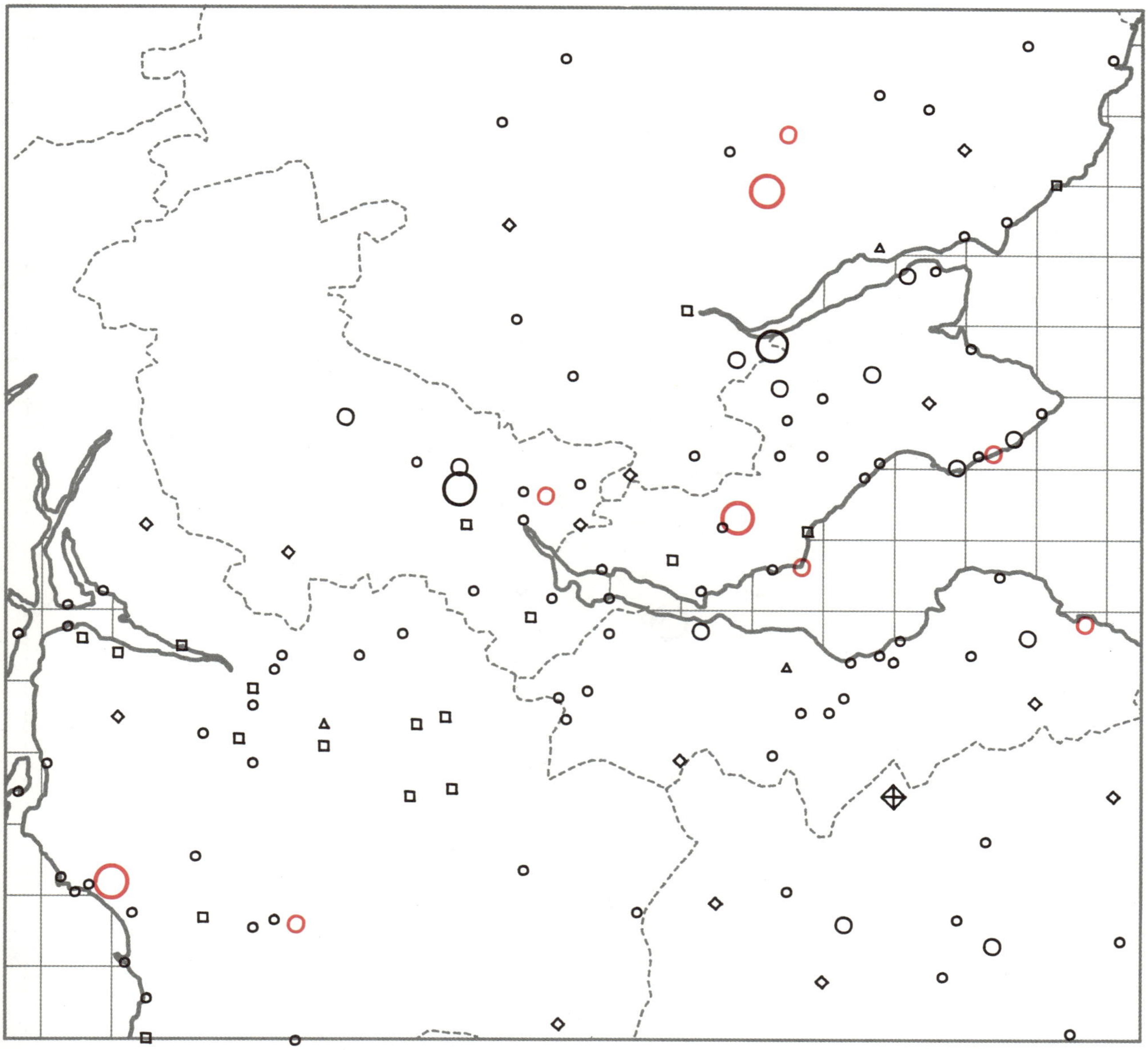

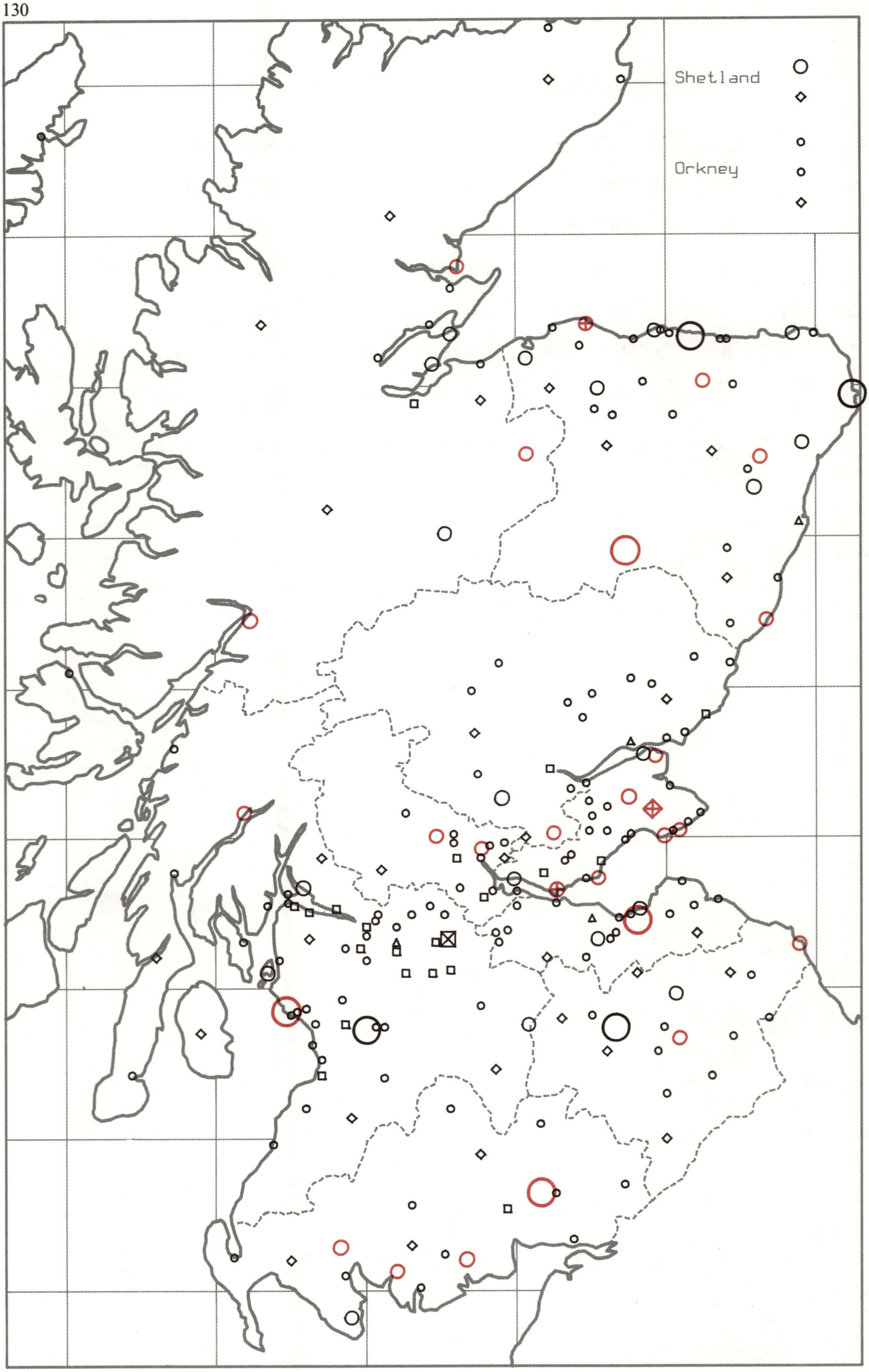
Shetland
Orkney

SEX RATIOS OF BIRTHS 1969-73

SMR significantly high ($p < 0.05$) and within the top tenth

SMR significantly high ($p < 0.05$) not within the top tenth

SMR not significantly high but within the top tenth

SMR not significantly high or low and not within the top or bottom tenth

SMR not significantly low but within the bottom tenth

SMR significantly low ($P < 0.05$) not within the bottom tenth

SMR significantly low ($P < 0.05$) and within the bottom tenth

City Large Burgh Small Burgh Landward Area

A SQUARE SYMBOL IS USED FOR THE DISTRICTS ON THE MAP OVERLEAF FOR 1979-83.

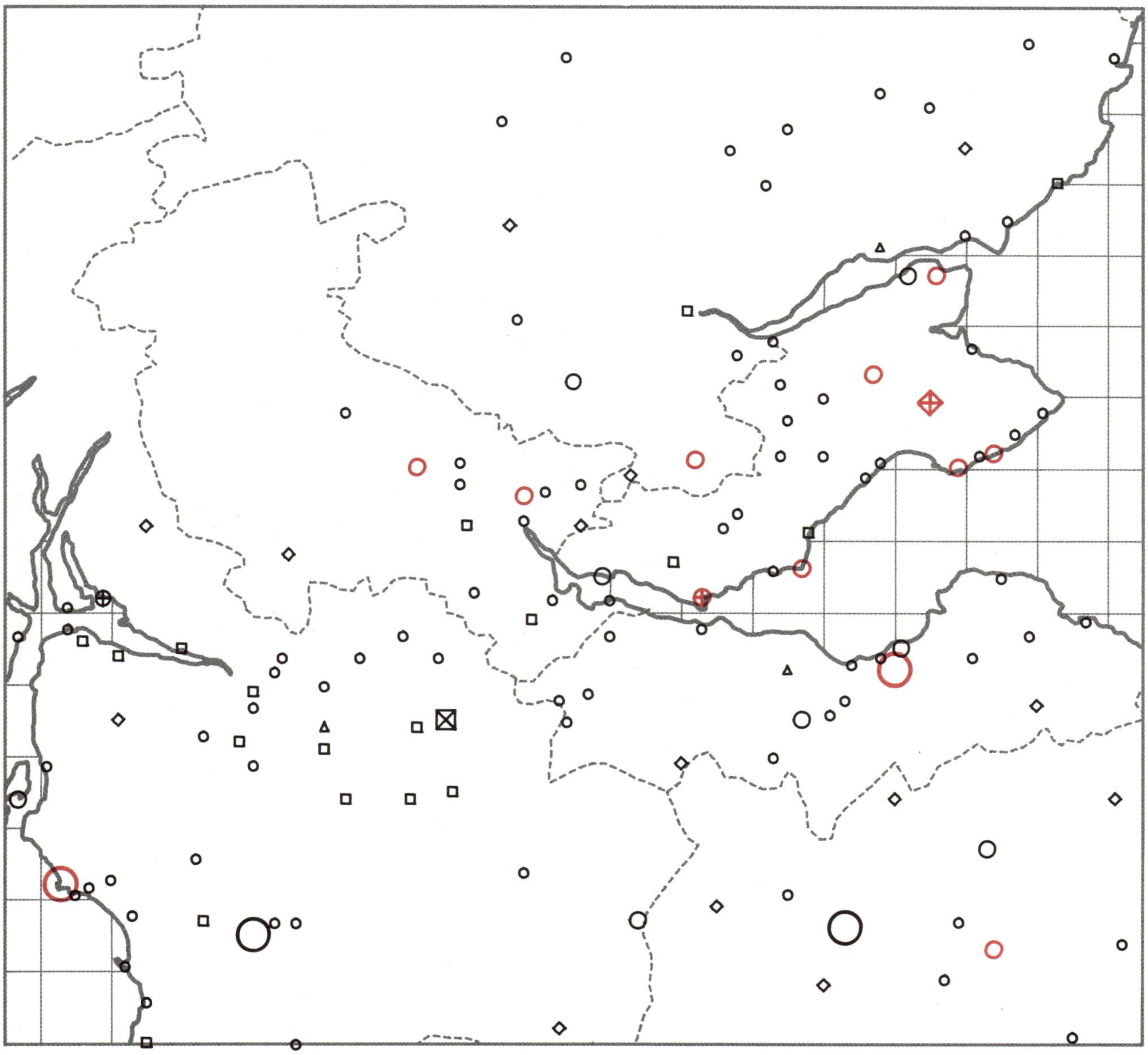

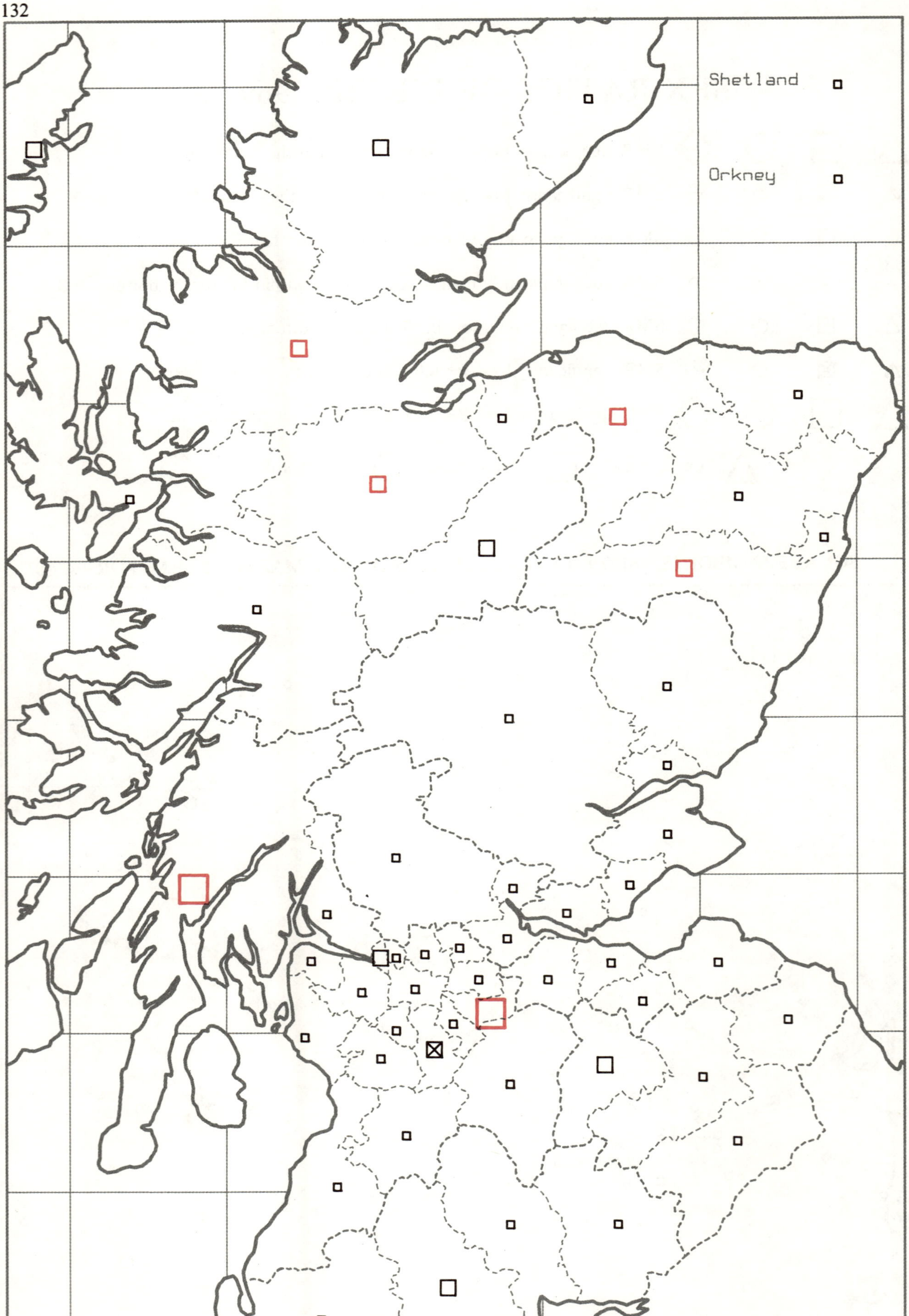
Shetland
Orkney

SEX RATIOS OF BIRTHS

In most human populations, more males than females are born. The number of males per 100 females at birth (the secondary sex ratio) in Europe is between 104 and 107. In Scotland over the last ten years, the ratio has been 106. Countries where sex ratios deviate from this norm include Hong Kong 109, Greece 113, Korea and Gambia 116, Aden 117, Chile 103 and the Asian people of the Republic of South Africa 101 [100].

Intrapopulation variations in sex ratios have been attributed to a large number of genetic, socio-economic and environmental factors. Disease, diet, occupational stress, pollution and differences in hormonal status have been alleged to have altered the usual sex ratio.

The Office of Population Censuses and Surveys listed the sex ratios of births for selected paternal occupations in England and Wales [101]. Noting that some occupations differed significantly in their sex ratios of births from the majority, the report commented on the 'possibility that some specific occupational exposures may influence the sex ratio, and given the remaining uncertainty over its determination, monitoring of the sex ratio may provide a useful warning of something requiring further investigation'. In a recent discussion on the effects of dibromochloropropane (DBCP), it was pointed out that the wives of production workers had an unusually high proportion of female children [102]. One of the conclusions reached was that the reproductive effects from new agents could be used as advance notice of their cancer producing qualities. Agents which cause cancer in humans take years or decades to manifest themselves, whereas reproductive effects may be identified in a much shorter time.

In Scotland, exploratory studies on two steel towns with high cancer rates demonstrated that sex ratios of births were high in the years immediately preceding a cancer epidemic [103,104]. These findings indicated that a systematic investigation of the ratios in other Scottish communities might reveal abnormal patterns.

In the period 1959-63, 50 percent of the towns with high sex ratios were on the Scottish coastline. The number of towns on the east coast is only twice the number on the west, yet there was a disproportionate frequency of towns with high sex ratios on the east coast, particularly along the shores of the Moray Firth. Diet may play an important role in the determination of sex [102-104], the consumption of salt foods producing an excess of male births; it is likely that fish was a staple food in the small towns of the Moray Firth in the early 1960s. (The possible link between fish consumption and sex ratio has been strengthened by the finding that census data for Newfoundland show an excess of male infants in communities along the east coast, where the fishing industry is concentrated.) Low sex ratios were infrequently present on the coastline, and the few found were mostly on the Tay and the Forth in places not strongly linked with fishing.

In 1969-73 the geographical patterns were not distinctive.

In 1979-83, high sex ratios were seen in six Districts; of these, Moray, Inverness and Ross and Cromarty border the Moray Firth; and a fourth, Kincardine and Deeside has its shores on the North Sea. The only District on the west was Argyll and Bute, which contains the important fishing port of Oban. Although Ross and Cromarty has a western coastline as well as an eastern, all the towns are on its eastern shores. The only landlocked District with high sex ratios was Motherwell and Wishaw, dominated by its steel industry; this association recalls the high ratios in the two other steel towns in Scotland, as described earlier.

Of the six Districts with low sex ratios in 1979-83, the three with coastlines are not associated in an important way with the fishing industry.

An imbalance in the sex ratio of births has been suggested as an indicator of the reproductive health of a community; a high sex ratio may mean excessive loss of the female fetuses, and a low ratio may result from the loss of males. If so, one would predict that some associations might be demonstrable with neonatal, perinatal and infant mortality. The high sex ratio which could be related to industrial pollution (in Motherwell and Wishaw) was associated firstly with infant mortality which was significantly high and in the top decile, secondly with perinatal mortality which was in the top decile but not significantly high, and thirdly with neonatal mortality which was significantly high but not in the top decile.

Low sex ratios were found in six Districts. A study of these Districts showed that infant mortality in Tweeddale and in Stewartry was significantly high; infant mortality in Badenoch and Strathspey was in the top decile although not significantly high; neonatal mortality in Tweeddale, Sutherland and Badenoch and Strathspey was in the top decile but not significantly high; and perinatal mortality in Tweeddale was in the top decile but not significantly high.

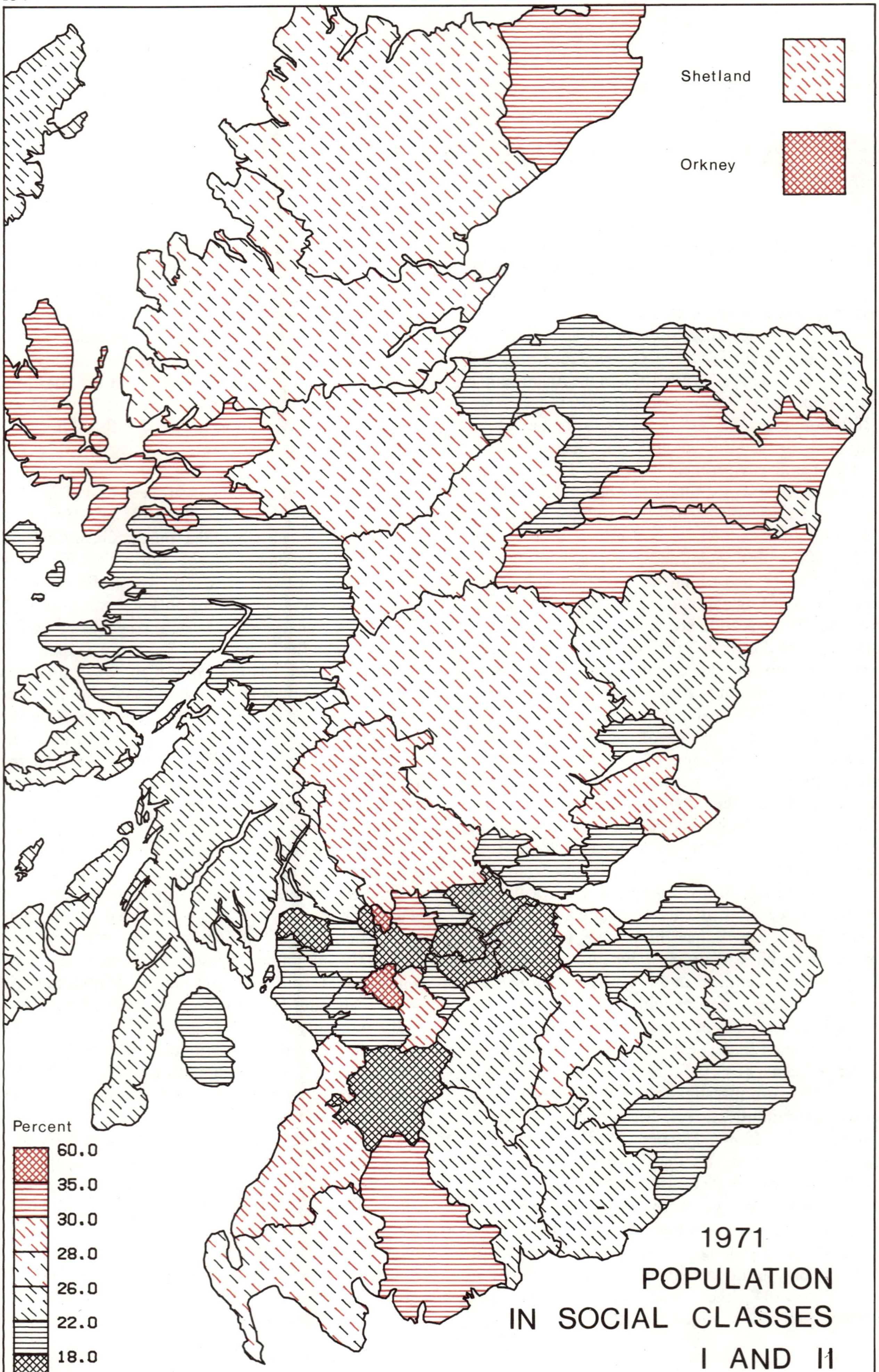
Shetland
Orkney
Percent
60.0
35.0
30.0
28.0
26.0
22.0
18.0
14.0
1971
POPULATION
IN SOCIAL CLASSES
I AND II

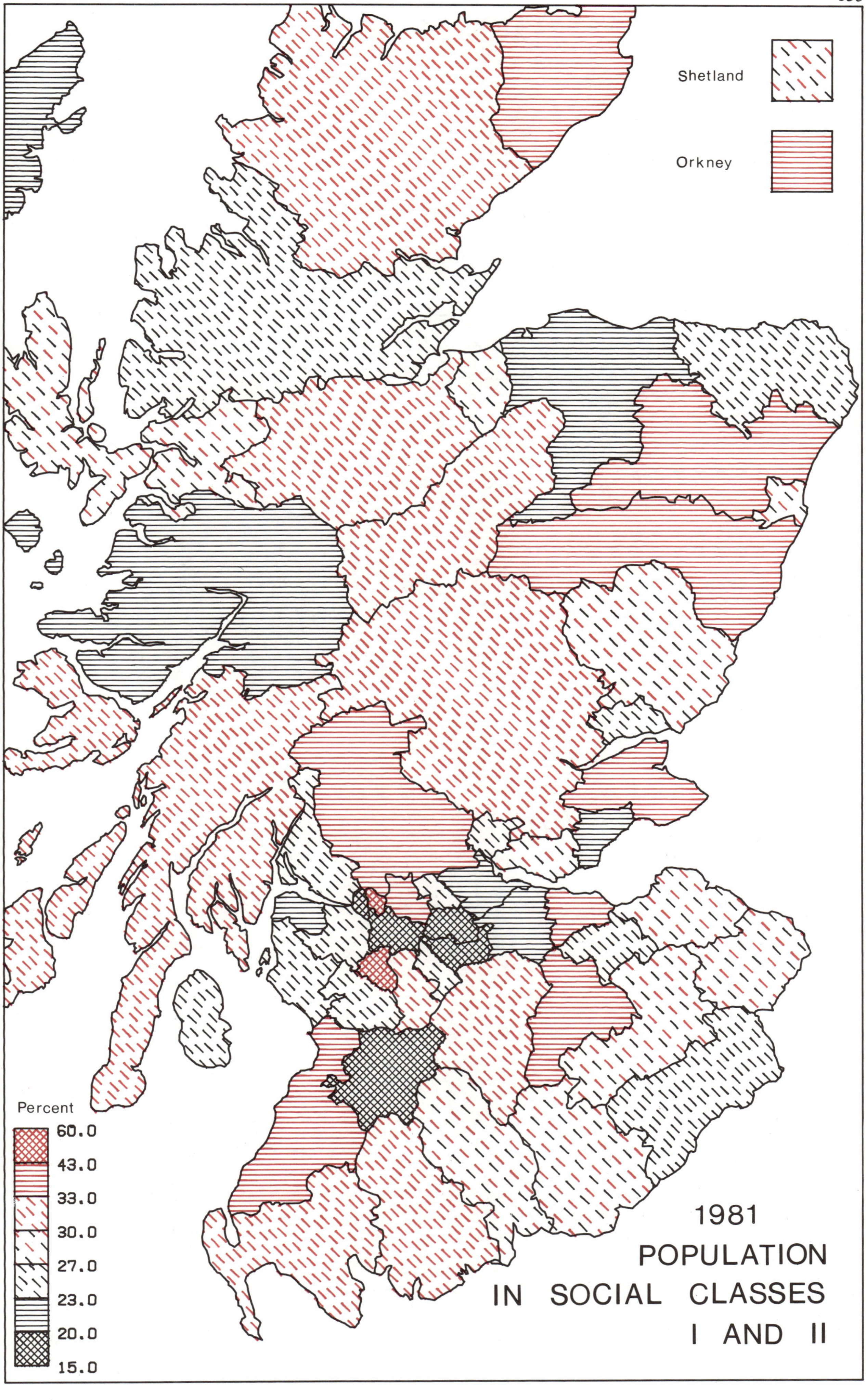
Shetland
Orkney
Percent
60.0
43.0
33.0
30.0
27.0
23.0
20.0
15.0
1981
POPULATION
IN SOCIAL CLASSES
I AND II

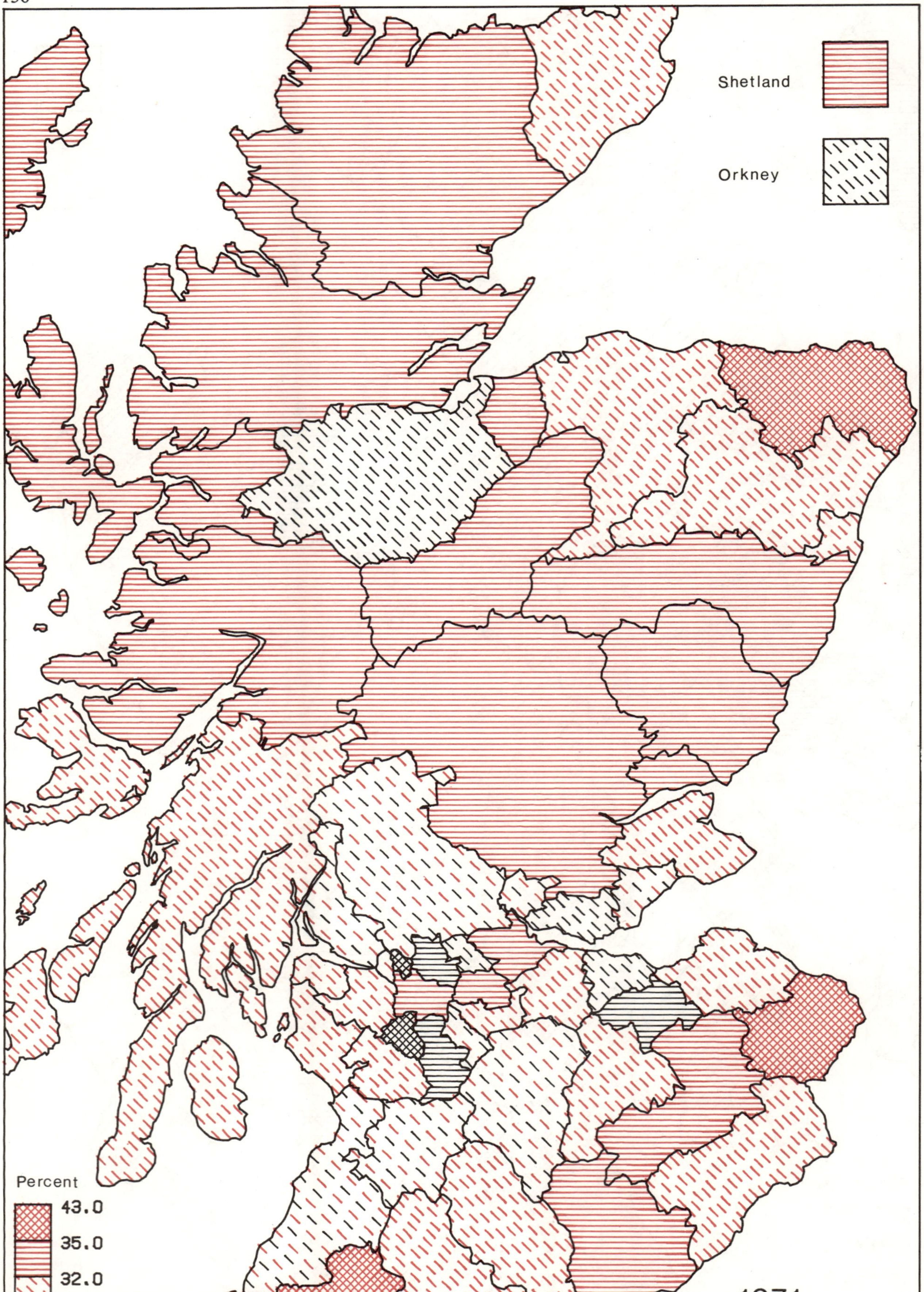
Shetland
Orkney
Percent
43.0
35.0
32.0
28.0
25.0
22.0
16.0
6.0
1971
POPULATION
IN SOCIAL CLASSES
IV AND V

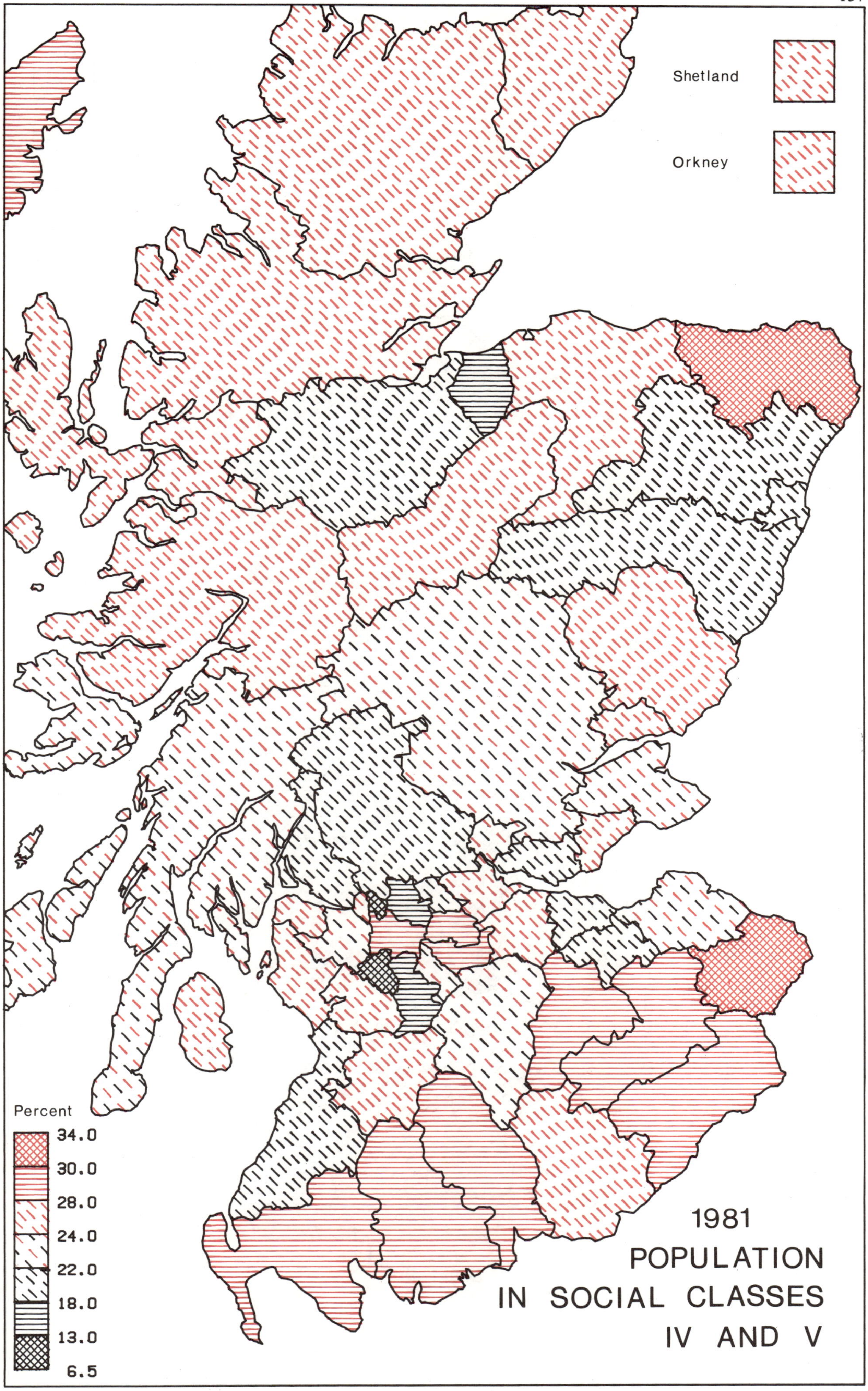
Shetland
Orkney
Percent
34.0
30.0
28.0
24.0
22.0
18.0
13.0
6.5
1981
POPULATION
IN SOCIAL CLASSES
IV AND V

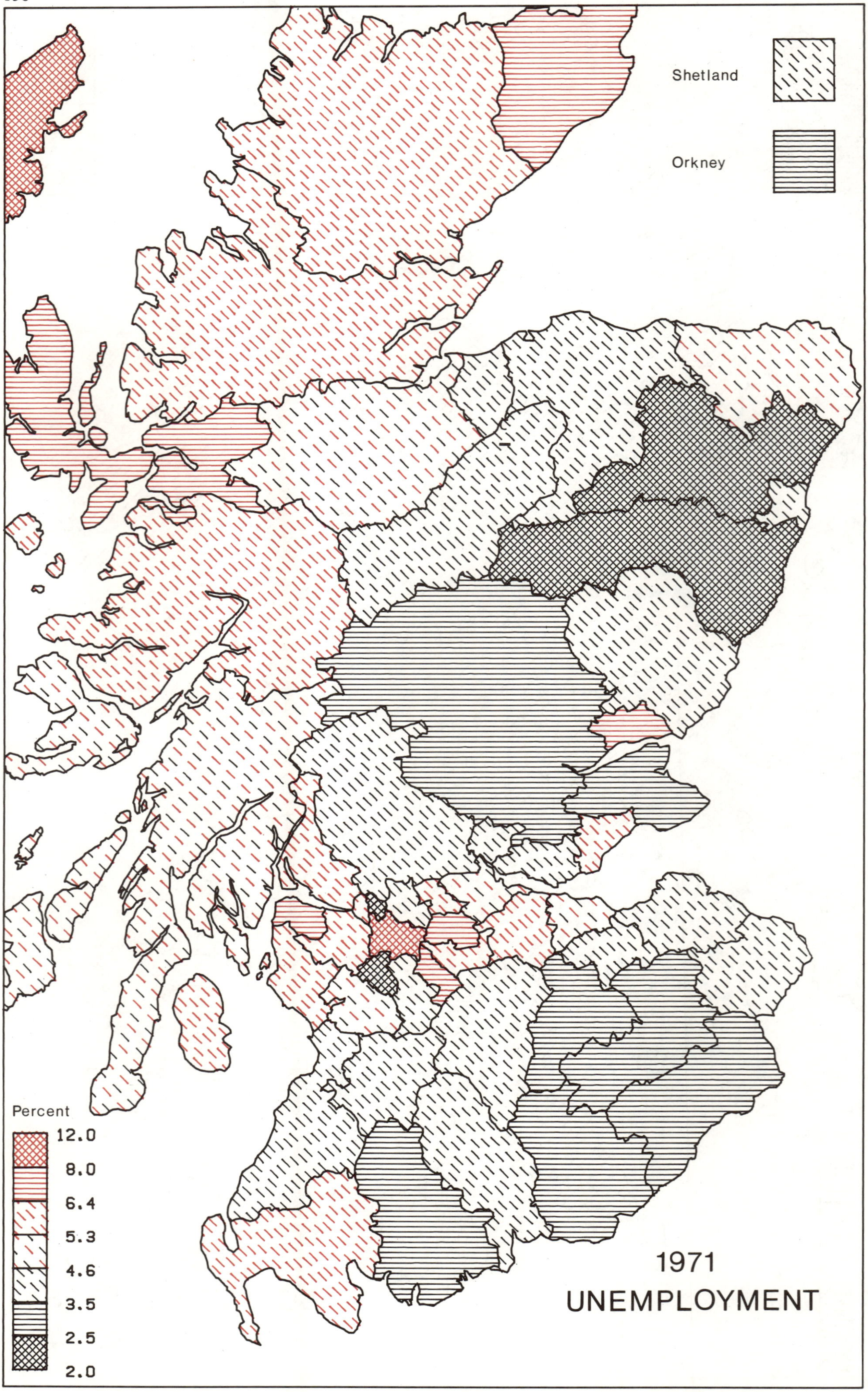
Shetland
Orkney
Percent
12.0
8.0
6.4
5.3
4.6
3.5
2.5
2.0
1971
UNEMPLOYMENT

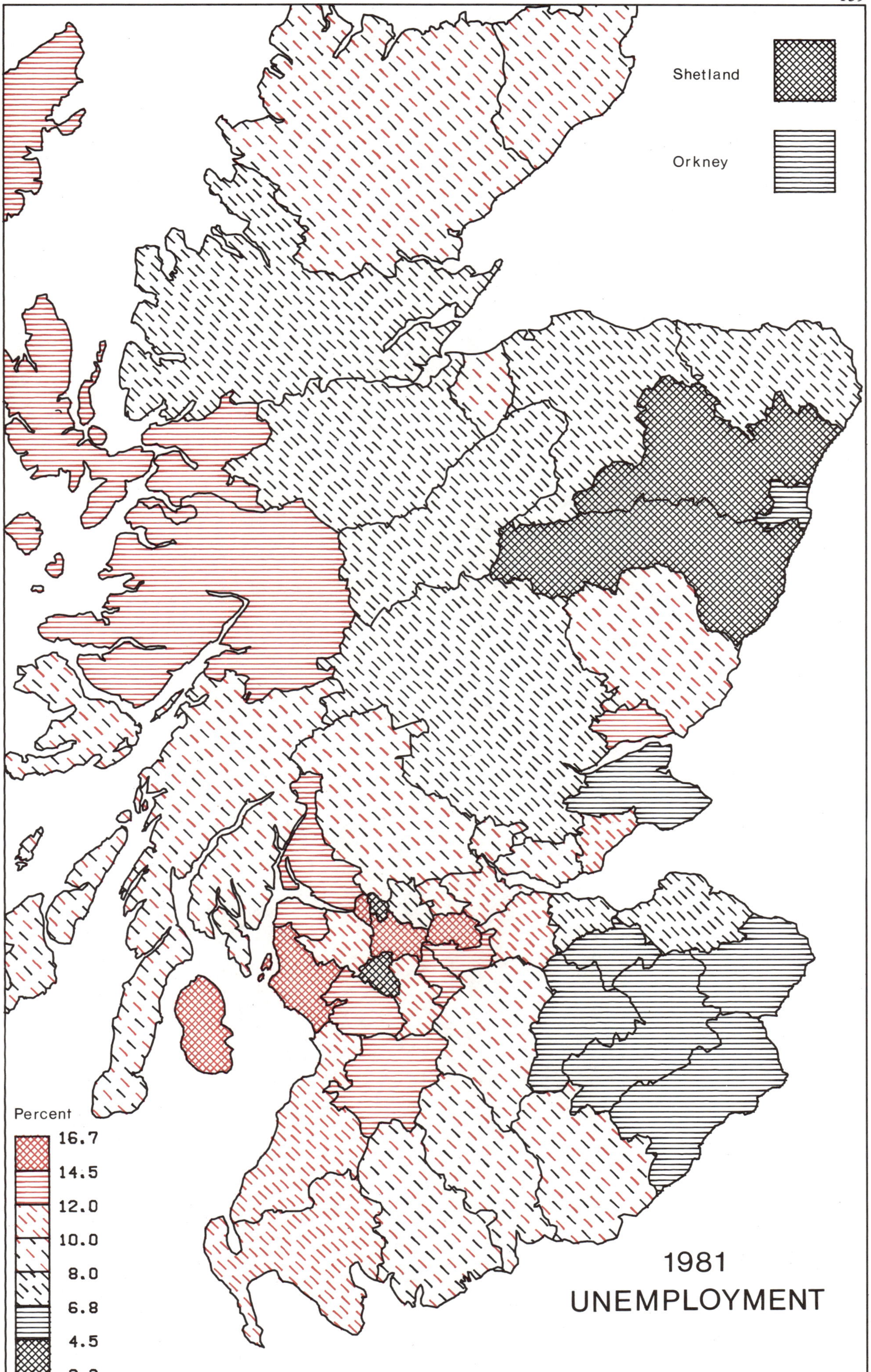

Shetland
Orkney
Percent
16.7
14.5
12.0
10.0
8.0
6.8
4.5
3.3
1981
UNEMPLOYMENT

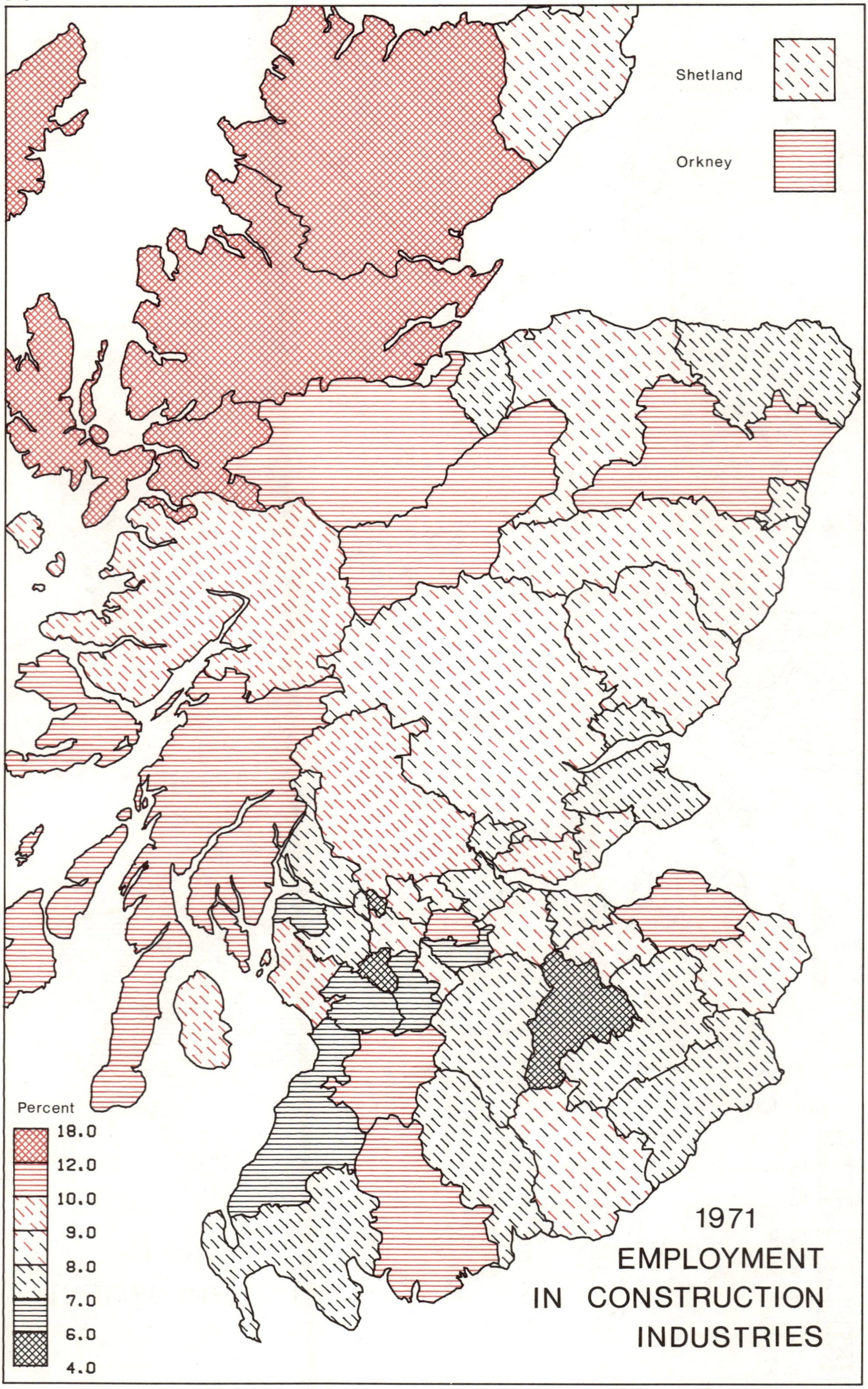
Shetland
Orkney
Percent
18.0
12.0
10.0
9.0
8.0
7.0
6.0
4.0
1971
EMPLOYMENT
IN CONSTRUCTION
INDUSTRIES

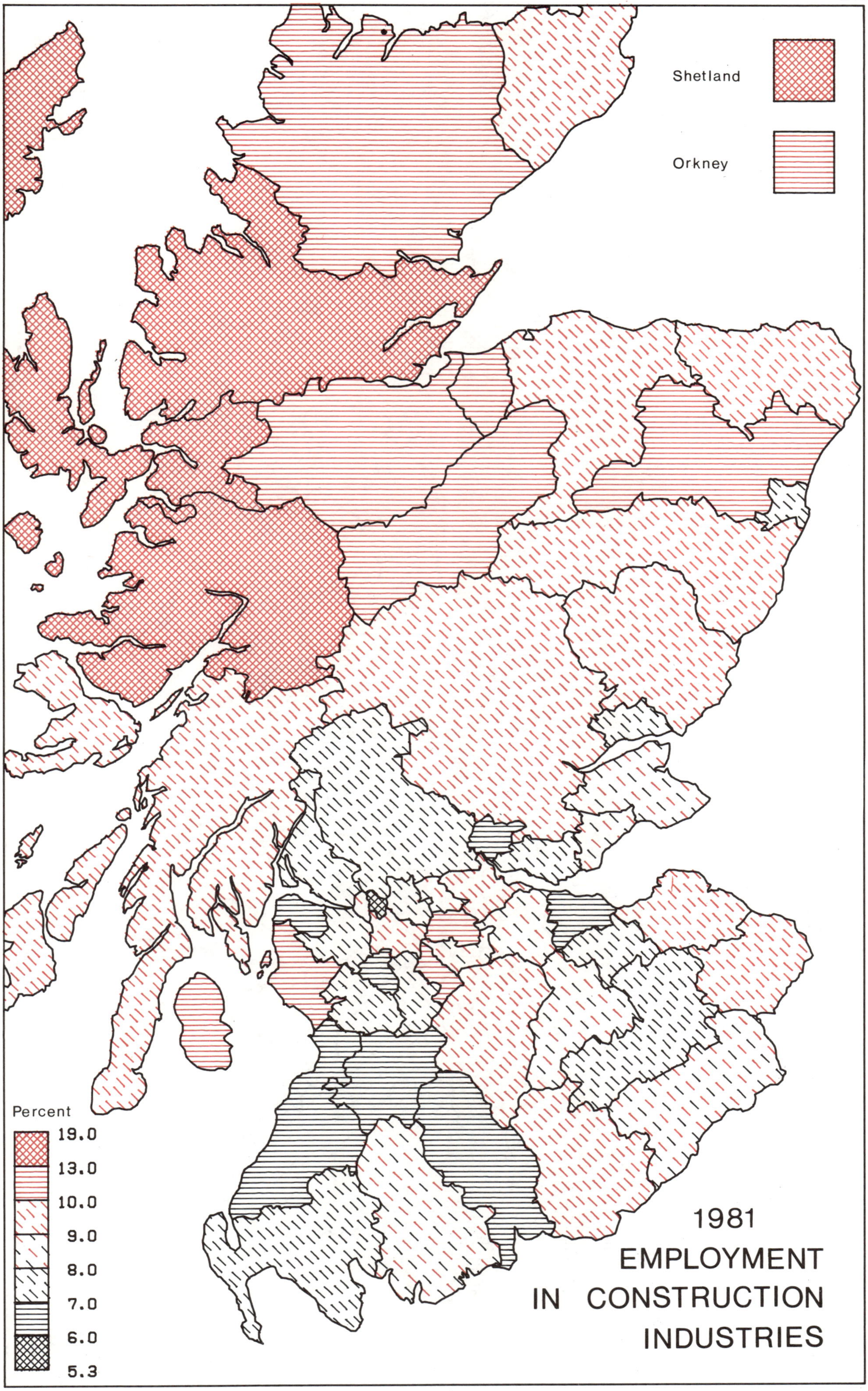
Shetland
Orkney
Percent
19.0
13.0
10.0
9.0
8.0
7.0
6.0
5.3
1981
EMPLOYMENT
IN CONSTRUCTION
INDUSTRIES

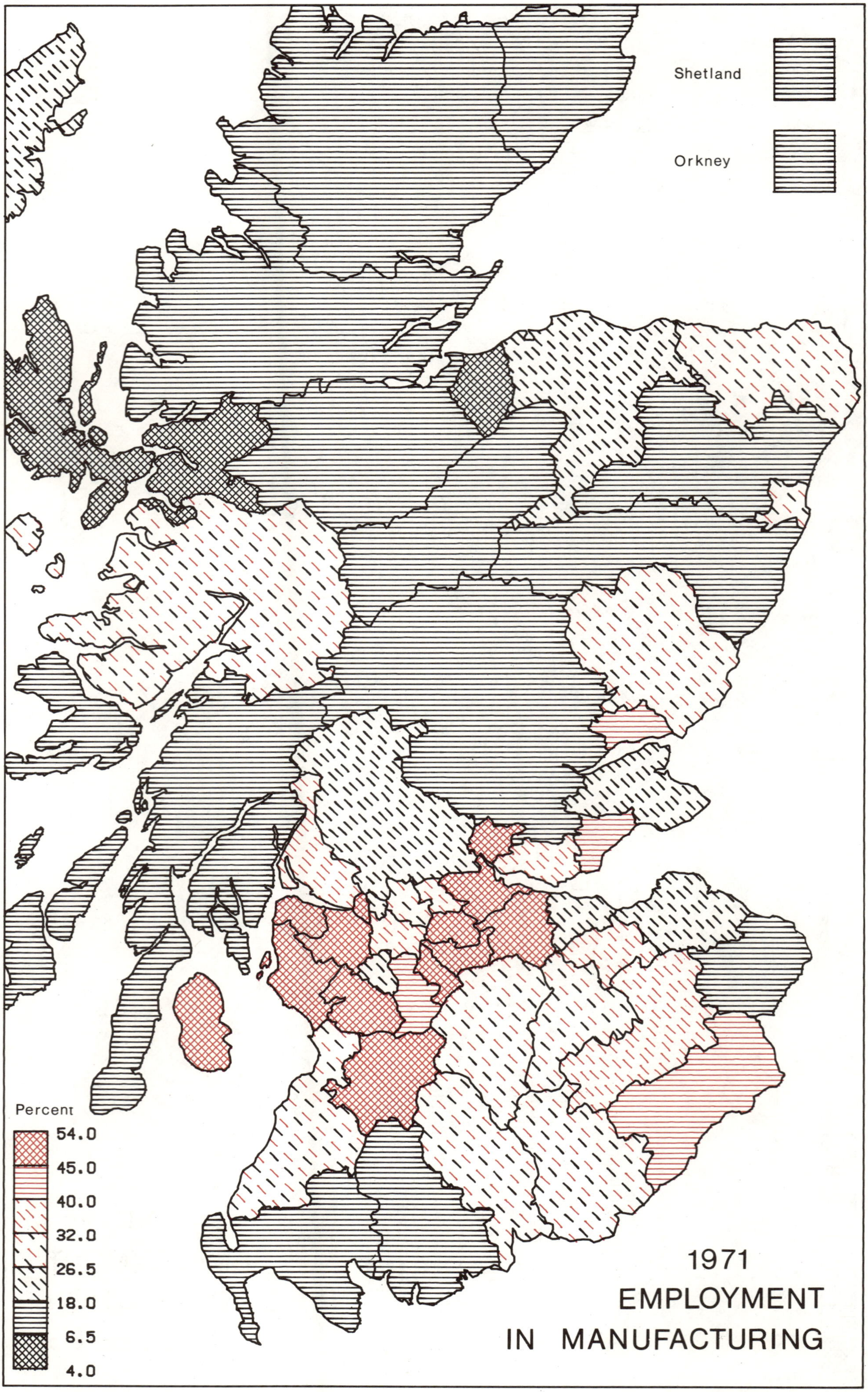
Shetland
Orkney
Percent
54.0
45.0
40.0
32.0
26.5
18.0
6.5
4.0
1971
EMPLOYMENT
IN MANUFACTURING

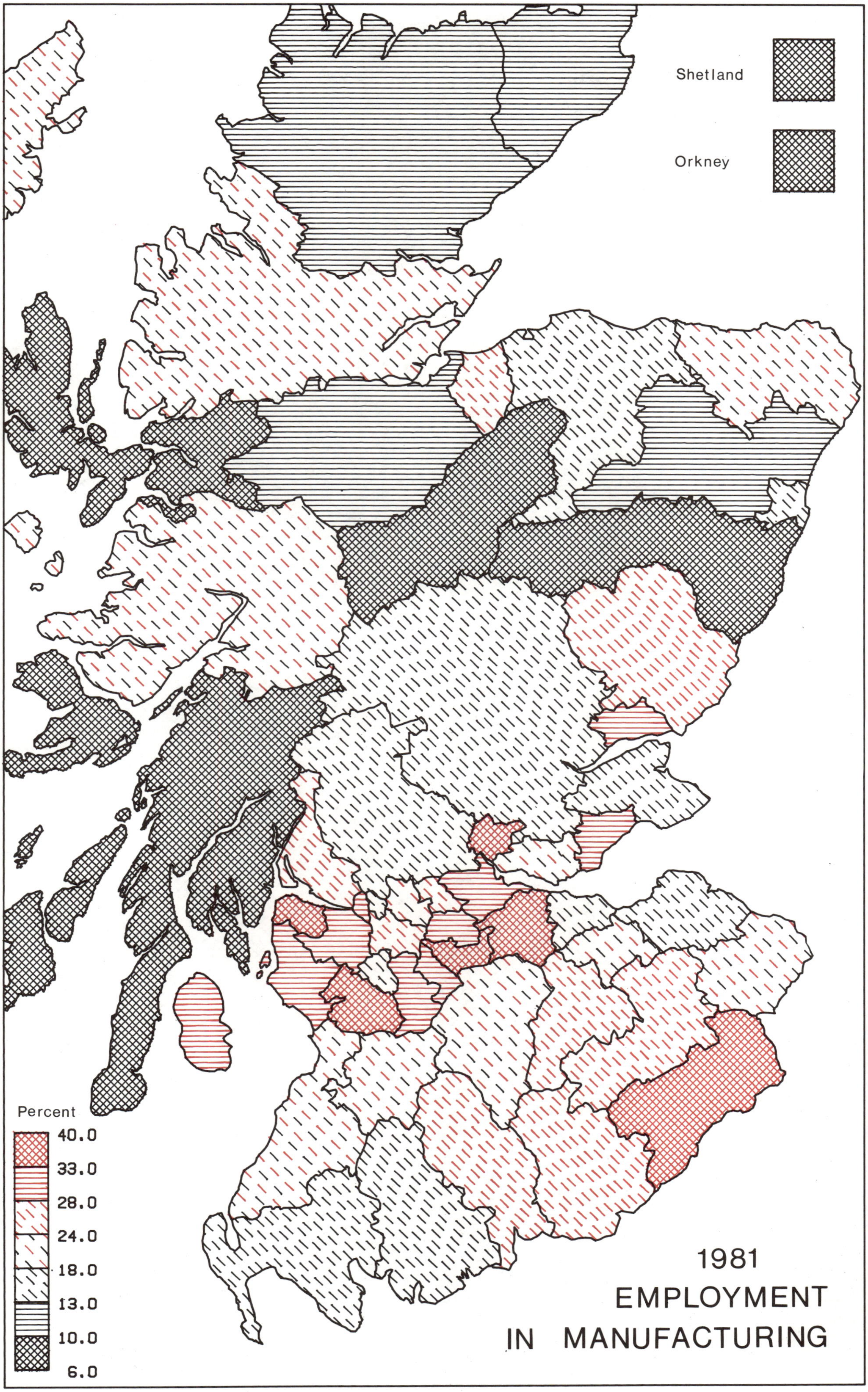
Shetland
Orkney
Percent
40.0
33.0
28.0
24.0
18.0
13.0
10.0
6.0
1981
EMPLOYMENT
IN MANUFACTURING

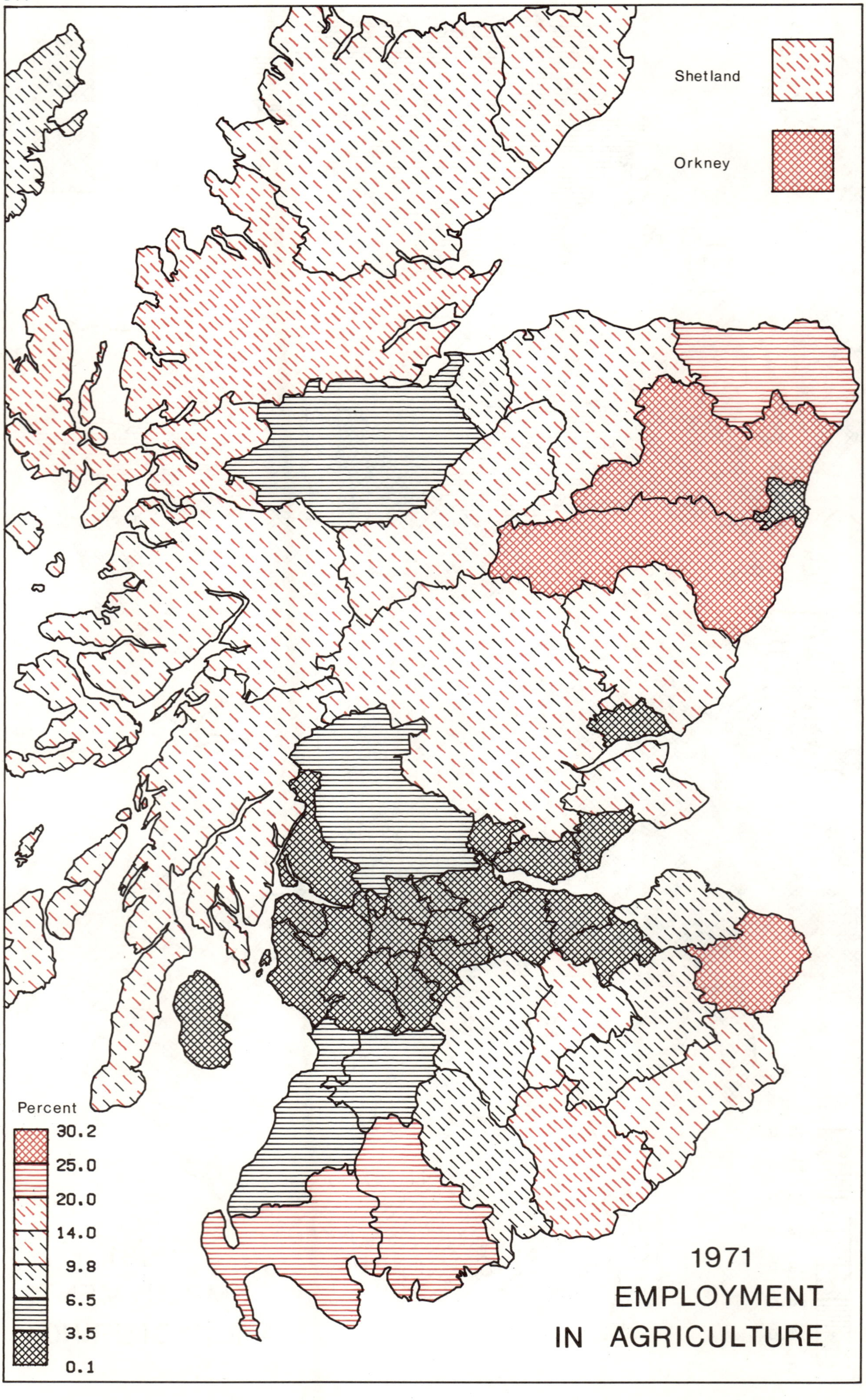
Shetland
Orkney
Percent
30.2
25.0
20.0
14.0
9.8
6.5
3.5
0.1
1971
EMPLOYMENT
IN AGRICULTURE

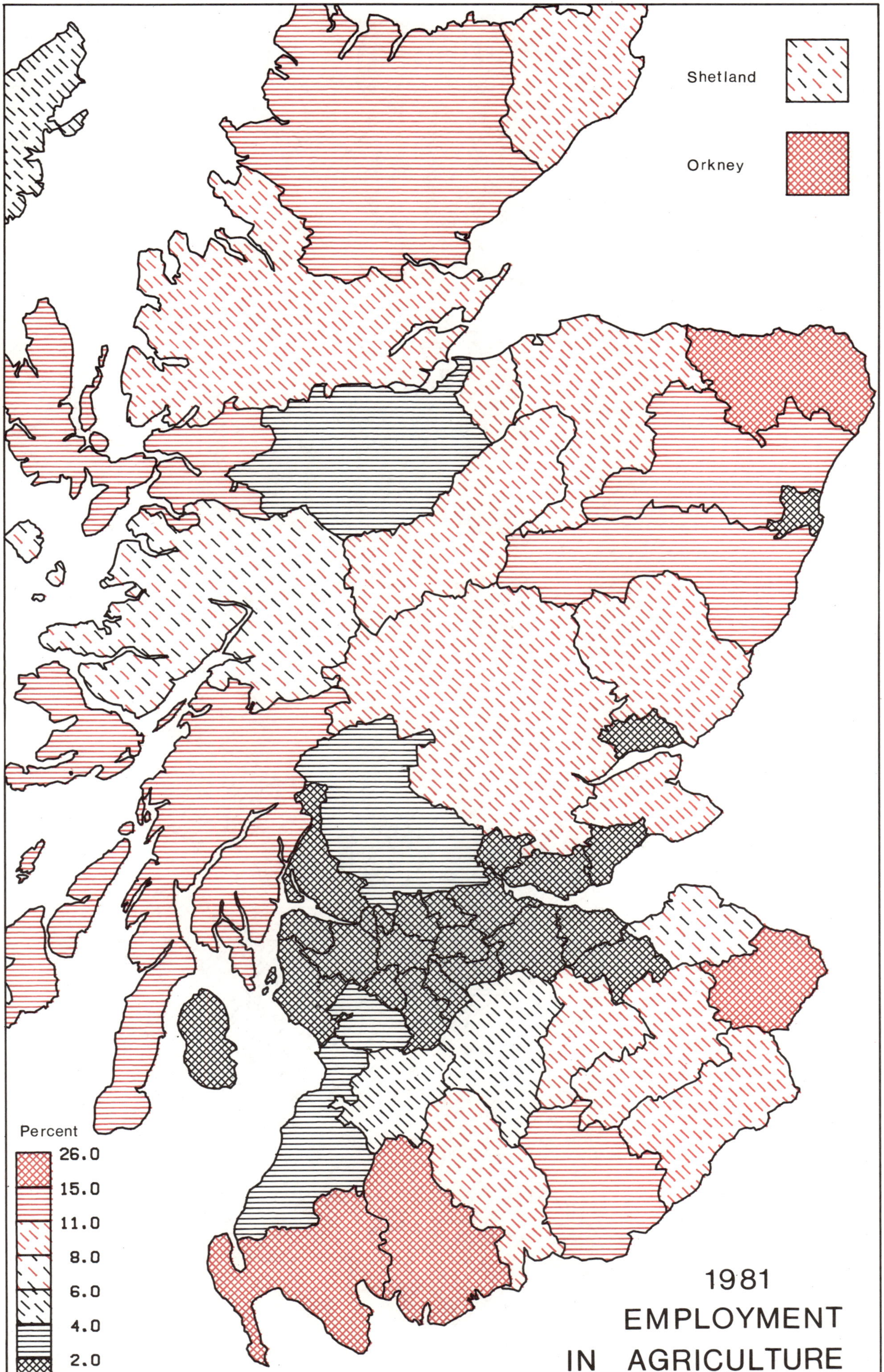
Shetland
Orkney
Percent
26.0
15.0
11.0
8.0
6.0
4.0
2.0
0.0
1981
EMPLOYMENT
IN AGRICULTURE

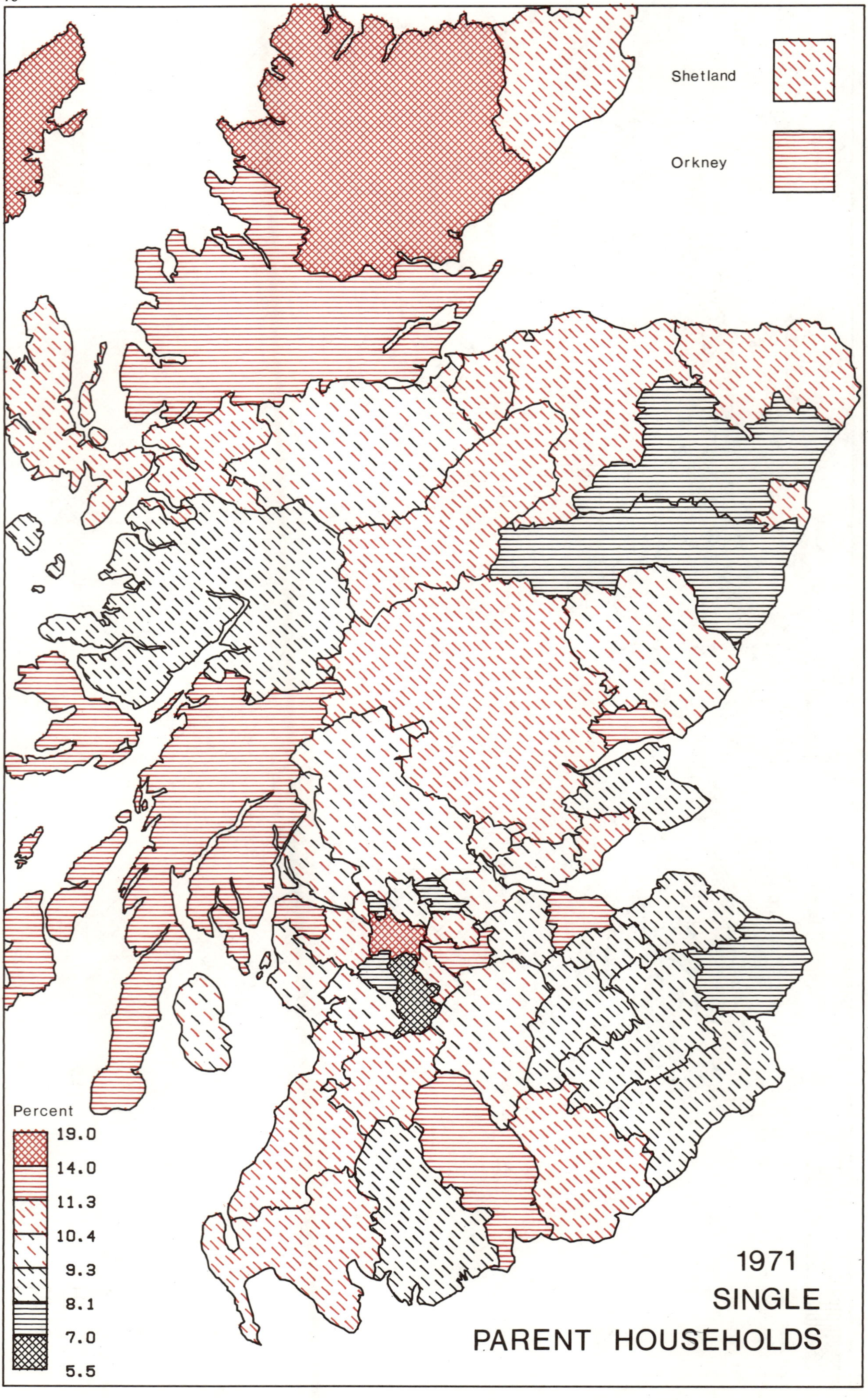
Shetland
Orkney
Percent
19.0
14.0
11.3
10.4
9.3
8.1
7.0
5.5
1971
SINGLE
PARENT HOUSEHOLDS

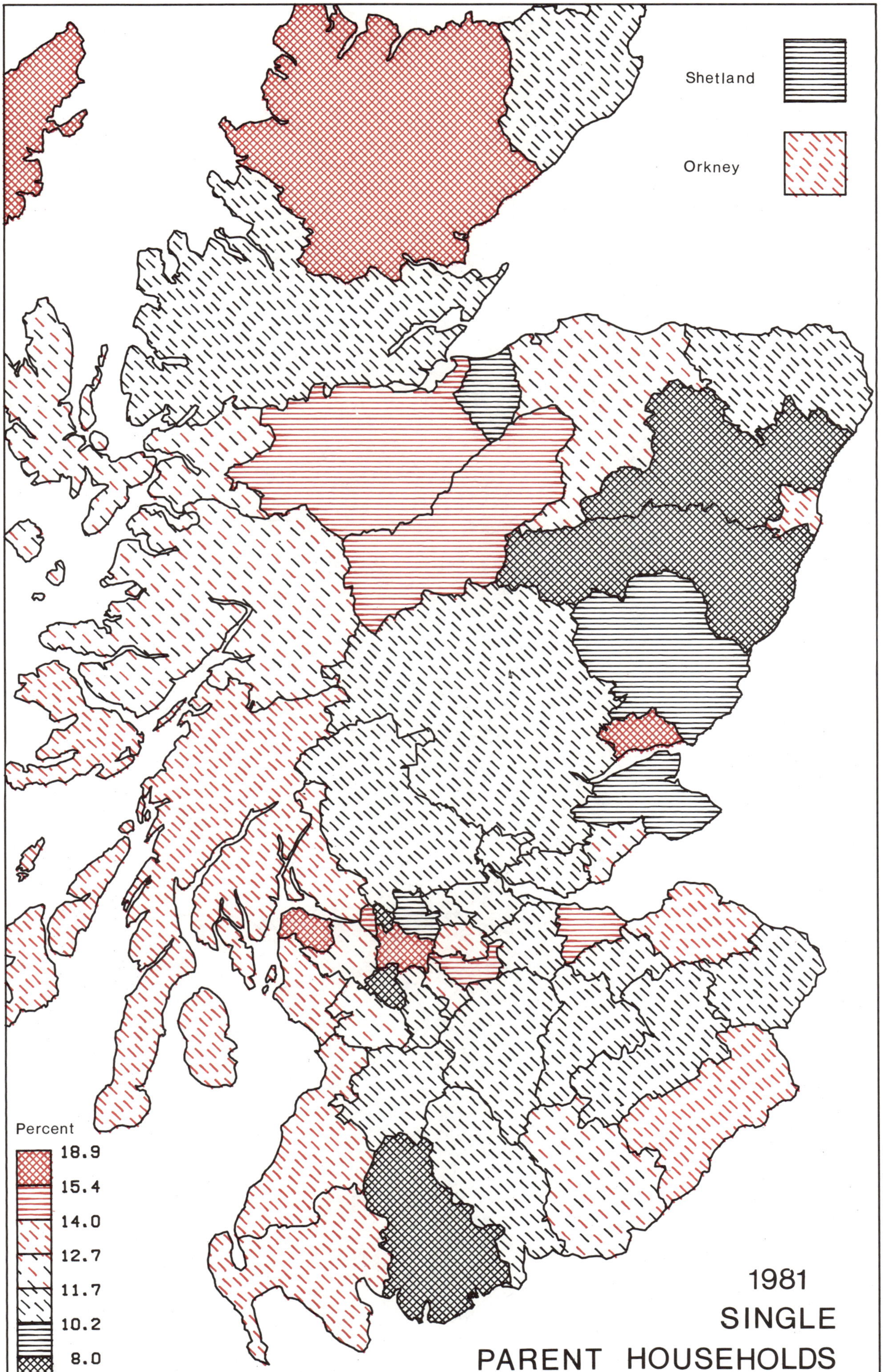
Shetland
Orkney
Percent
18.9
15.4
14.0
12.7
11.7
10.2
8.0
6.9
1981
SINGLE
PARENT HOUSEHOLDS

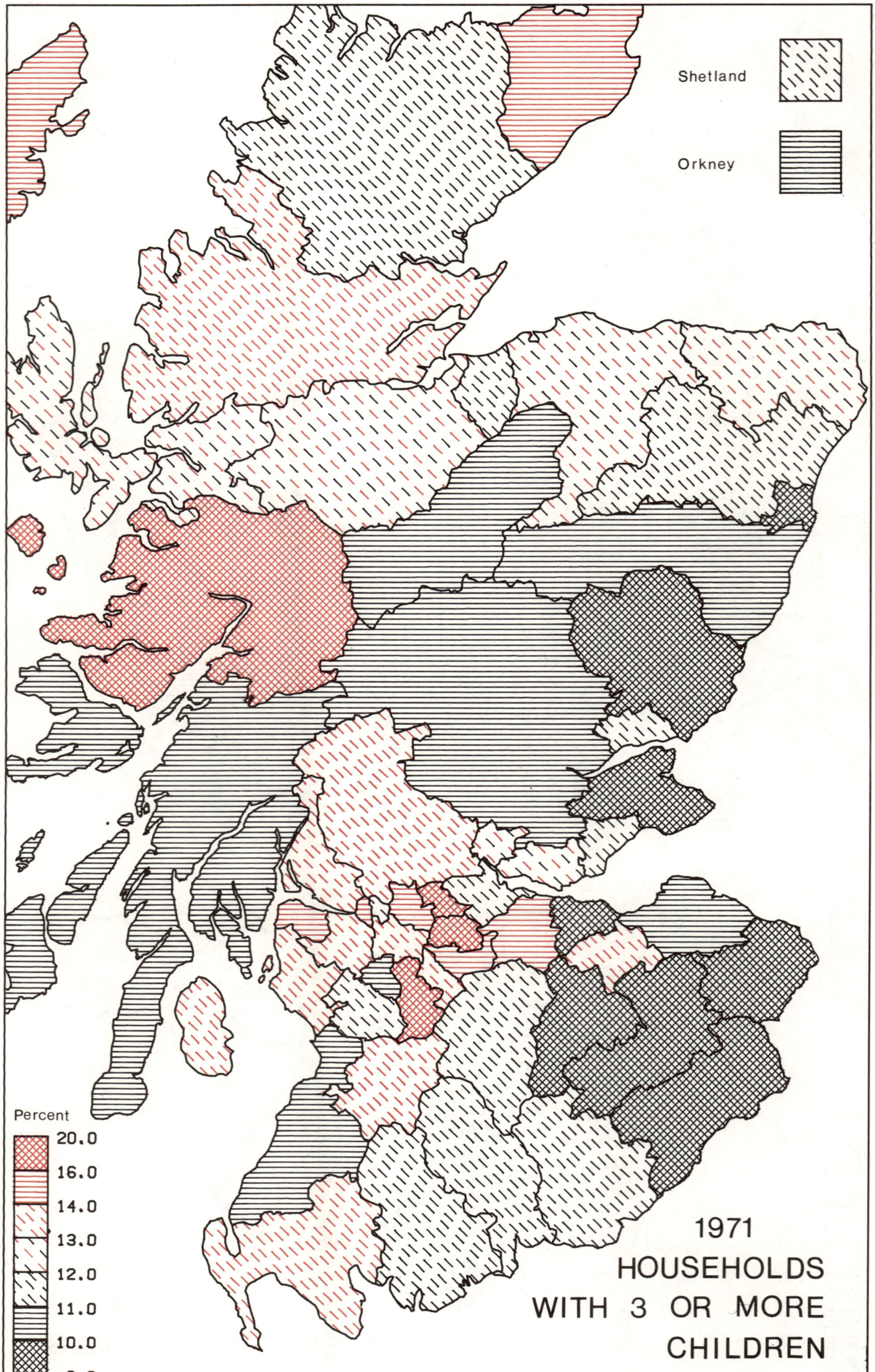
Shetland
Orkney
Percent
20.0
16.0
14.0
13.0
12.0
11.0
10.0
8.0
1971
HOUSEHOLDS
WITH 3 OR MORE
CHILDREN

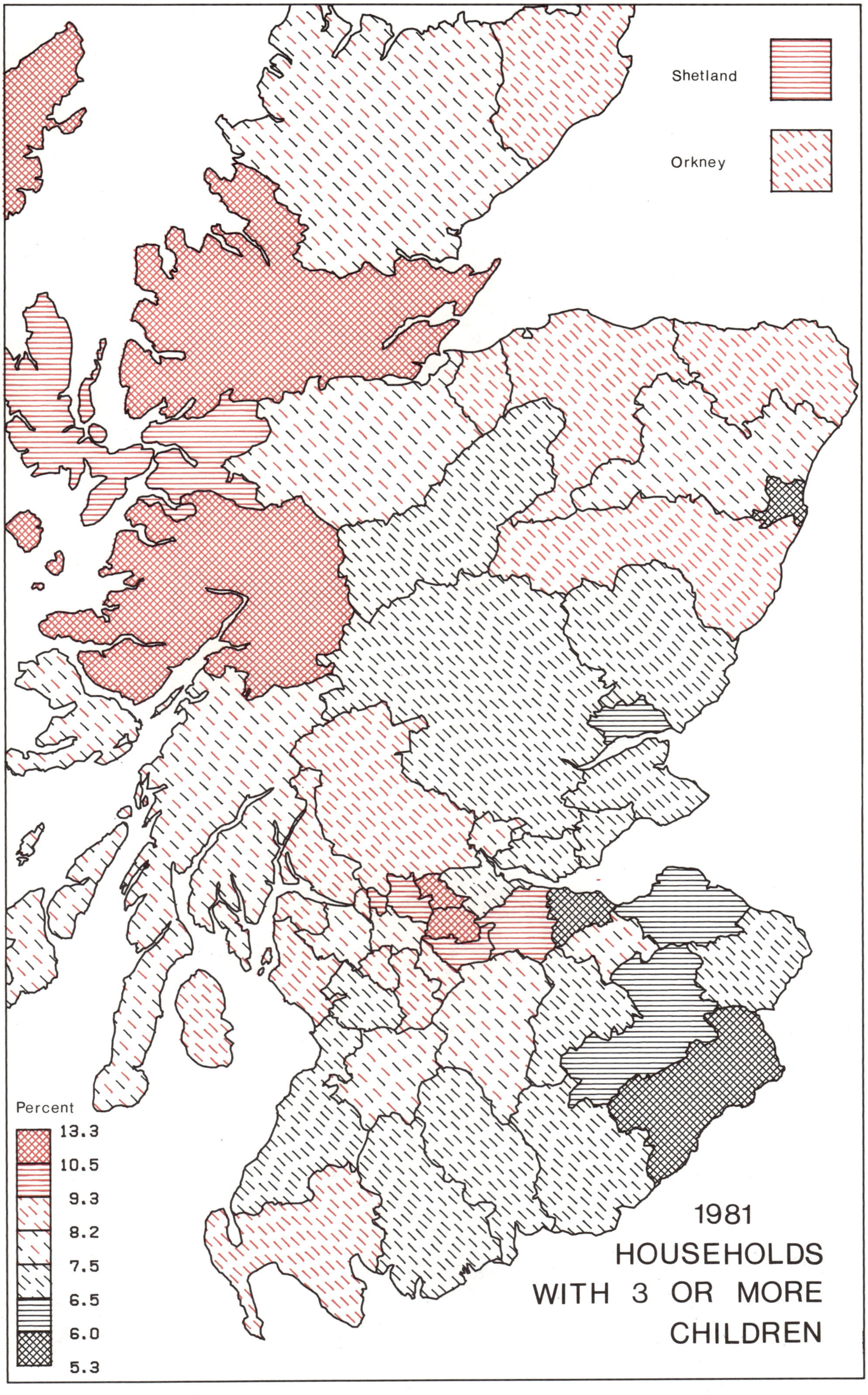
Shetland
Orkney
Percent
13.3
10.5
9.3
8.2
7.5
6.5
6.0
5.3
1981
HOUSEHOLDS
WITH 3 OR MORE
CHILDREN

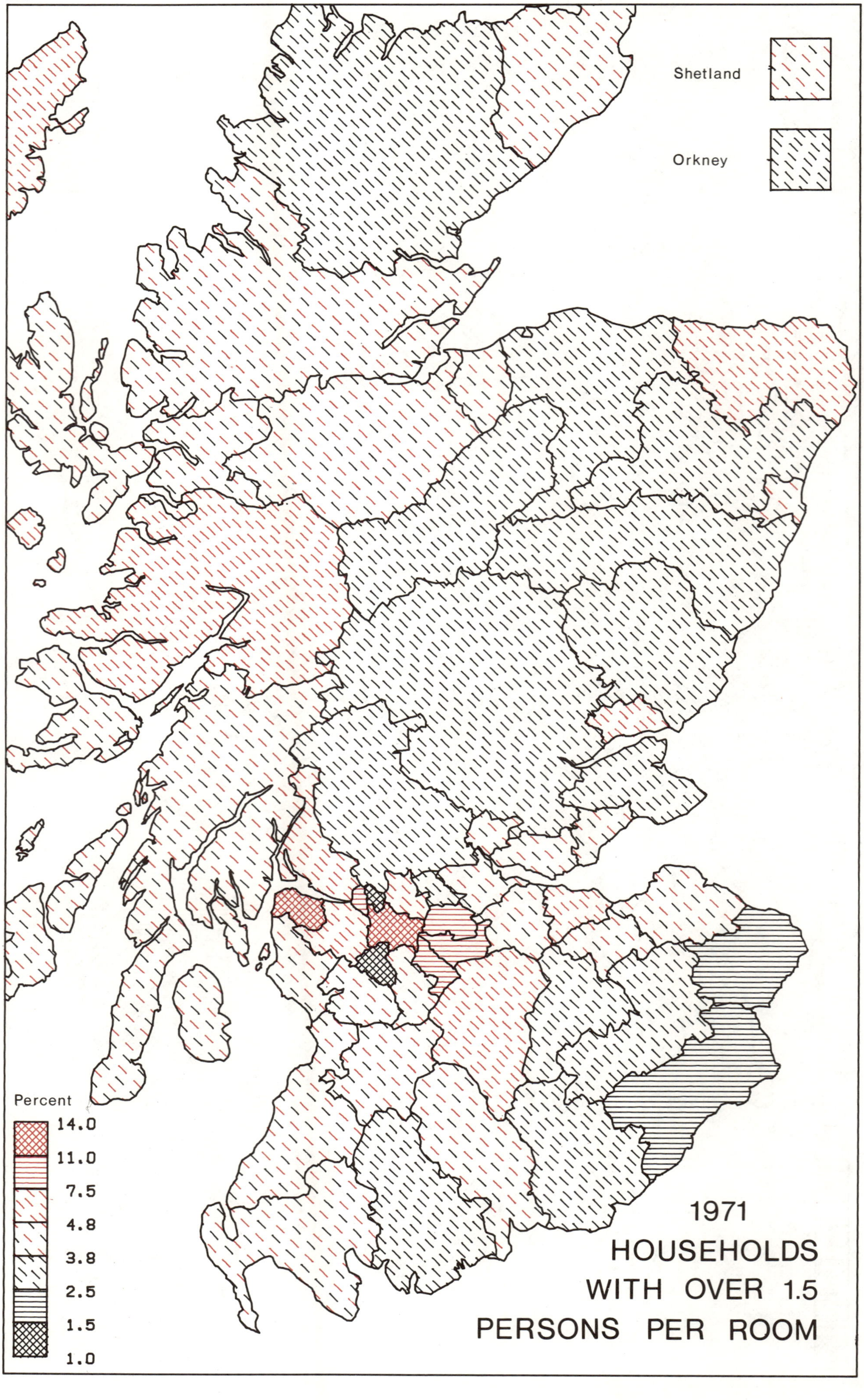
Shetland
Orkney
Percent
14.0
11.0
7.5
4.8
3.8
2.5
1.5
1.0
1971
HOUSEHOLDS
WITH OVER 1.5
PERSONS PER ROOM

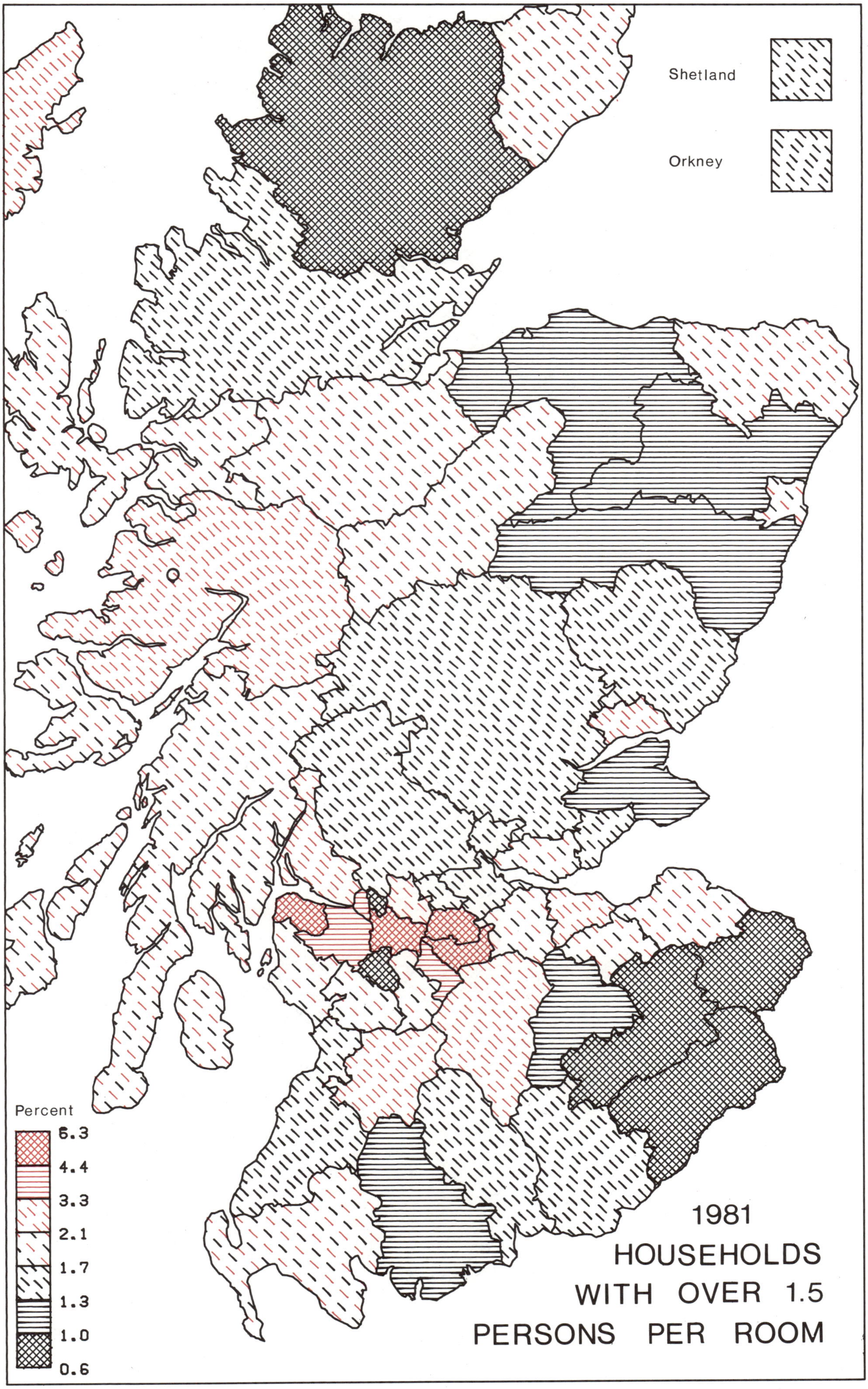
Shetland
Orkney
Percent
5.3
4.4
3.3
2.1
1.7
1.3
1.0
0.6
1981
HOUSEHOLDS
WITH OVER 1.5
PERSONS PER ROOM

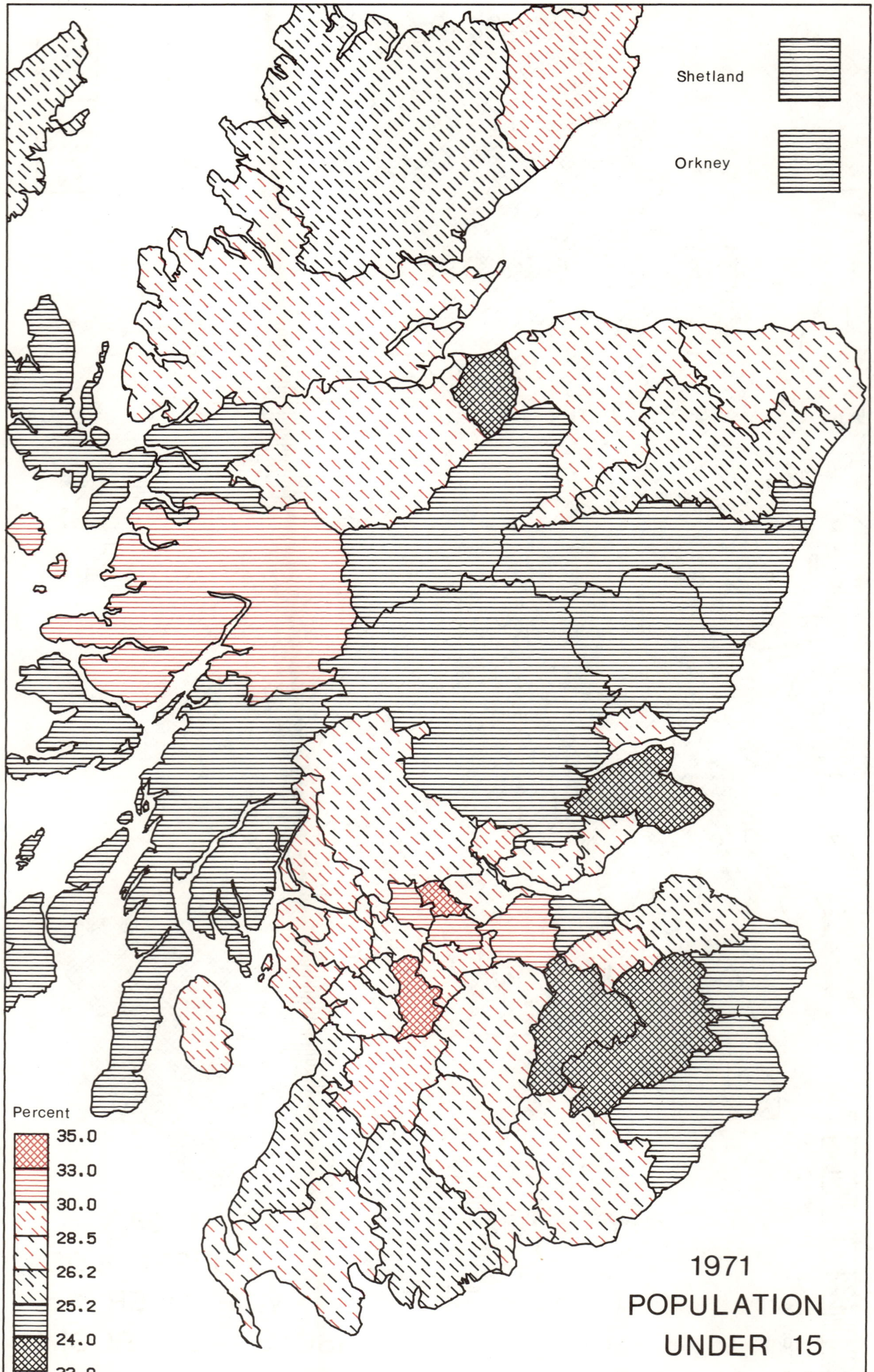
Shetland
Orkney
Percent
35.0
33.0
30.0
28.5
26.2
25.2
24.0
22.0
1971
POPULATION
UNDER 15

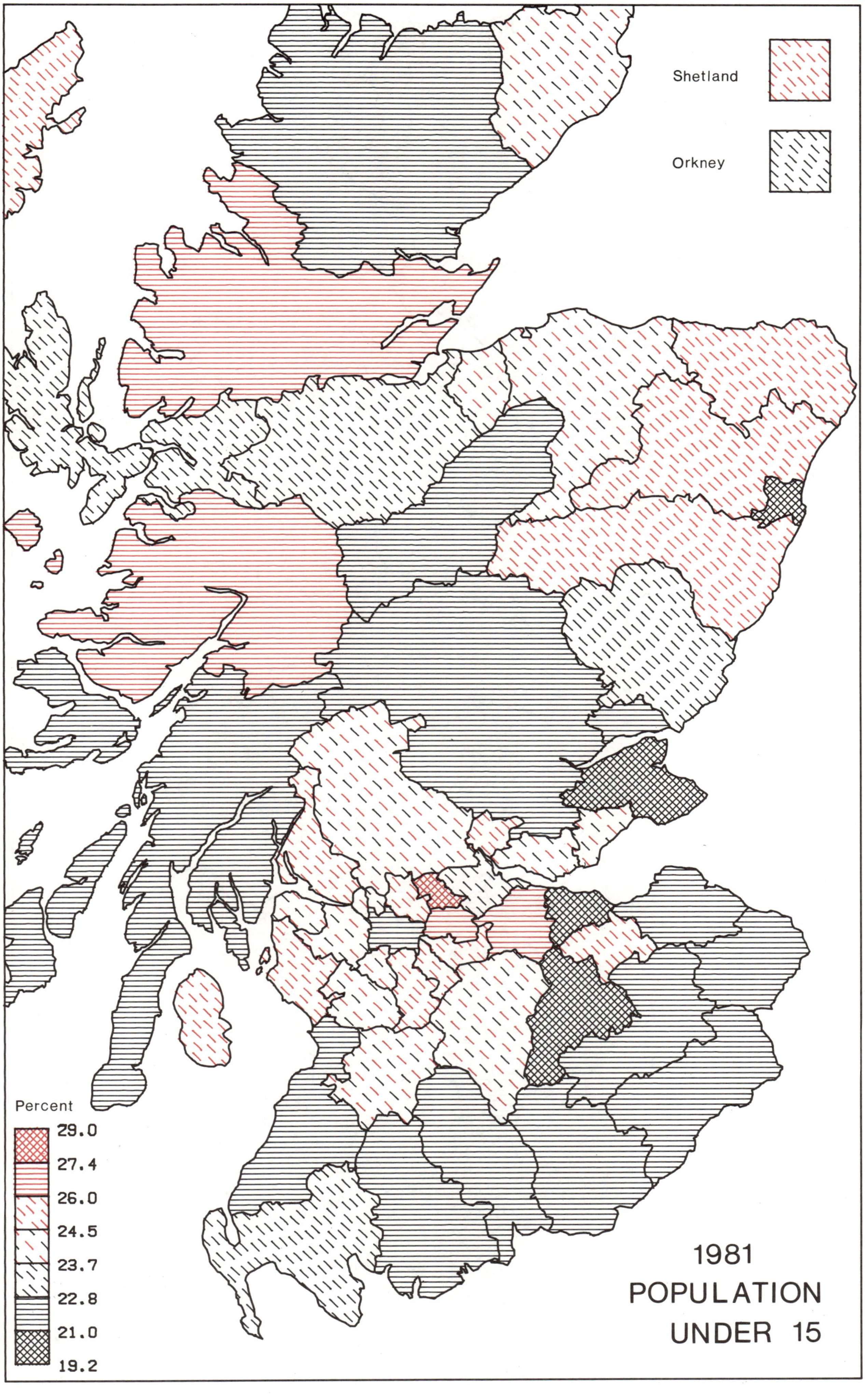
Shetland
Orkney
Percent
29.0
27.4
26.0
24.5
23.7
22.8
21.0
19.2
1981
POPULATION
UNDER 15

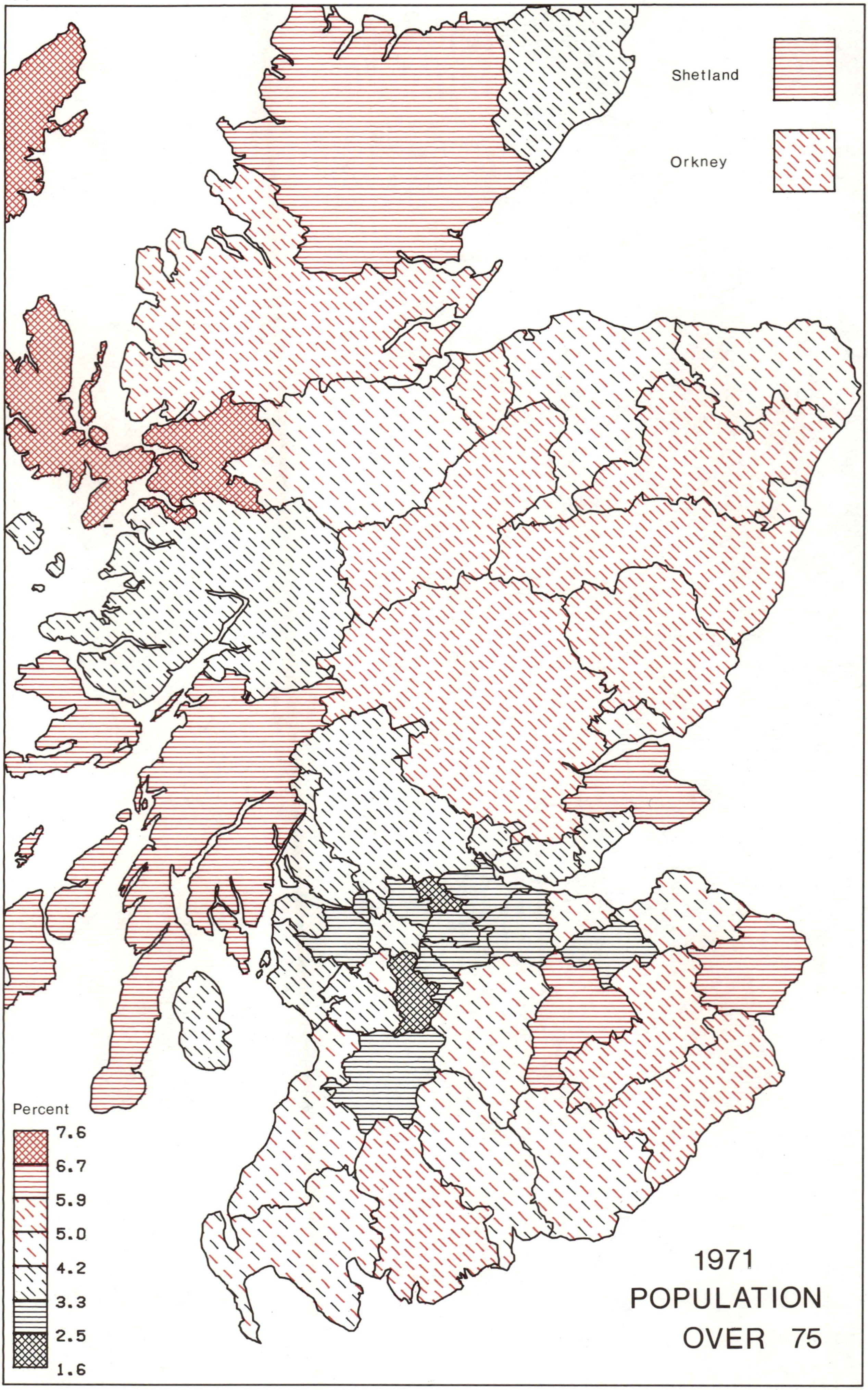
Shetland
Orkney
Percent
7.6
6.7
5.9
5.0
4.2
3.3
2.5
1.6
1971
POPULATION
OVER 75

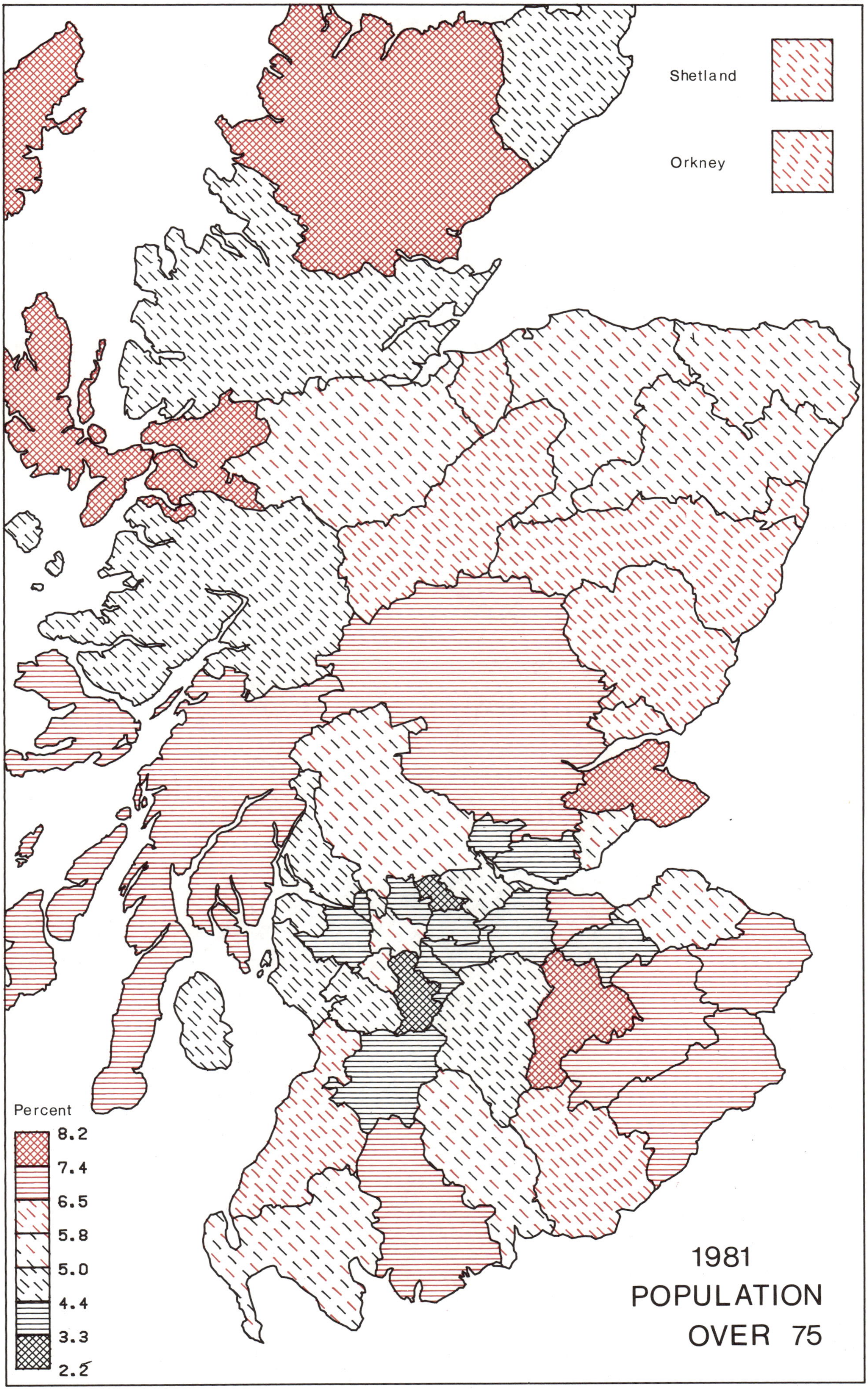
Shetland
Orkney
Percent
8.2
7.4
6.5
5.8
5.0
4.4
3.3
2.2
1981
POPULATION
OVER 75

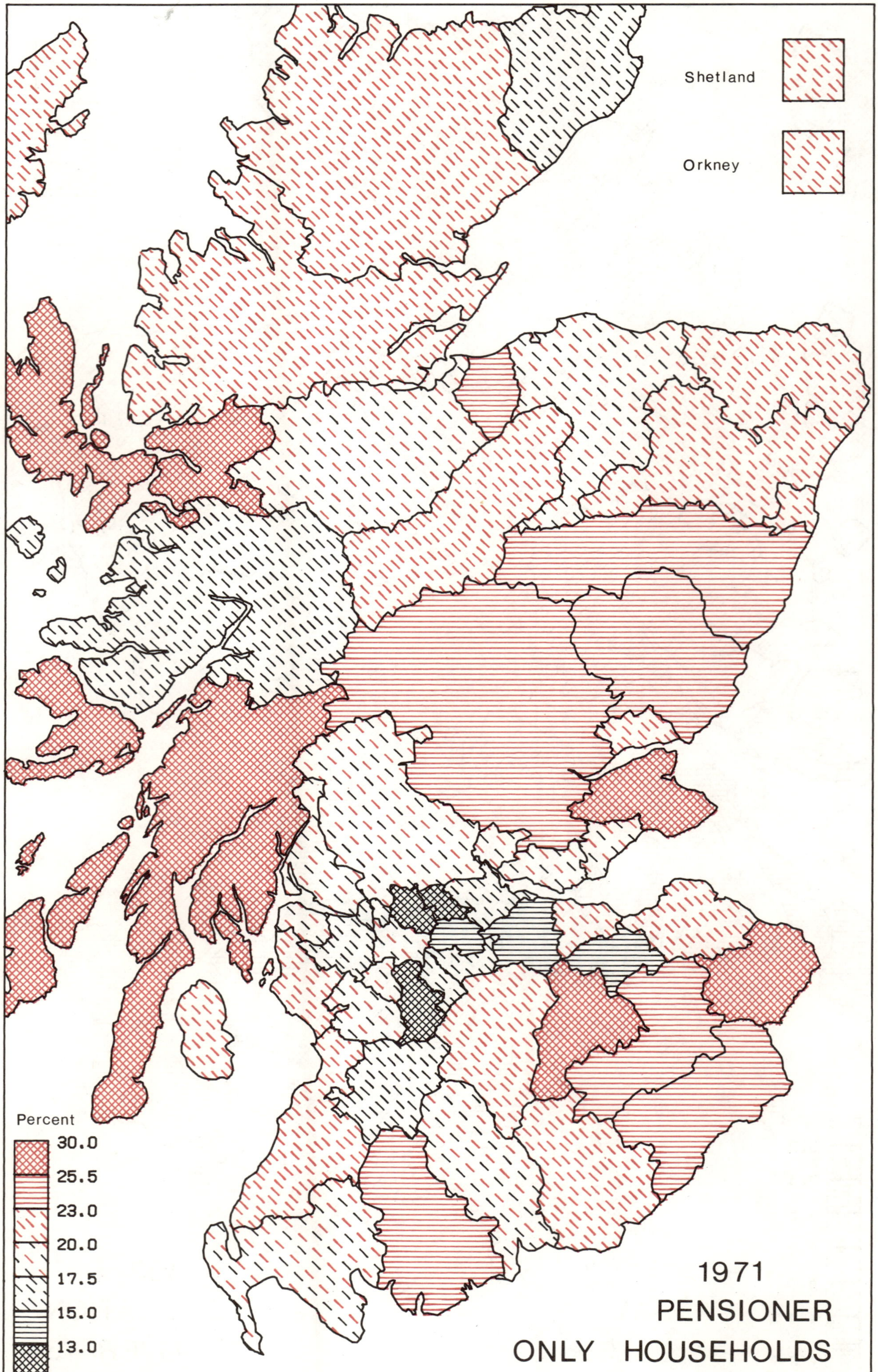
Shetland
Orkney
Percent
30.0
25.5
23.0
20.0
17.5
15.0
13.0
10.0
1971
PENSIONER
ONLY HOUSEHOLDS

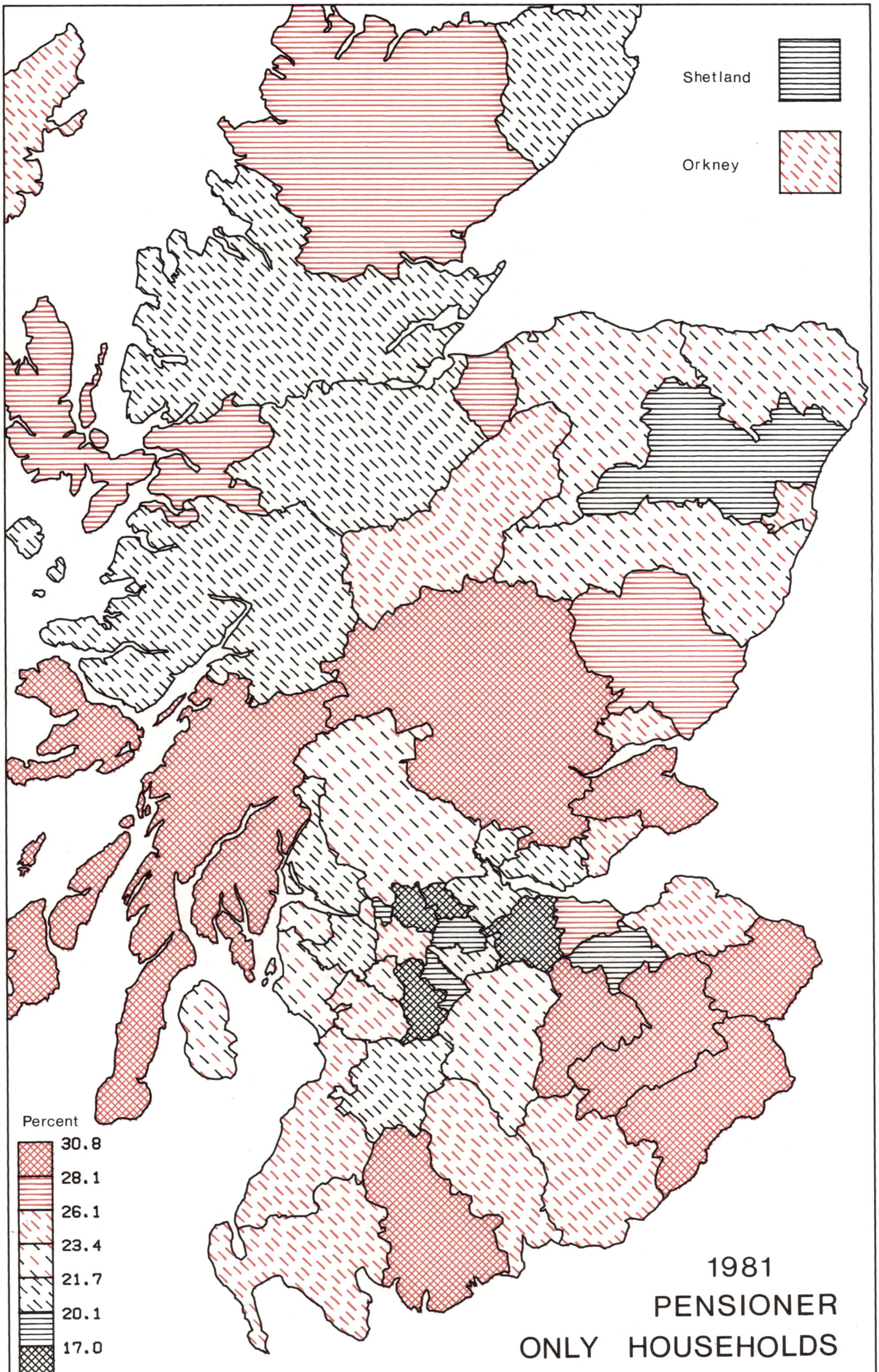
Shetland
Orkney
Percent
30.8
28.1
26.1
23.4
21.7
20.1
17.0
14.0
1981
PENSIONER
ONLY HOUSEHOLDS

SPATIAL VARIATIONS IN MORTALITY:

A CONTRIBUTION FROM MEDICAL SOCIOLOGY

The presentation of mortality data as maps has considerable potential for directing attention towards the possible aetiology of disease and for formulating policies for the reduction of premature or unnecessary death. However, when interpreting such maps, one must avoid drawing premature conclusions about the way mortality is unevenly distributed. For example, it is tempting to treat SMRs as if they were definitive and unproblematic statistics, caused directly by factors within the Districts in question. Additionally, almost anyone can see certain patterns which confirm some hunches or prejudices about what causes what; selective attention and interpretation can all too easily reflect the preoccupation of trained observers such as medical geographers, anthropologists or sociologists. Hence a range of issues must be considered before any firm conclusions can be drawn about patterns on maps.

Obviously, area of residence is only one parameter associated with the uneven distribution of mortality. Differences between men and women and between people in different age-groups, which necessitate the use of standardized death rates, are well-known. Less well-known are differences such as those linked to ethnic group and marital status. Married persons, for example, have lower SMRs than the divorced, who in turn show lower SMRs than the widowed or single [105]. However, the variable which has received most attention is social class, that slippery concept which seems to say so much and yet so little. Despite the controversies surrounding this concept, it is the most powerful social predictor of a range of health indicators. Unskilled workers (social class V), for example, have death rates two and a half times those of professional people (social class I) for most causes of death; and between these two extremes, mortality increases consistently with decreasing social class [106]. But, with these associations between social parameters and mortality, the problem lies in assessing correctly their biological significance. How do geographical patterns originate and for what reasons?

Explanations For Health Differentials

McIntyre provides a useful outline of three major types of explanation for health differentials [107]. The first explanation is artefact; this refers to factors which either singly or in combination produce an association which is at best only partial, at worst quite erroneous. For example, the apparent spatial association between Districts and SMRs may be the effect of a confounding variable, or it may be an artefact of the measurement process. We prefer to restrict the term 'artefact' to the latter and to allude to the former as compositional explanations. The second explanation is health selection, which refers to the social processes by which individuals achieve a particular social position by reason of their health status. Spatial or class differentials, for example, arise through different patterns of geographical or social mobility among the healthy and less healthy. The third and most common explanation is social causation, whereby a range of material, behavioural or attitudinal factors within a District or social class may 'cause' health differentials. These three explanations will be examined to illustrate how they might affect the spatial variations in mortality. Inevitably, the discussion will be tentative; our aim is to promote caution in interpretation, while suggesting avenues worth exploring in more detail. We shall focus on the mortality data for 1979-83, against which the socio-demographic data for the mortality data for 1981 can be juxtaposed for comparison.

Artefact. As mentioned in the text on Methods, inconsistent interpretations of the rules about allocating the underlying cause of death [108] can affect the spatial distribution of specific causes of death, particularly if these interpretations vary strongly between Districts.

A different concern is that geographical patterns of mortality can be affected by the way in which the address of the deceased is recorded. A small percentage of the population resides in large communal establishments at the time of death. Because of sickness, disability and terminal illness, such individuals may be transferred by the organizations of the health and social services from one District lacking the appropriate residential institution to another containing it. Since 1953, deaths in psychiatric and mental handicap hospitals, and in certain hospitals for the chronically sick, have been recorded by reference to the hospital if the patient has resided there twelve months or more, rather than to the area of residence prior to admission. Hence, variations in mortality between Districts may reflect the spatial distribution of institutions for residential care. The impact this can have on SMRs has been demonstrated in two studies in England [109,110].

In the absence of a comparable investigation in Scotland, it is difficult to gauge the extent to which this factor might affect the variations shown in this atlas. It may be of particular importance in the Scottish context because of the large rural land mass and extensive island areas, where facilities for residential care are few or absent. For example, long term psychiatric care is not available on the Orkney or Shetland Isles; residents requiring such care are transferred to psychiatric hospitals in Aberdeen City and in the Gordon District of Grampian Region. A similar transfer occurs from the Western Isles to Inverness. This outflow of people with a higher risk of mortality must reduce the SMRs for the Districts of origin and must weight unfavourably the predominantly urban Districts containing the residential institutions. The comparatively low SMRs for the Island Districts are consistent with this explanation, and suggest that the favourable picture is artefactual, at least in part. That none of the three receiving Districts cited has a high SMR also suggests that the mortality profiles of their settled populations may be better than they appear from the given SMRs.

Social Selection. Much of the work into the effect of social selection has been concerned with explaining social class differentials in health. Proponents argue that, unless the social class of origin of an individual is taken into account, a causal link may be inferred erroneously between social class and health. The association arises rather because healthier people are more likely to be socially upwardly mobile, with less healthy people being downwardly mobile; and that measuring social class by reference to achieved occupation (as in the atlas) does not reflect changes in position consequent on health status. This explanation is supported by evidence in the contexts of mental illness [111] and of height, a general indicator of health - taller women marrying into higher social classes more frequently than shorter women [112]. Although no comparable study has been conducted specifically to examine how mortality is affected by social mobility, the latter is generally held to be an important contributory explanation for the observed social class differentials.

The potential importance of social selection in contributing to spatial variations of mortality rests on a similar argument; it derives from the plausible hypothesis that people who migrate differ from those who do not in several qualities, of which one is health. Indeed, there is evidence that migrants are generally healthier than non-migrants, and hence an inflow of the former into a particular area will affect its health profile favourably at the expense of that of the area of origin, with its residue of less healthy people. In order to understand spatial variations in mortality, therefore, we ideally need information on the movements of people from District to District over the course of a lifetime.

Such data are not available in this atlas, and hence specific selection processes cannot be detected. However, when viewing the mortality patterns, three main processes of migration should be considered. Firstly, migration for better opportunities of employment typically results in rural to urban flows, and in urban to new town flows; in Scotland, migration is also related to centres of oil-related industries. Secondly, migration at retiral age takes place from urban areas to coastal or rural areas, or to Districts of birth. And thirdly, as mentioned previously, the sick and elderly migrate from rural to urban areas to obtain residential care. The age, social structure and health status of the migrant populations differ for each process, as do the directions of flow. There is no evidence in the atlas for the suggestion that rural to urban migration results in higher SMRs in rural Districts; in fact, almost without exception the rural Districts have lower SMRs. However, any 'healthy migrants' process which might exist may have been masked by the size and nature of the recipient populations, an illustration of how the detection of aetiological factors in local environments may depend partly on the scale of the analysis. In addition, a healthy migrant worker could be adversely affected by city life, thereby diminishing any health advantage present on arrival.

A pertinent pointer to the possible effects of spatial patterning of health selection may be seen in the comparison between the new towns and the major conurbations from which much of the populations of the former are drawn. The SMRs for total mortality of 107 and 94 in the new towns of Cumbernauld and East Kilbride respectively are both lower than that in their main source, Glasgow City (115), and are thus consistent with a health selection explanation. However, that Cumbernauld's SMR is still higher than average suggests this can only be a partial explanation.

An assessment of the effects of health selection for the spatial distribution of mortality is enormously complex in the absence of a study specifically designed to investigate it. To understand its full implications, we need to know much more about migration careers and the inter-relationship between geographic and social mobility. We need also to know who is migrating from urban to rural areas, the reverse of the more traditional direction. As it is, the available information is too crude for profitable analyses. In this atlas, indeed, the implications of the social selection explanation for the spatial patterns of mortality are precisely the reverse of the artefact explanation discussed earlier. The processes involved are extremely complex, but together they serve to warn us of the dangers of regarding mortality statistics as unproblematic facts.

Social Causation. This explanation rests on the proposition that factors in the social environment have a direct influence on health. Taking the example of social class, proponents of this explanation would argue that class encapsulates a wide range of material inequalities, behaviours and attitudes which, taken together, promote different degrees of vulnerability to disease, illness and death. The distinction sometimes made between 'enviromentalist' and 'lifestyle' explanations [113] draws attention to factors such as housing conditions and work settings on the one hand and behaviours such as smoking and drinking on the other. These variables are themselves associated with social class, and each is implicated directly in the aetiology of specific diseases.

In considering spatial variations in mortality, one of the first questions to arise concerns the distribution of such risk factors between the Districts. The difference between District A with lower than expected mortality and District B with higher than expected mortality may simply reflect the differences between the two in social class, housing or industrial composition. Unless the social compositions of the Districts are taken into account, we cannot properly infer that some specific factor within a District is responsible for the higher or lower mortality.

It is clear from the maps of social class that the proportions of social classes I + II and IV + V in the 56 Districts vary enormously. Eastwood, and Bearsden and Milngavie, both suburbs of Glasgow, represent the extremes of middle-class areas, with the adjacent Glasgow City representing the converse. The former have the lowest SMRs for total mortality in Scotland (79 and 81 respectively), the latter the second highest (115). The variation in mortality between Districts is possibly a partial consequence of differences in social class composition.

This hypothesis was assessed tentatively by calculating the correlation coefficient between the SMRs in each District and their proportions of the populations in social classes I + II and IV + V. The former showed a correlation of -0.71 ($p<0.001$, 95 percent confidence interval 0.55 to 0.82), the latter a lower figure of +0.37 ($p<0.005$, 95 percent confidence interval 0.12 to 0.58). In the first comparison, therefore, about one half of the total variation in mortality between Districts is accounted for by different proportions of social class I + II. The lower figure may simply reflect the considerable variation between urban and rural areas of the occupations in social class IV + V, whereas the occupations in social class I + II tend to be similar. Indeed, much stronger correlations between social classes IV + V and SMRs have been found when examining intra-urban variations within the Greater Glasgow area (unpublished work, Medical Sociology Unit).

This simple analysis reveals the importance of considering social class when attempting to interpret spatial variations in mortality. One must point out, nevertheless, that Districts such as Gordon and Moray have SMRs lower than their social class compositions would lead one to expect, and conversely Districts such as Glasgow City and Renfrew fare less favourably. In general, rural areas fare better than urban, with some exceptions such as Caithness and Wigtown where SMRs are higher than would have been expected from their social class composition.

Districts vary not only in social class but also in other social factors, many of which are acknowledged indicators of deprivation: overcrowding, single parent households and unemployment, for example. The distributions of these variables are shown in the atlas. As with the social class pattern, those Districts with deprivation indicators higher than average, such as Glasgow City, Inverclyde and Monklands, tend also to have high SMRs for major categories of death such as all cancers, ischaemic heart disease and cerebrovascular disease. Further analysis of the data is required to ascertain what contribution, beyond that due to social class, such factors make to the spatial variations of mortality.

A final way in which spatial differences could be accounted for is through the industrial composition of the Districts. As expected, the Central Belt of Scotland, together with Dundee City, is categorized as low in Agriculture and high in Manufacturing Industries; the exceptions are Edinburgh City and the Districts of Bearsden and Milngavie, and Eastwood. Again, most of the urban Districts in the Central Belt have higher SMRs for total mortality. What specific hazards there might be for employees and local residents remain a matter for speculation, but they might include exposure to general air and water pollution, or to specific substances such as asbestos, coal dust and certain chemicals, or to a high risk of accidental injury or death.

Social causation, therefore, may partly explain the spatial variations in mortality in terms of the composition of risk factors in each of the 56 Districts. Together with artefact and social selection, social causation must be considered when attempting to understand the patterns of mortality in the atlas.

Conclusion

We have drawn attention to the likelihood that the pattern of association between Districts and SMRs may have far more complex causes than at first sight. Health is obviously a social as well as a medical phenomenon in that it both affects, and is in turn influenced by, an individual's social position. Before making any tentative causal assertion, we must take account of geographical mobility, whether it be the result of sickness or health. We also require to consider whether or not spatial variations in mortality can be explained through the composition of factors such as social class. Only after excluding such effects can we begin to suggest that other factors in Districts may be associated causally with high or low SMRs.

The socio-demographic data in the atlas are not exhaustive. Housing tenure, car ownership, household amenities and other indicators of deprivation or privilege have exhibited associations with health status elsewhere, and are potentially relevant here. Thus, while most rural areas appear to fare better than urban areas on the basis of our simple analysis, the other unexamined compositional influences which have not been considered may have played a significant part in the picture.

Finally, with the geographical scale of the analysis by District provided by this atlas, any observed associations can only produce tentative hypotheses; these require further investigations in greater detail. The risk of the 'ecological fallacy' is ever present. For example, in an area with high mortality from breast cancer and high levels of unemployment, it is quite feasible that the individuals dying from breast cancer and those experiencing unemployment are within different sections of the population. No direct causal link should be made, therefore, where such large-scale associations are found. Even if the association between low social class and high mortality, for example, is documented on the same individuals, we do not know what range of factors is aetiologically implicated. As indicated, these could vary from material conditions such as work environments to behaviours such as smoking. Thus, this atlas should be seen as the starting line from which the search for 'real' causes can begin.

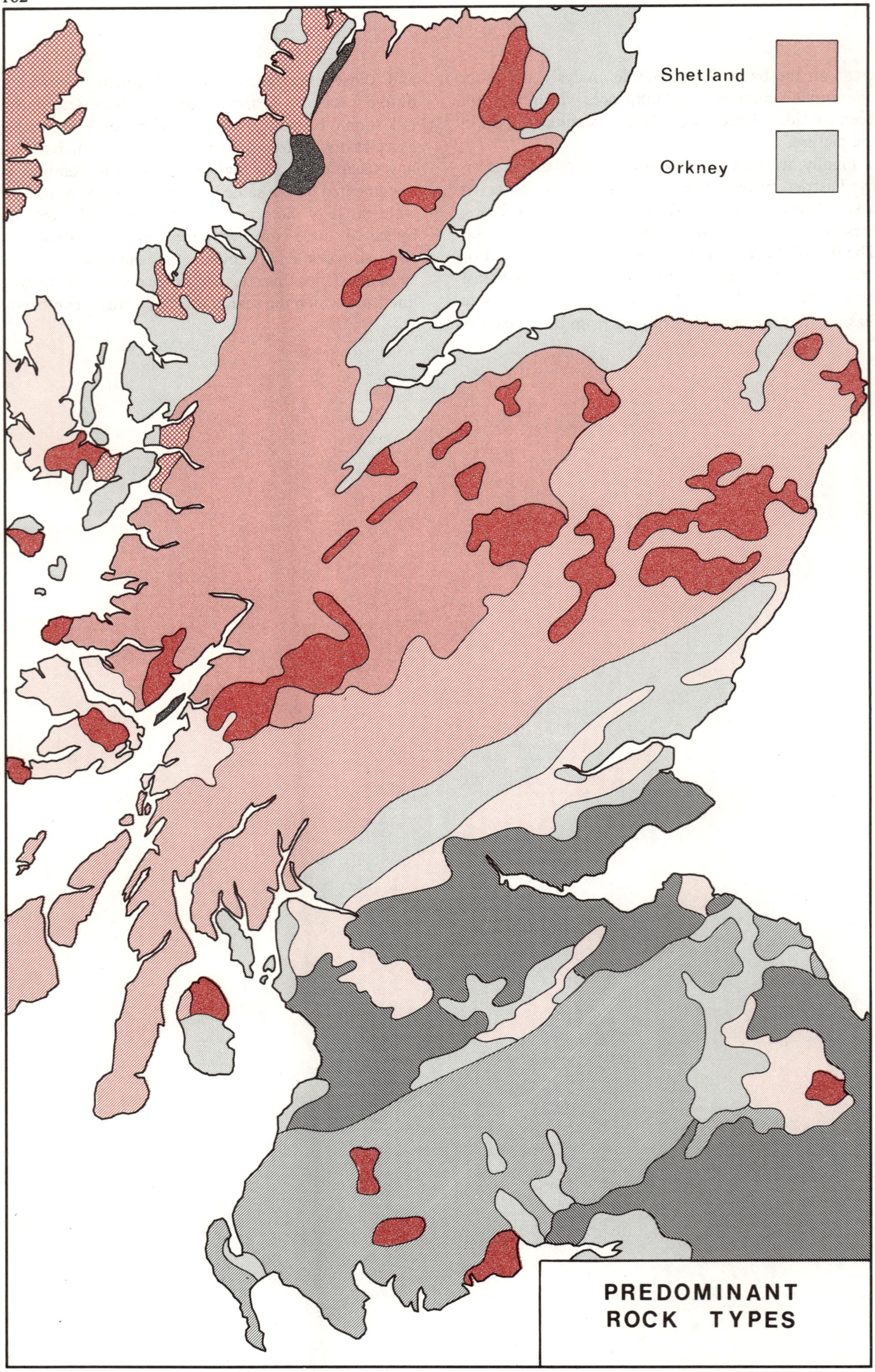
Shetland
Orkney
PREDOMINANT
ROCK TYPES

THE GEOLOGICAL ENVIRONMENT

Granites etc. (intrusive igneous rocks).

Gneiss.

Quartzose metamorphic rocks, metamorphic limestones, mica schists and other schists.

Quartzose metamorphic gneiss, with mica schists and other schists.

Volcanic rocks.

Hard sandstones.

Slates and hard muddy sandstones.

Mudstones, shales, sandstones and limestones.

Metamorphic limestones.

THE GEOLOGICAL ENVIRONMENT AND DISEASE

The geological environment (lithosphere) is one of five geochemical environments, the others being the pedosphere, hydrosphere, biosphere and atmosphere [114]. Most of the raw materials from which soils are formed, in which plants thrive, and from which water derives its inorganic constituents are supplied by bedrock [115]. Thus, the compositions of plant, animal, and human food and drink reflect, in part, the compositions of these source rocks or 'parent material'.

The disease ecology branch of medical geography is concerned with spatial associations between many environmental variables and human disease, but particular attention has been paid to geological variables [116]. The food chain affords direct contact between elements and tissue, providing a plausible biological mechanism between a geochemical stimulus and a human response [117]. Studies of the influences of soil chemistry upon the health of crops and livestock, which have predominated hitherto, are now gradually giving way to analyses of associations between geochemical variables and human health [118].

Rock Origin and Classification. The origin of the major rock types (igneous, sedimentary and metamorphic) is described by the rock-forming (geochemical) cycle [119]. Igneous rocks are formed from sub-crustal magma, the precise type being dependent on magma chemistry, temperature and pressure. Sedimentary rocks are formed in low pressure marine environments from the detrital, chemical and biological products of surface weathering [120]. The constituents of both igneous and sedimentary rocks can undergo chemical or physical rearrangement to produce metamorphic rocks.

Since most igneous rocks have low porosity and only slightly soluble constituent minerals, water from igneous catchments contains relatively few dissolved chemicals. By contrast, sedimentary catchments have a greater effect on the composition of the hydrologic discharge.

Structural Geology and Stratigraphy. The bedrock is varied and has exerted a profound influence on relief [121]. The three-fold division of the mainland into Highlands, Central Lowlands and Southern Uplands recognizes fundamental geological and geomorphological differences.

The Central Lowlands are delimited to the north by the Highland Boundary Fault (Helensburgh - Stonehaven) and to the south by the Southern Uplands Fault (Girvan - Dunbar). These major features run parallel in a SW-NE alignment. The mean altitude and relief amplitude of the Central Lowland 'rift valley' (100 kilometres wide) are low compared with those of the Highlands to the north and of the Southern Uplands to the south.

The ages of the geological units range from the oldest rocks (Pre-Cambrian and Cambrian) in the Highlands and Islands, through the younger rocks (Silurian and Ordovician) predominant in the Southern Uplands, to the youngest Scottish units (Old Red Sandstone and Carboniferous) forming extensive tracts in the Central Lowlands [122]. With the exception of restricted outcrops of Triassic and Jurassic age, Mesozoic or Cainozoic bedrock is absent.

The geography of the rock type formations, of the derived soil associations, and of the mineral assemblages possibly yields the greater potential for identifying spatial associations. The extent of intrusive and extrusive igneous and metamorphic formations in general, particularly in west and north-west Scotland, is greater than the outcrop of pure sedimentary units; in England and Wales, the converse is true. Most of the sedimentary basement in Scotland is south-east of the Highland Boundary Fault.

Evidence of Associations between Geology and Disease. The major and trace elements in soils and crops [123], in water [124], and in the atmosphere [125] known to be essential for, or toxic to, human [126,127] or animal [128] life have been summarized recently [118]. Although associations have been identified between many geological and disease variables, only a few - such as that between iodine and thyrotoxicosis [129] - are considered to be causal. Nevertheless, particular interest has been generated by possible geochemical influences on the aetiology of the major causes of adult mortality in Scotland - coronary heart disease [130] and cancer [131].

Cancer. Because the food chain provides a route and mechanism for the effects of micro-nutrient excess or deficiency to be manifest, epidemiological attention has focussed on site-specific cancers of the digestive tract: stomach, oesophagus and colorectum. In England and Wales, excess cancers of the stomach, buccal cavity, pharynx and larynx (males only) demonstrate a very general but reasonably consistent association with pre-Jurassic strata [7].

Gastric Cancer. Excess nitrate in drinking water has been suspected as a causal factor for gastric cancer [132]; another investigation of the association between nitrate in drinking water and stomach cancer mortality in England and Wales was inconclusive [133]. The evidence that nitrate is implicated in stomach cancer, therefore, is considered to be 'very weak' [21]. No geological variables have yet been shown to have a definite role in the aetiology of stomach cancer, and the contribution of such factors to its spatial distribution remains unclear [117].

Whereas the effects of alcohol and tobacco consumption are relatively easy to investigate by conventional case-control methods and present visible targets for intervention, micro-nutrient dietary imbalances are less amenable to investigation, intervention, or control.

The distribution of the communities in Scotland with excess gastric cancer (1969-73) essentially reveals an excess in the Central Lowlands. Furthermore, most of these communities are situated within sedimentary outcrops. Exceptions to both generalizations include Stornoway (gneiss) and Inverary and Aberfeldy (both quartzose, limestone and schists). Although situated outside the Central Lowlands, the towns of Kirkcudbright (slates and sandstones), Lauder (sandstones), and the Moray Firth trio of Burghead, Elgin and Buckie (all sandstones) are within broadly sedimentary areas.

All eight communities with significant excess (Greenock, Port Glasgow, Clydebank, Glasgow, Hamilton, Dundee, Arbroath and Burghead) have either coastal or riverine situations on sedimentary basements and, with the exception of Burghead, are within the Central Lowlands. The 'ribbon' of five communities strung out along the Clyde, from Hamilton downstream to Greenock, is within a single hydrologic catchment.

Of the 14 communities with significant deficit, six are within the Central Lowlands. Only one of these significantly low communities (Landward Renfrew) shares a common catchment - the Clyde basin - with the 'ribbon' group.

The general pattern during 1969-73 is replicated at District level for 1979-83. Seven out of eight significantly high Districts are within the Central Lowlands, five being within the Clyde catchment.

Oesophageal Cancer. The hypothesis that micro-nutrient dietary deficiencies offer a unifying explanation of the epidemiology of oesophageal cancer is now considered plausible [21]. An association between incidence and bedrock in South Africa indicates increased risk on sedimentary strata [134]. In England and Wales, spatial incidence [7] is inconsistent for both sexes but the values for females are generally higher on older strata. The incidence in Scotland is low, in common with most European countries [21].

Colo-Rectal Cancer. In England and Wales, significantly high areas for rectal cancers [7] are generally upon older sediments. In Scotland, Districts with significantly high or low SMRs were too few for any impression of spatial association to emerge.

Coronary Heart Disease. Identification of an association between water acidity and mortality from cerebrovascular accidents [135] triggered the continuing development of the 'water story'. The inverse relationship between water hardness and total cardiovascular mortality has since been investigated in clinical, pathological and statistical studies [21,48,136-140]. Although water hardness makes an independent contribution to coronary heart disease, its effect appears to be small.

With the exceptions of Oban (1959-63) and Dingwall, Inverness, Nairn and Rosehearty (1969-73), communities with significant excess mortality are south of the Highland Boundary Fault on sedimentary basements in west-central and south-west Scotland. North of the Fault, towns with excess mortality (except Oban) are on sediments bordering igneous/metamorphic complexes. The general pattern for 1979-83 is similar to those for the earlier periods.

Conclusion. Firstly, although conclusions drawn from comparisons of over-generalized spatial data have attendant caveats, these do not attenuate the necessity of mapping [141]. Secondly, solid geology does not necessarily predict the mineral content of the overburden. Where the superficial cover is exotic (glacial or alluvial), the mineralogic suites of the bedrock and overburden might be diametrically opposite. In Scotland, this has been made especially complex by extensive regional glaciation. Typically, there may be several differing soils within a single field. Even in locally till covered terrain there may be some directional smearing (up to ten kilometres) [142]. Similarly, urban or peri-urban geology might not reflect the geochemical status of a distant water supply. Thirdly, the confounding effects of modern food production (fertilisers and pesticides), processing (preservatives and additives) and widespread retail distribution, together with an initially heterogeneous soil base, make it particularly difficult to determine if any valid relationship exists except in culturally primitive or atypical societies [143].

Although there is evidence of association between geochemical variables and the prevalence of certain human diseases in the United Kingdom, few associations fulfil the criteria for causation [24]. Base-line data on trace elements of human tissue are limited, and regional studies in the United Kingdom are lacking. Despite an appeal to combine geological, pedological and epidemiological expertise and methods to examine associations between lithospheric and disease variables [144], adequate evidence of, or from, such concerted endeavours is lacking. Instead, what emerges from the rather limited effort of medical geology is an over-riding impression of largely unconnected and opportunistic investigations. So far, the gauntlet of trying to combine the research expertise of these separate traditions for preventive purposes remains on the ground.

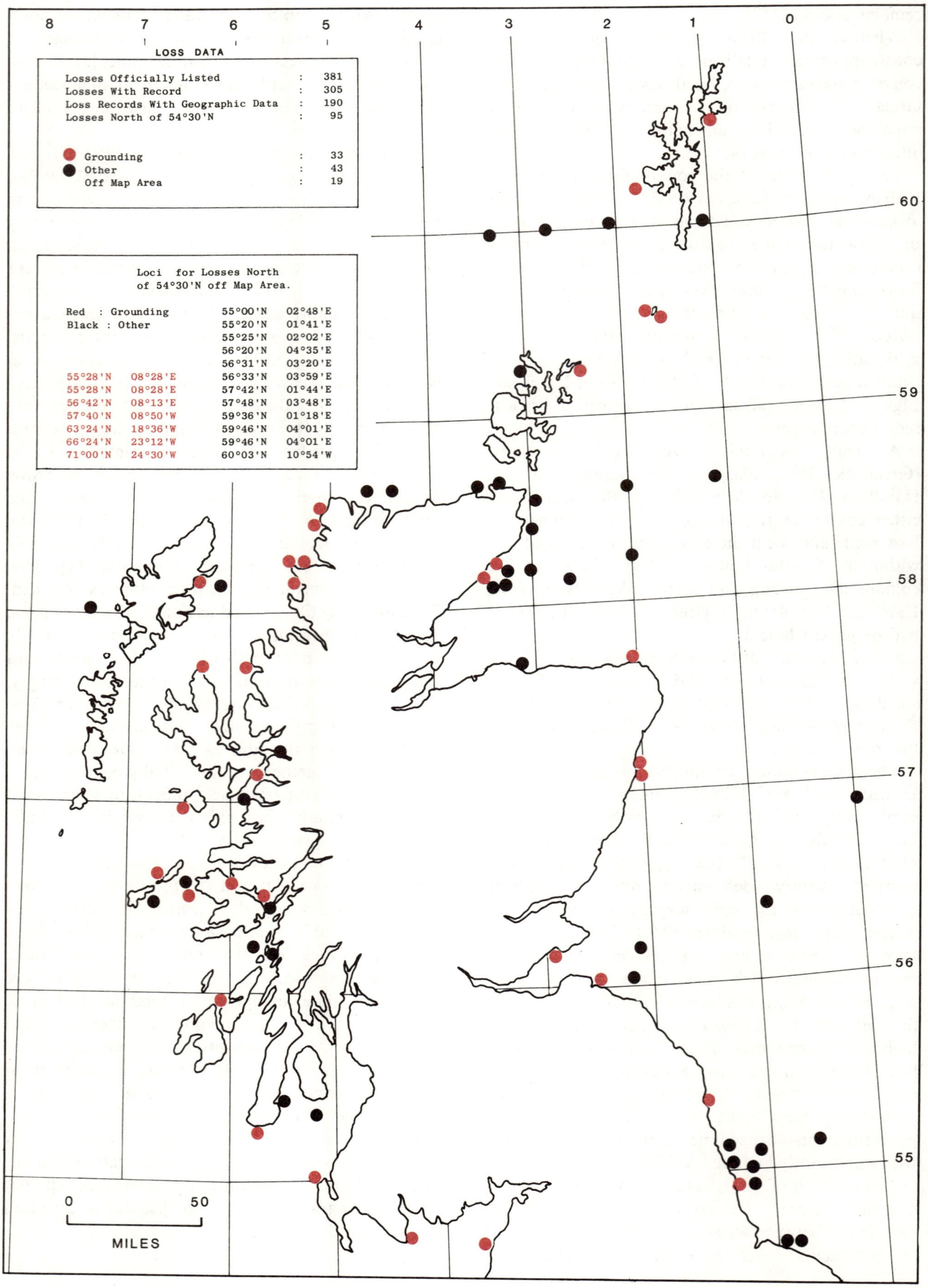

8
7
6
5
4
3
2
1
0
LOSS DATA
Losses Officially Listed : 381
Losses With Record : 305
Loss Records With Geographic Data : 190
Losses North of 54°30'N : 95
Grounding : 33
Other : 43
Off Map Area : 19
Loci for Losses North of 54°30'N off Map Area.
Red : Grounding
Black : Other
55°00'N 02°48'E
55°20'N 01°41'E
55°25'N 02°02'E
56°20'N 04°35'E
56°31'N 03°20'E
55°28'N 08°28'E
56°33'N 03°59'E
55°28'N 08°28'E
57°42'N 01°44'E
56°42'N 08°13'E
57°48'N 03°48'E
57°40'N 08°50'W
59°36'N 01°18'E
63°24'N 18°36'W
59°46'N 04°01'E
66°24'N 23°12'W
59°46'N 04°01'E
71°00'N 24°30'W
60°03'N 10°54'W
60
59
58
57
56
55
0
50
MILES

THE GEOGRAPHY OF FISHING VESSEL LOSSES

Unrestricted access to the beaches of Scotland and the seas beyond presents hazards and risks to those indulging in leisure activities or earning a living.

Fishermen. Of all groups exposed to maritime hazards, the occupational group at greatest risk of death or injury appears to be fishermen [145]. Numerically, United Kingdom fishermen represent the largest group engaged in the commercial exploitation of the sea, outnumbering the offshore oil and gas industry population by 50 percent.

Nationally, 19,050 men are employed in the catching sector of the fishing industry, with 40 percent based in Scotland [146]. Two-thirds of the UK catch is now landed in Scotland, with Peterhead, Fraserburgh and Aberdeen at the focal point, although Ullapool and Lerwick are also important centres.

Accident mortality and vessel loss. During 1961-85, 742 UK fishing boats were lost and at least 1021 fishermen died at sea. Eighty percent of these deaths were caused by accidents; the rest arose from sudden-onset illness - usually myocardial infarction.

Of the deaths due to accidents, 50 percent resulted from the total losses of boats from causes such as foundering, stranding, collision and fire. The other half was caused by accidents involving individual fishermen which generally occur as falls overboard, falls on deck or from one deck to another, and traumatic amputation of limbs precipitated by entanglement in unguarded machinery.

These facts not only emphasize the risks of an exceptionally hazardous occupation but also help to explain why both Tunstall and Schilling described the occupation as 'extreme' [147,148], and why Mair claimed that '...little or nothing...' had been done in respect of their occupational health [149]. Some support for each contention is provided by recent examination of the occupational accident and vessel loss rates. No improvements have taken place in total accident mortality since the 1960s, mean crude death rates having remained static for 20 years [150]. Fishermen are, on average, four times more likely to die in accidents at work than coal miners. As far as vessel losses are concerned, the incidence of loss (particularly from foundering) appears to have increased by 70 percent [151]. Naval architectural preoccupation with vessel stability, though important, seems to have diverted attention from achieving and maintaining adequate means of water clearance from the deck as well as from preserving the water-tightness of boats, some of which fish until overloaded [152,153].

So far, the process of elucidating risk factors common to fishing boat losses and fatal accidents is rudimentary and unsystematic. Quite possibly, the cause of accident investigation and prevention has been further retarded by the decline and recent cessation of Courts of Inquiry ('Formal Investigations') into the loss of hundreds of boats [154].

Geography of fishing vessel losses. Mapping losses at sea yields some potential for a better understanding of causes contributing to catastrophic events and for implementing preventive priorities - most notably collision avoidance procedures. The mapping of the global distribution of merchant shipping losses for 1978-79, for instance, and of the UK coastal distribution for 1970-79 has revealed several accident 'black spots' [155,156]. Although dot maps are crude and can not account for geographical variations in exposure to risk, in the absence of area-based incidence or frequency rates they continue to present worthwhile information.

In 1973, the Department of Transport (DTp) began to computerize records of fishing vessel losses. Using the geographical data from each record, a dot map of UK fishing vessel losses between 1st January 1973 and 31st December 1982 was compiled for the sea area around the Scottish mainland bounded by the prime meridian, the meridian at 8°00'W, and the parallels at 61°00'N and 54°30'N. During this ten-year period, 381 UK fishing vessels were listed officially as total losses of which the DTp had 305 traceable records. Of these loss records, only 190 had complete geographic data. Ninety-five of these occurred north of 54°30'N, of which 76 were within the map area.

Discrimination between groundings (on the coastline, rock outcrops or sand-banks) and other causes of loss (such as foundering, collision, capsize and fire) reveals the hazardous nature of the west coast. The promontories of the mainland and islands north of Islay, together with several difficult harbour approaches, represent a graveyard for several boats which have run aground with fatal consequences [157]. Groundings accounted for 58 percent of losses west of 4°W, whereas to the east of 4°W only 33 percent of boats were lost in this way.

Conclusion. Relatively major developments have occurred in certain aspects of fishing industry safety since publication of the Report of the Committee of Inquiry into Trawler Safety in 1969 [158] and subsequent legislation in 1975 [159]. Nevertheless, the implementation of preventive action has been intermittent and the pace of change lethargic.

Addressing the Royal Society of Medicine twenty years ago, Professor Schilling concluded his perspective with the words of Sir Walter Scott: 'Its no fish ye're buying, its men's lives'. These words are no less appropriate now than they were then.

ENVIRONMENTAL FACTORS INFLUENCING EMERGENCY SURVIVAL AT SEA

Emergencies at sea requiring rescue or medical evacuation commonly arise in one of three ways: hypothermia from capsize and man overboard incidents; traumatic injury; and rapid-onset medical conditions. In such circumstances many personal characteristics (such as age, sex, weight, injury severity, fitness, insulation, and training) of those immersed or injured are known to be fundamental to survival [160-165]. No less important are variables in the physical and human environment.

The physical (sea) environment. Immersion hypothermia and drowning are the most common emergency conditions precipitated by accidental immersion in the sea. If core body temperature drops sufficiently, loss of consciousness ensues, airway protection is lost, and drowning occurs [166]. Apart from personal characteristics, the likelihood of becoming hypothermic and at risk from drowning is determined by sea surface temperature, wind-chill and sea state [167].

Sea surface temperature. In Scottish waters, the mean sea surface temperature during February (the coldest month) varies between 4° and 10°C. [168]. In the North Atlantic, sea surface temperature decreases latitudinally, but this zonation changes abruptly to a longitudinal delineation on the west coast. In the northern North Sea, the zoning has both latitudinal and longitudinal dimensions; the latitudinal temperature gradient is reversed so that, paradoxically, it is warmer in the north becoming progressively colder further south. This phenomenon is caused by the eastward movement of 'lobes' of warmer water through the Faroe - UK gap and then southwards to heat up the colder northern North Sea, thereby

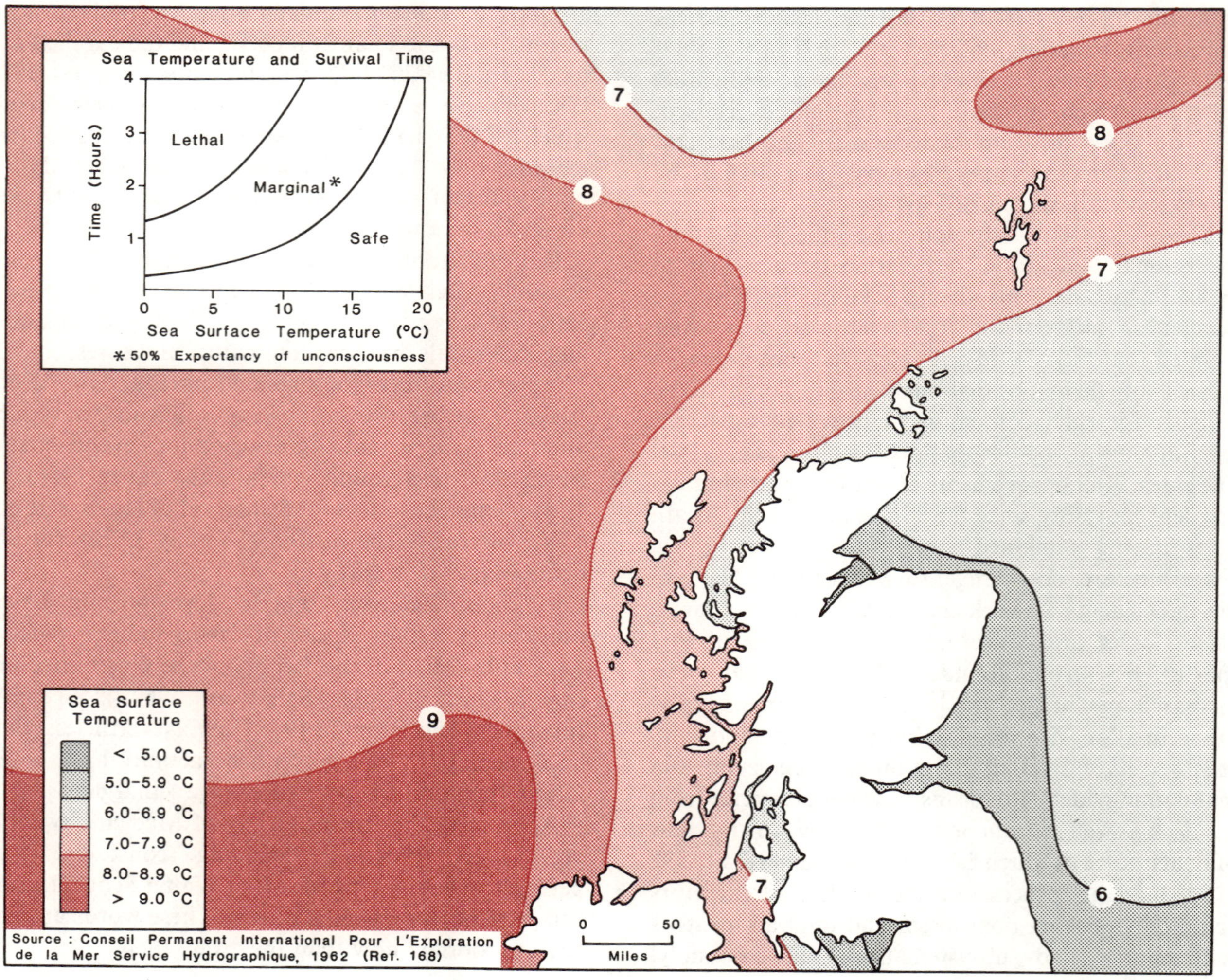

revealing the prevailing direction of sub-surface tidal currents and the thermal influence of the Gulf Stream. Neverthless, the east coast firths of Dornoch, Cromarty, Moray, Tay, and Forth (all below 5.5°C.) are among the coldest in the British Isles during the winter.

The relationship between sea surface temperature and survival time has been determined both experimentally and from observations of actual disasters. Much of this knowledge was gained from experience during the Second World War, from the ground work of Molnar, and from Royal Navy and other interests [169-172]. In the coldest water around Scottish shores, unprotected survivors will become hypothermic within 75 minutes, but usually much sooner. Longer survival is possible but extremely uncommon [173].

Wind-chill. The effects of wind speed on air temperature and on the rate of heat loss from the heads of immersed survivors, or from the unprotected bodies of those in uncovered liferafts, can be critical [174]. Survivors with wet clothing are at particular risk [175]. Even on a moderately warm summer day, with mean air temperatures around 15°C., danger exists at wind speeds exceeding 20 miles per hour if no wind-proof clothing is worn. Such wind speeds are common in the seas around the Scottish mainland.

Sea-state. Increasing roughness of the sea (State 6 and above) heightens the risk of drowning before the effects of hypothermia develop [166,167].

The human (rescue) environment. Serious illness or injury can rarely be treated satisfactorily at sea. The medical evacuation of the victims of sudden-onset incapacitating injury or illness presents frequent challenges to the helicopters and lifeboats of the UK marine Search and Rescue (SAR) organization [176].

Offshore (rigid-hull) and inshore (inflatable) lifeboats, which are owned and operated by the Royal National Lifeboat Institution, are located in Scotland primarily on the east coast mainland and in Orkney and Shetland. Military and civilian helicopters are stationed on the mainland at Leuchars (Royal Air Force), Lossiemouth (Royal Air Force), Prestwick (Royal Navy), and in the Shetland Isles at Sumburgh (HM Coastguard). Offshore SAR helicopters in the Brent and Forties oil production complexes operate on behalf of private oil companies, but may be used when other civilian needs arise.

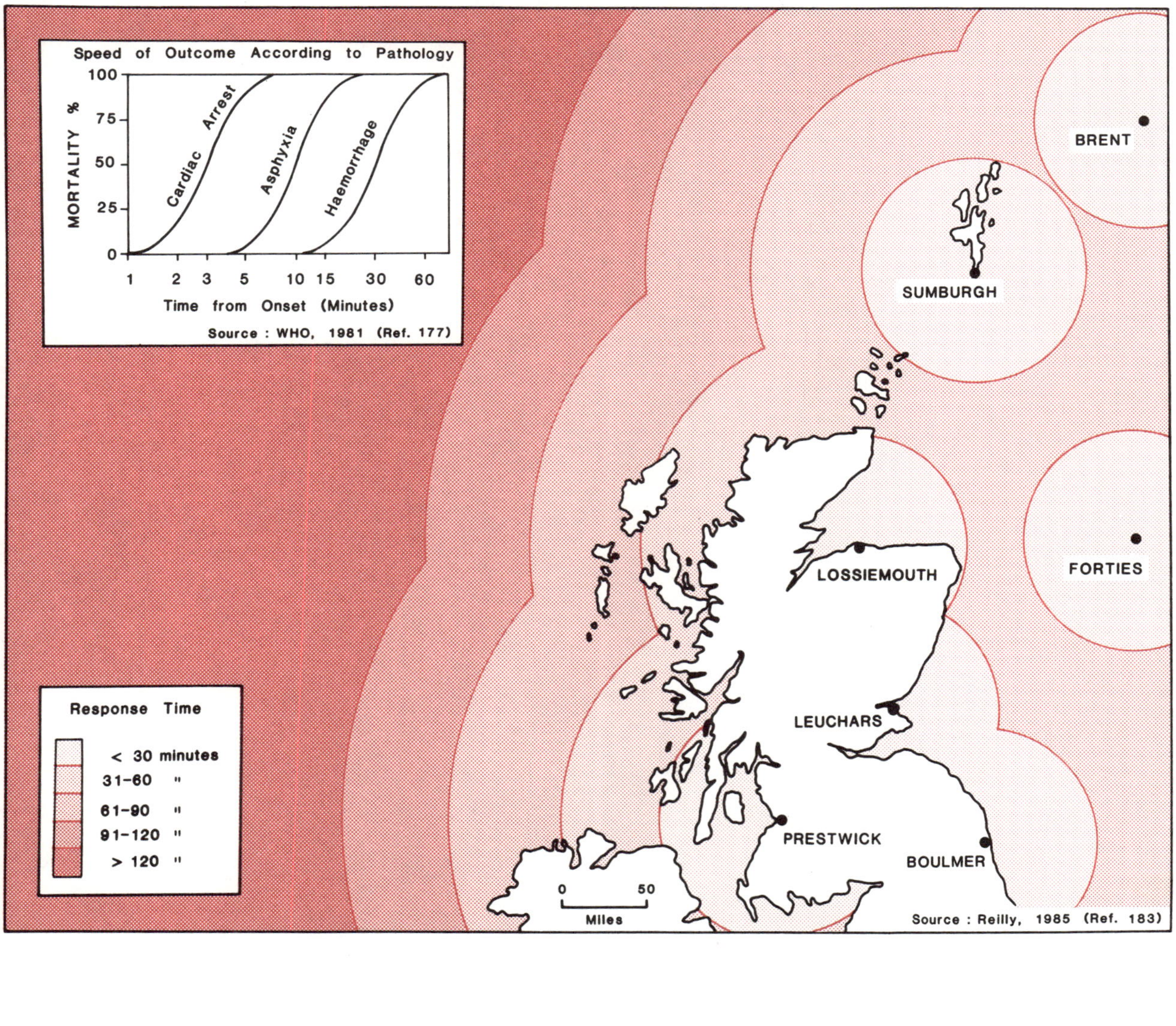

Response time and outcome. The delay between the onset of a medical emergency and subsequent rescue can determine the likelihood of survival or the severity of disability [177,178]. The geography of rescue facilities in relation to the ill or injured person, therefore, assumes crucial importance [179-181]. Previous evaluation of the marine SAR system has been concerned only with its structural organization [182]. Of more importance is the spatial efficiency of helicopter and lifeboat deployment. Mapping helicopter location and predicted response times for 1985 highlights areas deficient in cover [183]. On the map, each isochrone joins points of equal travel time from the nearest helicopter base. This map presents an optimal pattern because it assumes response without any delay as well as calm atmospheric conditions. In reality transit times will be greater particularly as the winds prevail from west south-west at this latitude.

Although most of the mainland coast of Scotland is served within an arbitrary 30 minute interval, many miles of the highly indented and rugged west coast, northwards from Oban and east to the Pentland Firth, are less well covered. Much of this area is known to present a greater than expected risk of grounding to fishing boats. The most poorly served district is the Outer Hebrides, where response times are greater than those for the central North Sea. This presents an added risk not only for west coast fishing but also for the critically injured in remote road traffic accidents, or for occasional obstetric cases requiring emergency transfer to mainland hospitals. After the deaths of six fishermen when a fishing boat grounded on rocks whilst approaching the port of Kinlochbervie in December 1985, the Department of Transport set up a Working Group to review SAR helicopter coverage with particular regard to trends in fishing activity off north-west Scotland [184]. This Group was due to report in December 1986.

Conclusion. Although the organization of SAR has been improved since 1970 (when it was last reviewed officially) [182], crucial gaps in helicopter coverage and deficiencies in response times still persist [183]. From what is known about survival following the onset of hypothermia, together with the effects of delays in providing emergency medical intervention, one conclusion is clear. Present helicopter coverage and response times are inadequate to the needs of emergencies involving not only fishing boats but also aircraft and ferries, for the Scottish west coastal zone north of Oban.

TOTAL MORTALITY: SMRs within the top tenth

COMMUNITY	OBS	SMR	p value
1959-1963			
Coldstream	132	134	0.001
Whithorn	88	132	0.013
Lauder	74	129	0.037
Abernethy	77	125	0.061
Prestonpans	174	125	0.004
Johnstone	960	121	0.000
Stromness	158	120	0.031
Buckhaven	1387	119	0.000
Stranraer	624	118	0.000
Inverary	238	115	0.033
Port Glasgow	1146	115	0.000
Glasgow	66876	115	0.000
Inverbervie	99	115	0.196
Irvine	922	114	0.000
Greenock	4700	113	0.000
Alva	297	112	0.056
Kilwinning	396	112	0.028
Kintore	72	112	0.380
Sanquhar	161	111	0.186
Coatbridge	2774	111	0.000
Newmilns	282	111	0.093
Galston	296	111	0.085
Aberchirder	76	110	0.423
1969-1973			
Doune	84	150	0.001
Whithorn	96	146	0.001
Galston	343	133	0.000
Armadale	506	132	0.000
Burghead	95	127	0.029
Coldstream	146	121	0.025
Alyth	150	121	0.028
Newmilns	302	121	0.002
Prestonpans	183	120	0.020
Kilwinning	472	119	0.000
Gatehouse	94	119	0.117
Tain	152	118	0.050
Rutherglen	1666	117	0.000
Ardrossan	656	117	0.000
Castle Douglas	327	117	0.008
East Linton	101	116	0.147
Nairn	503	116	0.002
Port Glasgow	1123	115	0.000
Alva	290	115	0.019
Johnstone	1028	115	0.000
Tillicoultry	266	114	0.033
Cowdenbeath	751	114	0.001
Newton Stewart	196	114	0.086
1979-1983			
Cumnock & Doon Valley	2822	116	0.000
Glasgow City	57920	115	0.000
Inverclyde	6564	112	0.000
Monklands	5918	112	0.000
Lochaber	1221	112	0.000
Motherwell	9228	111	0.000

TOTAL CANCERS: SMRs within the top tenth

COMMUNITY	OBS	SMR	p value
1959-1963			
Lauder	15	155	0.138
Moffat	48	148	0.012
Abernethy	15	146	0.194
Tain	31	139	0.091
Inverbervie	20	137	0.212
Coupar Angus	41	133	0.092
Tobermory	13	129	0.426
Ballater	24	129	0.261
Denny & Dunipace	93	129	0.021
Ardrossan	118	127	0.015
Dingwall	46	125	0.155
Aberfeldy	27	125	0.291
Blairgowrie	92	122	0.069
Tayport	51	122	0.185
Kirriemuir	67	121	0.134
Cove & Kilcreggan	20	119	0.494
Troon	158	119	0.037
Coldstream	21	118	0.501
Dalbeattie	48	118	0.285
Dalkeith	112	118	0.098
Dundee	2343	117	0.000
Port Glasgow	213	117	0.025
Ladybank	19	117	0.554
1969-1973			
Burghead	22	151	0.083
Armadale	111	141	0.001
Alyth	35	134	0.115
Castle Douglas	68	128	0.054
Innerleithen	46	127	0.129
Doune	14	127	0.446
Whithorn	16	123	0.481
Lossiemouth	76	122	0.104
Lauder	13	121	0.560
Glasgow	13120	121	0.000
Newton Stewart	40	121	0.275
Prestonpans	40	119	0.319
Cumbernauld	200	119	0.020
Bonnyrigg	96	119	0.114
Blairgowrie	103	118	0.106
Maybole	65	118	0.208
Galston	64	118	0.226
Crail	27	117	0.458
Banchory	47	117	0.311
Nairn	97	117	0.140
Barrhead	195	117	0.036
Kinross	38	116	0.405
Clydebank	587	115	0.001
1979-1983			
Glasgow City	13435	122	0.000
Clydebank	758	113	0.001
Lochaber	263	111	0.105
Monklands	1312	110	0.001
Cumbernauld & Kilsyth	543	108	0.074
Inverclyde	1389	108	0.008

LUNG CANCER: SMRs within the top tenth

COMMUNITY	OBS	SMR	p value
1959-1963			
Lauder	4	191	0.319
Auchtermuchty	7	185	0.180
Ladybank	7	184	0.183
New Galloway	2	178	0.618
Portsoy	9	176	0.151
Innerleithen	12	161	0.153
Glasgow	3823	150	0.000
Kirkcudbright	10	148	0.288
Kinghorn	10	145	0.323
Helensburgh	40	142	0.041
Tobermory	3	142	0.708
Penicuik	18	139	0.212
Port Glasgow	61	139	0.017
Abernethy	3	136	0.757
Rutherglen	85	135	0.009
Tain	6	134	0.589
Sanquhar	8	133	0.518
Dundee	586	131	0.000
Ardrossan	29	130	0.191
Musselburgh	60	129	0.067
Lochmaban	4	127	0.775
Cockenzie	11	124	0.552
Dumbarton	73	124	0.080
1969-1973			
Armadale	39	174	0.002
Kinross	14	154	0.155
Glasgow	4518	153	0.000
Pitlochry	18	148	0.137
Queensferry	16	143	0.210
Findochty	8	141	0.422
Maybole	21	141	0.159
Bonnyrigg	31	141	0.083
Doune	4	136	0.677
Port Glasgow	78	136	0.012
Clydebank	193	134	0.000
Burghead	5	134	0.638
Dufftown	8	133	0.511
Dunblane	22	132	0.247
Lossiemouth	21	130	0.281
Paisley	379	129	0.000
Castle Douglas	17	127	0.390
Moffat	11	124	0.557
Innerleithen	12	122	0.570
Greenock	269	122	0.002
Barrhead	54	121	0.186
Ladybank	6	120	0.774
Dundee	703	119	0.000
1979-1983			
Glasgow City	4765	148	0.000
Cumbernauld & Kilsyth	179	121	0.016
Clydebank	241	119	0.011
Inverclyde	424	112	0.030
Edinburgh City	2080	111	0.000
Aberdeen City	917	110	0.006

LYMPHATIC/HAEMATOPOIETIC CANCERS: SMRs within the top tenth

COMMUNITY	OBS	SMR	p value
1959-1963			
Whithorn	3	459	0.058
Cromarty	2	385	0.192
Aberfeldy	4	362	0.052
Ballater	3	329	0.130
Culross	1	296	0.573
Biggar	3	280	0.189
Landward Sutherland	3	251	0.238
Cupar	9	239	0.030
Tayport	5	227	0.145
Crail	2	219	0.463
Banff	5	218	0.166
Auchtermuchty	2	214	0.481
Moffat	3	193	0.410
Newburgh	3	190	0.421
Doune	1	188	0.825
Dingwall	4	188	0.334
Crieff	8	184	0.149
Milngavie	10	181	0.109
Haddington	6	171	0.286
Dunblane	4	171	0.419
Burntisland	7	170	0.249
Landward Roxburgh	20	168	0.039
Bo'ness	10	161	0.200
1969-1973			
Abernethy	5	712	0.002
Findochty	4	345	0.061
Invergordon	5	310	0.049
Laurencekirk	4	308	0.086
Kintore	2	280	0.321
Port Knockie	3	263	0.216
Kinross	5	260	0.092
Dollar	4	252	0.155
Cullen	3	242	0.258
Biggar	4	226	0.208
Leslie	6	226	0.107
Banchory	5	221	0.160
Grantown-on-Spey	3	211	0.343
East Linton	2	211	0.490
Lochmaban	2	210	0.492
Newburgh	4	206	0.266
Prestonpans	4	196	0.303
Innerleithen	4	194	0.307
Linlithgow	7	178	0.208
Kirkintilloch	25	172	0.015
Bishopbriggs	18	172	0.042
Girvan	10	170	0.153
Landward Zetland	18	168	0.052
1979-1983 LEUKAEMIA			
Berwickshire	13	202	0.029
Ettrick & Lauderdale	18	165	0.061
Cumnock & Doon Valley	17	141	0.205
West Lothian	44	140	0.038
Lochaber	7	134	0.548
Badenoch & Strathspey	4	132	0.718

REMAINDER CANCERS: SMRs within the top tenth

COMMUNITY	OBS	SMR	p value
1959-1963			
Inverbervie	17	159	0.089
Abernethy	12	159	0.164
Moffat	38	157	0.011
Lauder	11	154	0.216
Tain	24	145	0.103
Coupar Angus	32	143	0.062
Denny & Dunipace	69	138	0.013
Kirriemuir	56	137	0.030
Alyth	27	135	0.161
Tobermory	10	134	0.433
Coldstream	17	133	0.297
Aberfeldy	21	133	0.246
Blairgowrie	74	132	0.024
Findochty	18	132	0.295
Dornoch	11	131	0.447
Laurencekirk	20	131	0.279
Dingwall	34	130	0.164
Cove & Kilcreggan	16	128	0.390
Lockerbie	34	127	0.199
Ardrossan	82	125	0.054
Bo'ness	97	125	0.036
Banff	41	125	0.192
Stromness	20	124	0.387
1969-1973			
Whithorn	15	171	0.069
Burghead	17	171	0.052
Alyth	27	155	0.040
Gatehouse	16	148	0.164
Rosehearty	15	142	0.233
Lauder	10	138	0.389
Newton Stewart	31	137	0.113
Doune	10	134	0.442
Prestonpans	29	133	0.157
Armadale	68	133	0.030
Lochmaban	14	132	0.375
Castle Douglas	48	131	0.080
Ballater	20	127	0.334
Dornoch	13	127	0.456
Campbeltown	73	127	0.057
Crail	20	127	0.349
Cumbernauld	140	127	0.008
Nairn	71	126	0.064
Pittenweem	22	126	0.340
Banchory	34	125	0.227
Blairgowrie	75	125	0.067
Galston	45	124	0.178
Innerleithen	30	124	0.290
1979-1983			
Lochaber	191	118	0.026
Monklands	908	112	0.001
Glasgow City	8433	112	0.000
Clydebank	505	111	0.019
Dunbarton	695	108	0.038
Badenoch & Strathspey	104	108	0.489

BREAST CANCER: SMRs within the top tenth

COMMUNITY	OBS	SMR	p value
1969-1973			
Auchtermuchty	5	276	0.075
Whithorn	3	272	0.201
Dollar	6	250	0.071
Newtown Stewart	7	241	0.058
Fortrose	4	240	0.177
Rothes	3	223	0.308
Maybole	11	222	0.026
East Linton	3	214	0.333
Kilrenny	9	212	0.060
Ladybank	3	200	0.384
Invergordon	4	185	0.348
Banchory	6	182	0.235
Tain	4	176	0.390
Selkirk	13	175	0.081
New Galloway	1	174	0.874
Armadale	11	170	0.129
Nairn	12	169	0.115
Landward Clackmannan	28	164	0.019
Sanquhar	4	164	0.461
Landward Bute	14	160	0.123
Leslie	6	160	0.358
Inverary	1	153	0.958
Callander	4	152	0.544
1979-1983			
Inverness	85	140	0.004
Stewartry	39	129	0.147
Clackmannan	31	128	0.065
Dunbarton	105	127	0.023
Inverclyde	143	125	0.011
Strathkelvin	98	121	0.079

GASTRIC CANCER: SMRs within the top tenth

COMMUNITY	OBS	SMR	p value
1969-1973			
Burghead	7	460	0.002
Doune	3	257	0.227
Lauder	2	174	0.637
Cockenzie	8	174	0.191
Falkland	3	173	0.502
Kilwinning	13	157	0.157
Aberfeldy	5	154	0.453
Port Glasgow	31	152	0.034
Cumbernauld	24	152	0.066
Prestonpans	5	150	0.491
Arbroath	46	149	0.013
Stromness	4	148	0.573
Pittenweem	4	146	0.586
Kirkcudbright	6	146	0.462
Buckie	16	146	0.182
Stornoway	11	143	0.305
Ardrossan	16	138	0.260
Brechin	16	136	0.281
Clydebank	70	135	0.018
Inverary	1	135	0.999
Hamilton	63	132	0.038
Bonnyrigg	11	132	0.441
Elgin	29	131	0.179
1979-1983			
Monklands	118	132	0.004
Motherwell & Wishaw	183	130	0.001
Kilmarnock & Loudoun	104	129	0.015
Badenoch & Strathspey	14	127	0.446
Dundee City	252	126	0.001
Renfrew	225	121	0.007

COLORECTAL CANCER: SMRs within the top tenth

COMMUNITY	OBS	SMR	p value
1979-1983			
Lochaber	40	139	0.056
Bearsden & Milngavie	79	132	0.021
Tweeddale	41	132	0.104
Ross & Cromarty	89	129	0.022
Clydebank	99	124	0.039
Angus	206	120	0.011

CORONARY HEART DISEASE: SMRs within the top tenth

COMMUNITY	OBS	SMR	p value
1959-1963			
Whithorn	40	200	0.000
Coldstream	50	164	0.001
Kilwinning	157	157	0.000
New Galloway	15	148	0.184
Inverbervie	40	146	0.028
Stranraer	225	144	0.000
Doune	25	144	0.100
Auchtermuchty	51	141	0.023
Grangemouth	339	139	0.000
Stewarton	85	138	0.005
Johnstone	299	137	0.000
Duns	56	135	0.036
Langholm	84	130	0.023
Lanark	217	130	0.000
Buckhaven & Methil	445	130	0.000
Prestwick	356	130	0.000
Stevenston	195	128	0.001
Montrose	352	128	0.000
Troon	289	127	0.000
Oban	181	127	0.002
Hamilton	779	125	0.000
Airdrie	597	125	0.000
Findochty	41	124	0.196
1969-1973			
Doune	31	192	0.001
Whithorn	31	164	0.013
Coldstream	53	151	0.006
Rosehearty	33	145	0.049
Gatehouse	33	140	0.075
Newnmilns	101	139	0.002
Burghead	29	139	0.110
Galston	103	138	0.002
Dingwall	90	137	0.006
Rutherglen	535	132	0.000
Coatbridge	892	131	0.000
Tobermory	16	130	0.356
Castle Douglas	104	129	0.015
Wigtown	31	128	0.213
Girvan	184	128	0.002
Tillicoultry	84	127	0.038
Dollar	49	127	0.118
Nairn	154	127	0.005
Johnstone	312	127	0.000
Cumbernauld	258	126	0.000
Cumnock	110	126	0.024
Hamilton	798	125	0.000
Banchory	74	125	0.073
1979-1983			
Cumnock & Doon Valley	910	127	0.000
Monklands	1896	125	0.000
Renfrew	3752	118	0.000
Wigtown	673	118	0.000
Inverclyde	1937	115	0.000
Nithsdale	1194	115	0.000

CEREBROVASCULAR DISEASE: SMRs within the top tenth

Community	OBS	SMR	p value
1959-1963			
Prestonpans	36	191	0.001
Markinch	46	179	0.000
Stewarton	57	178	0.000
Kintore	19	177	0.028
Newmilns	65	160	0.001
Auchterarder	59	159	0.001
Coldstream	25	155	0.049
Dingwall	49	153	0.007
Ellon	30	152	0.037
Saltcoats	175	146	0.000
Stromness	33	145	0.051
Huntly	76	144	0.003
Whithorn	15	143	0.223
North Berwick	110	143	0.001
Galston	60	142	0.012
Annan	72	141	0.006
Aberchirder	17	141	0.207
Lossiemouth	67	140	0.010
Abernethy	15	140	0.254
Ladybank	20	140	0.180
Dufftown	29	139	0.109
Irvine	160	139	0.000
Stranraer	111	138	0.001
1969-1973			
Gatehouse	25	187	0.006
Whithorn	19	178	0.027
Tain	36	171	0.004
Galston	67	168	0.000
Wigtown	23	167	0.028
Tillicoultry	60	167	0.000
Sanquhar	38	165	0.005
Ardrossan	135	157	0.000
Leslie	55	155	0.003
Kingussie	32	153	0.029
Coldstream	31	152	0.035
Alyth	30	152	0.039
Kirkcudbright	48	151	0.009
Lockerbie	57	146	0.008
Lochgilphead	18	146	0.155
Ellon	39	145	0.034
East Linton	21	142	0.148
Kirkwall	74	142	0.005
Irvine	200	141	0.000
Callander	36	141	0.059
Bathgate	154	140	0.000
Aberlour	17	139	0.225
Saltcoats	175	139	0.000
1979-1983			
Cunninghame	1432	133	0.000
Ross & Cromarty	470	129	0.000
Roxburgh	500	127	0.000
Renfrew	1874	124	0.000
Dunfermline	1125	122	0.000
Kyle & Carrick	1344	122	0.000

BRONCHITIS, EMPHYSEMA AND ASTHMA: SMRs within the top tenth

COMMUNITY	OBS	SMR	p value
1959-1963			
Kintore	6	223	0.112
Glasgow	4169	177	0.000
Rutherglen	102	170	0.000
Gatehouse	5	168	0.359
Aberfeldy	8	164	0.242
Ardrossan	34	163	0.010
Eyemouth	10	154	0.243
Cumnock	17	151	0.132
Renfrew	60	150	0.004
Lochgelly	34	148	0.037
Whithorn	4	148	0.577
Port Glasgow	57	143	0.013
Hamilton	127	142	0.000
Dumbarton	80	142	0.004
Denny & Dunipace	23	141	0.138
Buckhaven & Methil	69	141	0.008
Motherwell	224	140	0.000
Falkirk	137	140	0.000
Paisley	291	134	0.000
Kingussie	5	126	0.731
Johnstone	40	125	0.185
Milngavie	27	124	0.321
Loanhead	15	121	0.527
1969-1973			
Port Glasgow	81	191	0.000
Grantown-on Spey	10	183	0.104
Kingussie	7	156	0.338
Glasgow	3538	153	0.000
Newmilns	17	152	0.124
Cromarty	4	149	0.568
Greenock	255	147	0.000
Biggar	10	144	0.325
Eyemouth	11	144	0.300
Ardrossan	34	141	0.068
Abernethy	4	140	0.638
Whithorn	4	139	0.648
Innerleithen	11	134	0.405
Hamilton	133	133	0.002
Motherwell	240	133	0.000
Rutherglen	80	131	0.023
Airdrie	99	131	0.011
Johnstone	50	131	0.077
Falkirk	141	130	0.003
Landward Stirling	304	130	0.000
Auchterarder	12	130	0.446
Maybole	15	129	0.386
Alloa	49	129	0.098
1979-1983			
Inverclyde	221	152	0.000
West Lothian	219	143	0.000
Renfrew	375	137	0.000
Cunninghame	257	131	0.000
Glasgow City	1604	129	0.000
Kirkcaldy	289	129	0.000

PNEUMONIA : SMRs within the top tenth

COMMUNITY	OBS	SMR	p value
1959-1963			
Aberchirder	9	308	0.006
Lauder	6	269	0.053
Annan	25	190	0.005
Coupar Angus	13	187	0.051
Whitburn	16	171	0.060
Moffat	14	171	0.081
Bo'ness	41	170	0.002
Airdrie	113	164	0.000
Old Meldrum	7	162	0.292
Loanhead	19	159	0.074
Haddington	24	153	0.060
Coatbridge	161	152	0.000
Newton Stewart	9	145	0.350
Glasgow	3192	138	0.000
Penicuik	17	138	0.241
Dundee	611	134	0.000
Armadale	16	134	0.300
Bathgate	36	134	0.105
Cockenzie	11	134	0.413
Culross	2	134	0.882
Stromness	7	133	0.558
Carnoustie	27	131	0.199
Tranent	17	128	0.370
1969-1973			
Tayport	22	226	0.001
Tobermory	3	203	0.373
Markinch	12	196	0.046
Tranent	29	192	0.002
Prestonpans	11	184	0.083
Inverary	3	178	0.478
Kinross	12	177	0.087
Macduff	20	174	0.029
Innerleithen	14	172	0.079
Buckie	41	167	0.003
Denny & Dunipace	31	167	0.010
Moffat	15	167	0.083
Callander	11	165	0.154
Dundee	811	162	0.000
Lochmaban	5	157	0.436
Armadale	26	156	0.042
Castle Douglas	21	155	0.071
Doune	4	155	0.520
Kirriemuir	28	155	0.037
Penicuik	25	152	0.059
Portknockie	7	152	0.370
East Linton	6	151	0.426
Cromarty	5	150	0.484
1979-1983			
Strathkelvin	333	149	0.000
Cumbernauld & Kilsyth	154	139	0.000
Monklands	401	138	0.000
Clydebank	225	137	0.000
Glasgow City	3997	132	0.000
Dundee City	958	128	0.000

OTHER RESPIRATORY DISEASES:
SMRs within the top tenth

COMMUNITY	OBS	SMR	p value
1959-1963			
Tobermory	6	692	0.001
Prestonpans	7	348	0.009
Alva	11	305	0.003
Kingussie	4	290	0.103
Kilsyth	21	270	0.000
Cumnock & Holmhead	10	259	0.013
Lauder	2	256	0.370
Lochgilphead	3	245	0.252
Landward Lanark	596	243	0.000
Landward Stirling	168	237	0.000
Buckhaven & Methil	39	231	0.000
Newmilns	8	228	0.055
Kelso	10	206	0.054
Armadale	9	202	0.077
Tranent	9	199	0.083
Gatehouse	2	197	0.539
Irvine	22	190	0.008
Airdrie	45	187	0.000
Lochmaban	2	178	0.617
Markinch	4	177	0.388
Stornoway	8	173	0.197
St Monance	3	172	0.509
Cockenzie	5	170	0.351
1969-1973			
Rothes	4	330	0.070
Kilsyth	27	311	0.000
North Berwick	19	301	0.000
Old Meldrum	5	292	0.061
Sanquhar	6	285	0.041
Burghead	3	280	0.187
Tranent	14	274	0.002
Alva	10	271	0.010
Dollar	5	261	0.090
Cowdenbeath	24	246	0.000
Ballater	4	238	0.181
Whithorn	2	209	0.497
Lochgelly	15	200	0.021
Stewarton	7	198	0.138
Kingussie	3	195	0.400
Macduff	7	191	0.158
Kirkcudbright	5	185	0.276
Leslie	6	183	0.231
Bathgate	20	182	0.018
Langholm	5	179	0.303
Gatehouse	2	179	0.617
Loanhead	9	177	0.147
Armadale	10	175	0.130
1979-1983			
Glasgow City	1974	171	0.000
Monklands	170	139	0.000
Aberdeen City	409	132	0.000
Sutherland	33	129	0.184
Strathkelvin	117	128	0.011
Cumbernauld & Kilsyth	63	128	0.068

REFERENCES

1) Howe GM. *National atlas of disease mortality in the United Kingdom*. London: Nelson, 1963.
2) Kemp I, Boyle P, Smans M, Muir C (Eds). *Atlas of cancer in Scotland 1975-1980. Incidence and epidemiological perspective*. Lyon: IARC Scientific Publications No 82, 1985.
3) Howe GM. The mapping of disease in history. In: Clarke E (Ed). *Modern methods in the history of medicine*, chapter 20. University of London, Athlone Press, 1971.
4) Segi M. *Cancer mortality statistics in the world; commemorative publication for Professor Mitsuo Segi*. Eds. Kurihara M, Aoki K, Tominaga S. University of Nagoya Press, 1984.
5) Becker N, Frentzel-Beyme R, Wagner G. *Atlas of cancer mortality in the Federal Republic of Germany*. Berlin: Springer-Verlag, 1984.
6) Waterhouse J, Muir C, Correa P, Powell J. *Cancer incidence in five continents, Vol 3*. Lyon: IARC Scientific Publications No 15, 1976.
7) Gardner MJ, Winter PD, Taylor CP, Acheson ED. *Atlas of cancer mortality in England and Wales 1969-78*. Chichester: John Wiley, 1983.
8) Gardner MJ, Winter PD, Barker DJP. *Atlas of mortality from selected diseases in England and Wales 1968-1978*. Chichester: John Wiley, 1984.
9) Liddell FDK. Simple exact analysis of the standardized mortality ratio. *J Epidemiol Community Health 1984; 38:* 85-8.
10) Alderson MR, Bayliss RIS, Clarke CA, Whitfield AGW. Death certification. *Br Med J 1984; 287:* 444-45.
11) Fulton M, Adams W, Lutz W, Oliver MF. Regional variations in mortality from ischaemic heart and cerebrovascular disease in Britain. *Br Heart J 1978; 40:* 563-68.
12) Muir C, Boyle P, Smans M. The plans for a European cancer atlas: discussion. In: *Maps and cancer*. Southampton MRC Environmental Epidemiology Unit. 1983.
13) Black D. Medical aspects of death certification. *J R Coll Physicians Lond 1982; 16:* 206-18.
14) Brinkley D, Haybittle JL, Alderson MR. Death certification in cancer of the breast. *Br Med J 1984; 289:* 465-67.
15) Busuttil A, Kemp IW, Heasman MA. The accuracy of medical certificates of cause of death. *Health Bull (Edin) 1981; 39:* 146-52.
16) Percy C, Stanek E, Gloeckler L. Accuracy of cancer death certificates and its effect on cancer mortality statistics. *Am J Public Health 1981; 71:* 242-50.
17) Gardner MJ. Mapping cancer mortality in England and Wales. *Br Med Bull 1984; 40:* 320-28.
18) Uemura K, Pisa Z. Recent trends in cardiovascular disease mortality in 27 industrialised countries. *Wld Hlth Statist Quart 1985; 38:* 142-62.
19) Beckman L. The Ronnskar smelter: occupational and environmental effects in and around a polluting industry in Northern Sweden. *Ambio 1978; 7:* 226-31.
20) Muir CS, Parkin DM. The world cancer burden: prevent or perish. *Br Med J 1985; 290:* 5-6.
21) Doll R (Ed). The Geography of Disease. (Various authors). *Br Med Bull 1984; 40.*
22) Schottenfield D, Fraumeni JF Jr. *Cancer epidemiology and prevention*. Philadelphia: WB Saunders, 1982.
23) Symington T, Carter RL. (Eds). *Scientific foundations of oncology*. London: Heinemann, 1976.
24) Hill AB. *Principles of medical statistics*. London: Lancet, 1971.
25) Martin MH, Coughtrey PJ. *Biological monitoring of heavy metal pollution*. London: Applied Science Publishers, 1982.
26) Gailey FAY, Lloyd OLL. Methodological investigations into low technology monitoring of atmospheric metal pollution; parts 1,2,3. *Environmental Pollution (Series B) 1986; 12:* 41-59, 61-74, 85-109.
27) Lloyd OLL, Gailey FAY. Techniques of low technology sampling of air pollution by metals: *Br J Ind Med;* (in press).
28) Lloyd OLL, Williams FLR, Gailey FAY. Is the Armadale epidemic over? *Br J Ind Med 1985; 42:* 815-23.
29) Veys C. The rubber industry: reflections on health risks. In: Ward Gardner A (Ed). *Current approaches to occupational health*. Bristol: John Wright, 1981.
30) Alderson M. *Occupational cancer*. Surrey: Butterworths, 1985.
31) Lloyd OLL, Barclay R, Lloyd MM, Armadale Group Practice. Lung cancer and other health problems in a Scottish industrial town. *Ambio 1985; 14:* 322-28.
32) Fielding JE. Smoking: health effects and control. *New Engl J Med 1985; 313:* 491-98.
33) Black D. (Chairman). *Investigation of the possible increased incidence of cancer in West Cumbria*. Report of the Independent Advisory Group. London: HMSO, 1984.

34) Boice JD, Fraument JF (Eds). *Radiation carcinogenesis. Epidemiology and biological significance*. Raven Press, 1984.
35) Bruzzi P. Epidemiological approach to breast cancer etiology. pp 479-97. In: *Epidemiology and quantitation of environmental risk in humans from radiation and other agents*. (Ed Castellani A). NATO Advanced Science Institute Series. Plenum Press, 1985.
36) Logan WPD. *Cancer mortality by occupation and social class 1851- 1971*. Lyon: IARC Scientific Publications, No 36, 1982.
37) Wynder EL, Hyams L, Shigematsu T. Correlations of international cancer death rates. *Cancer 1967; 20:* 113-26.
38) Pfeiffer CJ, Threlfall W. Seabirds - a possible environmental factor in gastric cancer in Newfoundland. *Digestion 1977; 16:* 1-9.
39) Marie R. *L'infarctus du myocarde et ses conséquences*. Paris, 1896.
40) Hart TJ. Coronary disease. *Br Med J 1982; 285:* 345-48.
41) Turner RWD. Coronary heart disease. The size and nature of the problem. *Postgrad Med J 1980; 56:* 538-47.
42) Ball KP. *The heart patient 1: Epidemiology*. Update Publications 1979.
43) National Heart Foundation of Australia. Dietary fat and CHD. *Med J Aust 1974; 575:* 1133-43.
44) Anonymous. Clofibrate: a final verdict. *Lancet 1978; 2:* 1132.
45) Brisson CJ. *Lipids in human nutrition*. pp 84-85. Lancaster: MTP Press, 1982.
46) Mitchell JRA. An association between ABO blood group distribution and geographical differences in death rates. *Lancet 1977; 1:* 295-97.
47) *Complete atlas of the British Isles*. Readers Digest Association. p 119. London, 1965.
48) Pocock SJ, Shaper AG, Cook DG et al. British Regional Heart Study: geographic variations in cardiovascular mortality, and the role of water quality. *Br Med J 1980; 280:* 1243-48.
49) *Annual Report of the Registrar General for Scotland*. 1959. Edinburgh: HMSO.
50) Wood C. Europe looks at heart disease. *New Scientist. 1982, June 3rd.*
51) Thom TJ, Epstein FH, Feldham JJ, Leaverton PE. Trends in total mortality and mortality from heart disease in 26 countries from 1950-78. *Int J Epidemiol; 1985; 14:* 510-20.
52) *Cerebrovascular Diseases. Prevention, treatment, rehabilitation*. Report of a WHO meeting (Technical Report Series No. 469). Geneva: WHO, 1971.
53) Heasman MA, Lipworth L. Accuracy of certification of cause of death. *Studies on medical and population subjects No. 20*. London: General Registry Office 1966.
54) Yates PO. A change in the pattern of cerebrovascular disease. *Lancet 1964; 1:* 65-9.
55) Florey C du V, Senter MG, Acheson RM. A study of the validity of the diagnosis of stroke in mortality data. A certificate analysis. *Yale J Biol Med 1967; 40:* 148-63.
56) Corwin LI, Wolf PA, Kannel WB, McNamara PM. Accuracy of death certification of stroke: the Framingham study. *Stroke 1982; 13:* 818-21.
57) Garraway WM, Whisnant JP, Furlan AJ et al. The declining incidence of stroke. *N Engl J Med 1979; 300:* 449-52.
58) Garraway WM, Whisnant JP, Drury I. The changing pattern of survival following stroke. *Stroke 1983; 14:* 699-703.
59) Kannel WB, Wolf PA. Epidemiology of cerebrovascular disease. pp 1-24. In: Ross Russell RW (Ed). *Vascular disease of the central nervous system*. Edinburgh: Churchill Livingstone, 1983.
60) Veterans Administration Co-operative Study Group on Antihypertensive Agents. Effect of treatment on morbidity in hypertension. I: Results in patients with diastolic blood pressure averaging 115 through 129 mmHg. *JAMA 1967; 202:* 1028-34.
61) Veterans Administration Co-operative Study Group on Antihypertensive Agents. Effects of treatment on morbidity in hypertension. II: Results in patients with diastolic blood pressures averaging 90 through 114 mmHg. *JAMA 1970; 213:* 1143-52.
62) Hypertension Detection and Follow-up Program Co-operative Group. The effect of treatment on mortality in 'mild' hypertension. *N Engl J Med 1982; 307:* 976-80.
63) Australian National Blood Pressure Study Management Committee. The Australian therapeutic trial in mild hypertension. *Lancet 1980; 1:* 1261-67.
64) Medical Research Council Working Party. MRC trial of treatment of mild hypertension: principal results. *Br Med J 1985; 291:* 97-104.
65) European Working Party on High Blood Pressure in the Elderly. Mortality and morbidity results from the EWPHE trial. *Lancet 1985; 1:* 1349-54.
66) Rose G. Strategy of prevention: lessons learned from cardiovascular disease. *Br Med J 1981; 292:* 1847-51.
67) Anon. 'Binge' drinking and stroke. *Lancet 1983; 2:* 660-61.

68) Roberts CJ. Water and health pp 43-58. In: Bennett AE (Ed). *Recent Advances in Community Medicine 1*. Edinburgh: Churchill Livingstone, 1978.
69) Williams DRR. Diet and cerebrovascular disease. pp 117-29. In: Smith A (Ed). *Recent Advances in Community Medicine 3*. Edinburgh: Churchill Livingstone, 1985.
70) Collaborative group for the study of stroke in young women. Oral contraceptives and increased risk of cerebral ischaemia or thrombosis. *N Engl J Med 1973; 288:* 871-78.
71) Lee DA, Winslow NR, Speight ANP, Hey EN. Prevalence and spectrum of asthma in childhood. *Br Med J 1983; 286:* 1256-58.
72) Speight ANP, Lee DA, Hey EN. Underdiagnosis and undertreatment of asthma in childhood. *Br Med J 1983; 286:* 1253-56.
73) Waldron HA, Vickerstaff L. *Intimations of quality. Ante-mortem and post-mortem diagnoses*. Nuffield Provincial Hospitals Trust, 1977.
74) Fletcher CM, Peto R, Tinker CM, Speizer FS. *The natural history of chronic bronchitis and emphysema*. London: Oxford University Press, 1976.
75) Doll R, Hill AB. Mortality in relation to smoking: ten years observations of British doctors. *Br Med J 1964; 1:* 1399-410.
76) Lawther PJ, Waller RE, Henderson M. Air pollution and exacerbation of bronchitis. *Thorax 1970; 25:* 525-39.
77) Fairbairn AS, Reid DD. Air pollution and other local factors in respiratory disease. *Br J Prev Soc Med 1958; 12:* 94-103.
78) Holland WW, Reid DD. The urban factor in chronic bronchitis. *Lancet 1965; 1:* 445-48.
79) Daly C. Air pollution and causes of death. *Br J Prev Soc Med 1959; 13:* 14-27.
80) Gardner MJ, Crawford MD, Morris JN. Patterns of mortality in middle and early old age in the County Boroughs of England and Wales. *Br J Prev Soc Med 1969; 23:* 133-40.
81) Chinn S, Florey C du V, Baldwin IG, Gorgol M. The relation of mortality in England and Wales 1969-73 to measurements of air pollution. *J Epidemiol Community Health 1981; 35:* 174-79.
82) Holland WW, Spicer CC. The influence of weather on respiratory disease. *Biometeorology II. Proceedings of Third International Biometeorological Congress*. Oxford: Pergamon Press, 1966.
83) Holland WW, Kasap HS, Colley JRT, Cormack W. Respiratory symptoms and ventilatory function: a family study. *Br J Prev Soc Med 1969; 23:* 77-84.
84) Office of Population Censuses and Surveys. *Occupational Mortality 1970-72. England and Wales*. Decennial Supplement. Series DS No 1, 1978.
85) Burrows B, Knudson RJ, Lebowitz MD. The relationship of childhood respiratory illness to adult obstructive airways disease. *Am Rev Resp Dis 1977; 115:* 751-60.
86) Kiernan KE, Colley JRT, Douglas JWB, Reid DD. Chronic cough in young adults in relation to smoking habits, childhood environment and chest illness. *Respiration 1976; 33:* 236-44.
87) Reid D, Grist NR, Pinkerton IWP. In: *Infections in current medical practice*. London: Butterworths/Update, 1986.
88) Urquhart AM, Grist NR, Pinkerton IW, Reid D. Influenza. *Update 1983; 26:* 616.
89) World Health Organization. *Viral Respiratory Diseases; report of a WHO Scientific Group*. WHO Technical Report Series, no. 642, 1980.
90) Grist NR, Kennedy D, Emslie JAN, Reid D. Respiratory infections. *Update 1982; 25:* 1835.
91) Hull D. Symposium on respiratory disorders in childhood; chairman's introduction. *Prescribers Journal 1980; 20:* 29.
92) Spence J, Walton WS, Miller FJW, Court SDM. *A thousand families in Newcastle-upon-Tyne*. London: Oxford University Press, 1954.
93) World Health Organization. Cardiovascular diseases in the developed world, respiratory diseases in the developing. *World Health 1984, Aug/Sept, 30*.
94) Buchan KA, Reid D. Epidemiological aspects of influenza in Lewis. *Health Bulletin 1972; 30:* 183.
95) World Health Organization. Influenza in the World; October 1969 - March 1970. *Weekly Epidemiological Record 1970; 45:* 409.
96) Graunt J. (1662) National and Political Observations upon Bills of Mortality, London. Cited by Brockington F. *The health of the developing world*. Lewes, Sussex. The Book Guild Ltd., 1985, pp15-18.
97) Walker CHM (Ed). *Tayside Infant Morbidity and Mortality Study*. Dundee: Tayside Health Board, 1985.
98) Heady JA, Heasman MA. *Studies on medical and population subjects 15. Social and biological factors in infant mortality*. HMSO, 1958.
99) Walker CHM. Computing in child health: significant progress. *Br Med J 1983; 287:* 1400-1.
100) Drew JS, London WT, Lustbader ED, Hesser JE, Blumberg BS. Hepatitis B virus and sex ratio of offspring. *Science 1978; 201:* 687-92.
101) Office of Population Censuses and Surveys. *Occupational Reproductive Epidemiology. Studies on Medical and Population Subjects 50*. London: HMSO, 1985.

102) Goldsmith JR. *Environmental epidemiology: epidemiological investigation of community environmental health problems.* pp 215-23. Florida: CRC Press, 1986.
103) Lloyd OLL, Lloyd MM, Holland Y, Lyster WR. An unusual sex ratio of births in an industrial town with mortality problems. *Br J Obstet Gynaecol 1984; 91:* 901-7.
104) Lloyd OLL, Smith G, Lloyd MM, Holland Y and Gailey F. Raised mortality from lung cancer and high sex ratios of births associated with industrial pollution. *Br J Ind Med 1985; 42:* 475-80.
105) Fox AF, Goldblatt PO. *Longitudinal Study; socio-demographic mortality differentials, 1971-75.* Series LS, No. 1, London, HMSO, 1982.
106) Townsend P, Davidson N. *Inequalities in health: the Black Report.* Harmondsworth, Penguin, 1982.
107) MacIntyre S. Social position and health: directions for sociological research. *Soc Sci and Med.* (in press).
108) Bloor MJ, Samphier ML, Prior L. Artefact explanations of inequalities in health: an assessment of the evidence. *Sociology of health and illness.* (in press).
109) Hewitt D. Vagaries of local mortality rates under the 1953-54 rules for the transfer of deaths. *Br J Prev Soc Med 1956; 11:* 45-9.
110) Gardner MJ, Winter PD. Mapping small area cancer mortality: a residential coding story. *J Epidemiol Community Health 1984; 38:* 81-4.
111) Goldberg FM, Morrison SL. Schizophrenia and social class. *Brit J Psychiat 1963; 109:* 785.
112) Knight I. *The heights and weights of adults in Great Britain.* OPCS. London: HMSO, 1984.
113) Doyal L. *The political economy of health.* London: Pluto Press, 1979.
114) Fitzpatrick EA. *An introduction to soil science.* Edinburgh: Oliver and Boyd, 1974.
115) Tourtelot HA. Chemical compositions of rock types as factors in our environment. In: Cannon HL, Hopps HC (Eds). *Environmental geochemistry in health and disease.* American Association for Advancement of Science Symposium, Dallas, Texas, December 1968. Geological Society of America Memoir 123: Boulder, Colorado: 1971.
116) Armstrong RW. Medical geography and its geologic substrate. In: Cannon HL, Hopps HC (Eds). *Environmental geochemistry in health and disease.* American Association for Advancement of Science Symposium, Dallas, Texas, December 1968. Geological Society of America Memoir 123; Boulder, Colorado: 1971.
117) Coggon D, Acheson ED. The geography of cancer of the stomach. In: Doll R (Ed). The geography of disease. *Brit Med Bull 1984; 40:* 335-41.
118) Stevenson R, Thompson K. Environmental geochemistry - a multidisciplinary effort. *Chem Br 1985; 21:* 893-95.
119) Zumberge JH, Nelson CA. *Elements of physical geology.* New York : John Wiley, 1976.
120) Pettijohn EJ. *Sedimentary rocks.* New York: Harper and Row, 1975.
121) Sissons JB. *Scotland* (from the series The Geomorphology of the British Isles). London: Methuen, 1976.
122) Rayner DH. *The stratigraphy of the British Isles.* Cambridge: Cambridge University Press, 1976.
123) Mitchell RL, Burridge JC. Trace elements in soils and crops. In: Environmental geochemistry and health. *Phil Trans R Soc Lond 1979; B288:* 15-24.
124) Wilson AL. Trace metals in waters. In: Environmental geochemistry and health. *Phil Trans R Soc Lond 1979; B288:* 25-40.
125) Peirson DH, Cawse PA. Trace elements in the atmosphere. In: Environmental geochemistry and health. *Phil Trans R Soc Lond 1979; B288:* 41-50.
126) Moynahan EJ. Trace elements in man. In: Environmental geochemistry and health. *Phil Trans R Soc Lond 1979; B288:* 65-77.
127) Underwood EJ. Trace elements and health: an overview. In: Environmental geochemistry and health. *Phil Trans R Soc Lond 1979; B288:* 5-14.
128) Mills CF. Trace elements in animals. In: Environmental geochemistry and health. *Phil Trans R Soc Lond 1979; B288:* 51-64.
129) Greig WR, Thomson JA, McGirr EM. The environment and thyroid disorders (Chapter 12) In: Howe GM, Lorraine JA (Eds). *Environmental medicine.* London: William Heinemann Medical Books, 1976.
130) Perry HM. Trace elements related to cardiovascular disease. In: Cannon HL, Hopps HC (Eds). *Environmental geochemistry in health and disease.* American Association for Advancement of Science Symposium, Dallas, Texas, December 1968. Geological Society of America Memoir 123; Boulder, Colorado: 1971.
131) Furst A. Trace elements related to cancer. In: Cannon HL, Hopps HC (Eds). *Environmental geochemistry in health and disease.* American Association for Advancement of Science Symposium, Dallas, Texas, December 1968. Geological Society of America Memoir 123; Boulder, Colorado: 1971.
132) Hill MJ, Hawksworth GM, Tattersall G. Bacteria, nitrosamines and cancer of the stomach. *Br J Cancer 1973; 28:* 562-67.

133) Fraser P, Chilvers C. Health aspects of nitrate in drinking water. *Sci Total Environ 1981; 18:* 103-16.
134) Kibblewhite MG, Van Rensburg SJ, Laker MC et al. Evidence for an intimate geochemical factor in the etiology of esophageal cancer. *Environ Res 1984; 33:* 370-78.
135) Koyayashi J. On geochemical relationship between the chemical nature of river water and death rate from apoplexy. *Ber Ohara Instlandwirtschaft Biologie 1957; 11:* 12-21.
136) Masironi R. Geochemistry and cardiovascular diseases. In: Environmental geochemistry and health. *Phil Trans R Soc Lond 1979; B288:* 193-200.
137) Stitt FW, Clayton DG, Crawford MD et al. Clinical and biochemical indicators of cardiovascular disease among men living in hard and soft water areas. *Lancet 1973; 1:* 122-26.
138) Crawford T, Crawford MD. Prevalence and pathological changes of ischaemic heart disease in a hard-water and in a soft-water area. *Lancet 1967; 1:* 229-32.
139) Morris JN, Crawford MD, Heady JA. Hardness of local water supplies and mortality from cardiovascular disease in the county boroughs of England and Wales. *Lancet 1961; 1:* 860-62.
140) Crawford MD, Gardner MJ, Morris JN. Mortality and hardness of local water supplies. *Lancet 1968; 1:* 827-31.
141) Reilly M. Maps, disease, and epidemiology. *Lancet, 1981; 2:* 90.
142) Webb JS. *The Wolfson geochemical atlas of England and Wales.* Oxford: Clarendon Press, 1978.
143) West TS. Soil as the source of trace elements. *Phil Trans R Soc Lond 1981; B294:* 19-39.
144) Shaper AG. Epidemiology for geochemists. In Environmental geochemistry and health. *Phil Trans R Soc Lond 1979; B288:* 127-36.
145) Reilly MSJ. Safety at sea - a forgotten frontier? (Editorial) *Br J Ind Med 1986; 43:* (in press).
146) Ministry of Agriculture, Fisheries and Food. *Sea fisheries statistical tables.* 1984. London: HMSO, 1985.
147) Tunstall J. *The fishermen.* London: MacGibbon and Kee, 1962.
148) Schilling RSF. Trawler fishing: an extreme occupation. *Proc Roy Soc Med 1966; 59:* 405-10.
149) Mair A. The health, welfare, and safety of fishermen in the North Sea littoral. In: Cumming RP, Taylor W (Eds). *Aspects of health and safety in oil development.* Proceedings of a symposium on occupational medicine at Lerwick Health Centre and Gilbert Bain Hospital, Lerwick, Shetland. 17th-18th March 1973. Shetland: The Shetland Times Limited, 1973.
150) Reilly MSJ. Mortality from occupational accidents to United Kingdom fishermen, 1961-80. *Br J Ind Med 1985; 42:* 806-14.
151) Reilly MSJ. The safety of United Kingdom fishing vessels, 1961-80. *Journal of Navigation* 1984; 37: 60-82.
152) Department of Trade. *Dangers associated with bulk fishing.* (Merchant Shipping Notice No. M. 974) London: HMSO, 1981.
153) Department of Trade. *Freeboards of fishing vessels.* (Merchant Shipping Notice No. M. 975) London: HMSO, 1981.
154) Reilly MSJ. Have 'formal investigations' into fishing vessel losses ceased? *Br J Ind Med 1986; 43:* (in press).
155) Coupar AD (Ed). *The Times atlas of the oceans.* London: Times Books, 1983 p164-65.
156) Read JF. *Shipping casualties around the British Isles 1970-1979.* (Report 106, NMI) London: National Maritime Institute, 1981.
157) Department of Trade. *Bridge manning, watchkeeping and the command of fishing vessels* (Merchant Shipping Notice No. M. 997) London: HMSO, 1981.
158) Holland-Martin D. *Trawler Safety - final report of the committee of inquiry into trawler safety.* London: HMSO, 1969.
159) *The Fishing Vessels (Safety Provisions) Rules 1975, SI 1975 No. 330* London: HMSO, 1975.
160) Brown C, Brengelmann G. Energy metabolism and temperature regulation. Chapters 53 and 54. In: Ruch TC, Patton HD (Eds). *Physiology and Biophysics.* Philadelphia: WB Saunders, 1966. (19th Edition).
161) MacLean D, Emslie-Smith D. *Accidental hypothermia.* Oxford: Blackwell Scientific Publications, 1977.
162) Adam JM (Ed). *Hypothermia ashore and afloat.* Proceedings of the Third International Action for Disaster Conference, Aberdeen. Aberdeen: Aberdeen University Press, 1981.
163) Pearn J. The management of near drowning. *Br Med J, 1985; 291:* 1447-52.
164) Smith GB, Hames EF. Estimation of tolerance times for cold water immersion. *Aerospace Medicine 1962; 33:* 834-40.
165) Bull JP. Injury severity scoring systems. *Injury 1982; 14:* 2-6.
166) Golden FSC, Rivers JF. The immersion incident. *Anaesthesia 1975; 30:* 364-73.
167) Air Standardization Co-ordinating Committee. A technical basis for specifying the insulation of immersion protective clothing. *AIR STD 61/40;* September 1984.

168) Conseil Permanent International Pour L'Exploration de la Mar Service Hydrographique. *Mean Monthly temperature and salinity of the surface layer of the North Sea and adjacent waters from 1905 to 1954*. Charlottensund Slot, Danemark, 1962.

169) Molnar GW. Survival of hypothermia by men immersed in the ocean. *JAMA 1946; 131:* 1046-50.

170) Keatinge WR. Death after shipwreck. *Br Med J 1965; 2:* 1537-41.

171) Golden FSC. Recognition and treatment of immersion hypothermia. *Proc Roy Soc Med 1973; 66:* 1058-61.

172) Harvey GR. Physiological changes encountered in hypothermia. *Proc Roy Soc Med 1973; 66:* 1053-58.

173) Keatinge WR, Coleshaw SRK, Millard CE et al. Exceptional case of survival in cold water. *Br Med J 1986; 292:* 171-72.

174) Adam JM. Cold weather: its characteristics, danger and assessments (Chapter 1). In: Adam JM (Ed). *Hypothermia ashore and afloat.* Proceedings of the Third International Action for Disaster Conference, Aberdeen. Aberdeen: Aberdeen University Press, 1981.

175) *Report of Court No. 8066 mv Lovat (On 360735)* London: HMSO, 1977.

176) Department of Transport. *United Kingdom search and rescue (UKSAR) handbook.* London: HMSO, 1985.

177) World Health Organisation. *Planning and organisation of emergency medical services.* Report on a WHO Technical Group, Toulouse, 24th-28th February 1979. Copenhagen: WHO, 1981 (EURO Reports and Studies 35).

178) Myrick JA. *An evaluation of emergency medical services based on patient outcome.* Ph D thesis, University of Missouri-Columbia, 1974.

179) Willemain TR, Larson RC. *Emergency medical systems analysis. Papers on the planning and evaluation of services.* Urban Public Safety Systems (Volume 4). Lexington and Toronto: DC Heath, 1977.

180) Mayer JD. Emergency medical service - delays, response time and survival. *Medical Care 1979; 17:* 818-27.

181) Mayer JD. Geographical patterns of cardiac arrests: an exploratory model. *Soc Sci Med 1981; 15D:* 329-34.

182) Board of Trade. *Marine search and rescue organisation - report of the committee to review the marine SAR organisation of the United Kingdom.* London: HMSO, 1970.

183) Reilly MSJ. The evaluation of maritime search and rescue: how does the system perform? In: *Proceedings of the Fourth Annual Offshore Search and Rescue Communications Conference, Leith Nautical College, Edinburgh.* 29th September - 1st October 1985.

184) *Official Report of Commons Debates.* 6th series; 96: 406-7, 1986.

PLACE NAME INDEX